# Making Babies

The Definitive Guide to Improving your
Fertility and Reproductive Health

## Jason Jackson N.D.

MAKING BABIES: THE DEFINITIVE GUIDE TO IMPROVING YOUR FERTILITY AND
REPRODUCTIVE HEALTH
Copyright © JASON JACKSON 2009

First published by Zeus Publications 2009
http://www.zeus-publications.com
P.O. Box 2554
Burleigh M.D.C.
QLD. 4220
Australia.

The National Library of Australia Cataloguing-in-Publication

Jackson, Jason, 1970-

Making babies : the definitive guide to improving your fertility and reproductive health

ISBN: 978-1-921406-68-3 (pbk.)

Subjects: Fertility, Human
Reproductive health.
Human reproduction technology.

Dewey Number: 301.321

This book is a work of non fiction.

The author asserts his moral rights.

# Contents

# Acknowledgements

Firstly I would like to thank all of my patients that have honoured me with their continual confidence over the years and have put their faith and trust in my hands to help to care for their health needs and wellbeing. Their encouragement for me to put pen to paper to write this book has been a source of inspiration and has created an everlasting bond between us. To my clinic team of dedicated practitioners, thank you for your support over the years. Special thanks must go to my office managers Erica (Black) French, Colleen Bendl, Kathy Burns and Maria Conias whose assistance has been priceless.

Working on the "*Making Babies*" project has been a true journey of discovery. The blood, sweat and tears that go into this type of venture are both agony and ecstasy at the same time. The effort I feel has been well worth it and I hope that the information I have compiled will also be of benefit to many others.

I would like to pay tribute to my colleagues in the natural health and medical industries, particular mention must go to individuals that have been pioneers and mentors of their respective fields who have led by sterling example. The following people have had tremendous influences to my practice and education of healthcare:

Glen Gillard (Natural therapist, mentor and Director of NRG), Henry Oseiki (Renowned nutritionist and Director of Bioconcepts), David McCloud (former president of the National Herbalist Association of Australia), Kerry Bone (World renowned Herbalist, Head of research and development for Mediherb, and Principal of the Australian College of Phytotherapy), Francesca Naish (Author on Infertility, Director of the Jocelyn Centre), Janette Roberts (Author and Foresight representative in Australia), Ruth Sharkey (Author and Herbalist), Catherine Chan (Author and Naturopath), Ruth Trickey (Author and Herbalist), Dr Warren De Ambrosis and Colleagues at the Queensland Fertility Group (QFG), Dr Schull and team at Monash IVF, and Professor Robert Jansen (Author, renowned specialist and Director at Sydney IVF).

These individuals, whom I greatly admire, have worked tirelessly to forge new pathways of awareness, understanding and treatment of reproductive disorders. To Ian 'king of the night' Maurice, (entertainer, TV and radio personality) I am very grateful for your friendship and allowing me the opportunity to spread the word of natural medicine over the air waves on talkback 4BC radio.

I would like to extend a heartfelt thanks to all who have contributed to the production of "Making Babies" and for their professional, supportive guidance and unwavering belief in this project. To the editors and publisher at Zeus who were also kind when wielding the axe to streamline the content of the book and for their expert help with the final presentation.

The ultimate accolade must go to my devoted wife, Nicole, and loving family, Ben, Corey, Amelia, Samuel, Jacob, and extended family members. This book is dedicated to you for providing me with the motivation and determination that drives me day-in-day-out to do the work that I do and for your tolerance that has allowed me to complete this project that I am so passionate about. This has been a labour of love!

Best wishes and good luck to you all!

# Foreword

It is with great pleasure and delight that I present this foreword for this marvellous book researched and written by my friend and colleague, Naturopath and Herbalist extraordinaire, Jason Jackson. He has all the presence of a very ordinary bloke because he is totally down to earth. When you look into his achievements as a profoundly caring and dedicated therapist, you find Jason has pushed himself to develop better protocols for treating many health conditions with such outstanding success that often eludes conventional therapy, especially in the field of infertility.

Jason lives up to the basic premise and ethic of a practising natural therapist. Note the symptoms and relieve them as best you can; however, firmly seek out the cause of an illness and devise natural treatments that harness the body's innate healing force to bring the person being treated to a state of balance where symptoms diminish without force or adding burdens that may be more toxic than the body can handle and have potential to produce ongoing rebound problems and/or permanent harm.

In our modern age, especially where those of normal fertility ages are exposed to a myriad of pollutants and stresses that can cause a lowering of health and viable fertility, a solution has to be sought to detoxify and de-stress the body for the hormonal system to restore. Other top natural fertility experts I have met also endorse this principle as they treat the person as a biochemical individual. Most often the herbal formulas and nutritional support are different for every patient.

Jason is a master at discerning the individual needs as he combines the principles of Ayurvedic, traditional Chinese and Western herbalism in his special herbal mixtures to bring the hormones and glands back to vital balance. Jason has a phenomenal record for bringing more than five thousand bonny babies to couples (who were told they would have little to no chance of conceiving) since he took up the challenge over twelve years ago to focus his specialty in this field.

Reproductive disorders are just one of the areas of health he excels at. He treats citizens of all ages, from newborn babies to the elderly, and he has many elite sportsmen and women under his wing relying on his expertise to stay at their peak.
Jason is often a guest on Queensland evening talk-back radio programmes giving free advice to the many who call in. He has a large family of his own and

manages to stay fit and give valuable time to all who seek him out for his encyclopaedic knowledge of health care.

I hope that one day the World Health Organisation knocks on his door to find out from him how to stabilise the decline in fertility levels in modern society before we phase ourselves out of existence due to the misguided concepts of having to use chemicals to grow food and stabilise water. We must move to reduce air pollution through reduction of polluting fuels as viable non-polluting options do exist and need to be fostered, not suppressed for the sake of big business. Governments need to put resources behind the growing of organic food so that it is affordable for all who seek it.

Remember, to avoid catastrophe we have to treat the cause of disease and if the earth is diseased so does our disease parallel that of the earth.

We need many more people in our community with the wisdom and vision of Jason Jackson. I am so glad he can spread the ripple with this excellent and very important book for our current times. Many couples wanting to conceive, whether fertile or experiencing difficulties, will gain much benefit and inspiration from this book.

Yours in support of a healthier planet and society,

Glen Gillard

Clinical Ecologist and Natural Therapist


"There is only one good, knowledge, and only one evil, ignorance."
- Socrates

"A man should consider that health is the greatest of human blessings."
- Hippocrates

"A true teacher is not the one with the most knowledge but the one who causes the most others to have knowledge."
- Neale Donald Walsh

"Optimism is the faith that leads to acheivement. Nothing can be done without hope and confidence."
- Helen Keller

# Introduction

Over the thousands of years that humans have been able to reproduce, it has only been in the last fifty years or so in the industrialised world, with its nutrient-depleted foods, genetically engineered agriculture, chemical processing, drugs, radiation and pollution, that we are now observing massive impacts on our ability to bear offspring, particularly in affluent Western societies.

Male sperm counts alone during this time have decreased by up to fifty percent. Industrialisation, technology and science have brought with them many advances in the way we live today, but this is a double-edged sword; along with the good has also come the bad. Modern living has set in motion a potent chain of events that pervades and moulds our very existence, which we haven't yet begun to understand and deal with.

Most people grow up assuming that one day when they are ready to start a family, it will automatically just happen within a short period of time. We often take our fertility very much for granted, not imagining that it may be a difficult process to conceive a child.

Chances are if you have selected this book to read you may be experiencing problems with conception or have had difficulty carrying a baby to term.

Perhaps you or your partner have been diagnosed with one of the many reproductive disorders that exist, and already know that conceiving will be a little more complicated for you. By reading this book you will find answers from both aspects of natural and orthodox medicine. From the natural side of things you will discover that by starting a pre-conception care program 3-6 months prior to trying to fall pregnant you will have a very good chance of correcting any imbalances that you may have.

For those couples thinking of starting reproductive medical procedures, such as IVF, or have been through several cycles of IVF, using natural therapies as a supportive role while undergoing these procedures would be very beneficial.

From the medical side of things, I have discussed all the procedures that are currently available, including all the drugs that are a part of these procedures and the pros and cons of using them.

Unfortunately, in this day and age we see more and more couples suffering from infertility. More than one in six couples is classed as infertile. This is a very disturbing number, considering not all couples experiencing infertility will seek medical assistance. We will never really know the exact figures. With that in mind, for those couples out there who may feel too embarrassed, or maybe for financial reasons think that they cannot possibly afford some of the more expensive orthodox medical procedures available, I have listed several things that you can do to increase your fertility without it costing a fortune.

When people come to me seeking my help for their infertility, it is usually as a last resort.

Couples who have been through several invasive medical procedures and are still unable to conceive, seemingly for no apparent reason, are referred to as 'unexplained' infertility; approximately 20 per cent of all infertility comes under this heading.

From a natural point of view, when a couple is experiencing infertility for this reason, I generally look thoroughly at their medical history, searching for clues that could have been previously missed. In natural therapies, when the practitioner treats the patient as a whole, by starting from the basics and correcting a person's health in general, quite often their unexplained infertility is corrected.

In this modern era women are focusing on their careers in their 20s, and leaving motherhood until they reach their 30s, when this is the time that her fertility starts to decline. A female's fertility is at its peak during her early to late 20s. This is the ideal time for her to start a family. As you are probably aware timing is very important. It is heart breaking for many couples that have decided to start a family later on in life, when they discover that their fertility has dropped dramatically. Although it may take a little bit longer to conceive when you are in the mid 30s to 40s, over the years I have had great success in helping many couples achieve their dream, when modern medicine has been unsuccessful.

You may be wondering what it is that I can do for you that is different from other practitioners. This question is asked frequently by new patients of mine, and it's a difficult one to answer, as I am not aware of what all naturopaths' treatment programs consist of.

Due to the complexity of infertility, I tend to spend a great deal of time trying to find out the medical history of my patients, therefore enabling me to design and tailor a treatment plan specifically for them. From my experience, having consulted with thousands of couples, it's not always the most obvious problem that is the actual cause, but rather the less obvious factors that are the ultimate culprit. It's the little details that can sometimes make the difference!

Each patient is unique; even if the medical condition is the same, the herbal formulas and nutritional supplements prescribed are still made differently, as there are many unique and individual factors that need to be taken into consideration. For example, patients presenting with PCOS (Poly Cystic Ovarian Syndrome) can greatly differ from each other. As there are several different levels of the condition, one can often require more or varied adaptation to treatment than another.

The purpose of this book is to help empower and prepare you for your journey in the pursuit of better reproductive health and restoration of fertility.

Depending on your particular circumstances and what stage you are at on this journey, having a reliable guide by your side can help answer your questions, regardless of whether you are pursuing pregnancy from a medically assisted program or from using natural therapy as a supportive protocol.

The more you know about infertility and the various treatment options that you can resource, the more able you will be to manage it successfully.

***Some of the questions that you may have in mind may include:***

- What are the causes and conditions that can contribute to infertility?

- What kind of external influences are known to affect fertility?

- Are there alternative/natural therapies I can use that could improve reproductive health? What are they and how do they work?

- What types of medical tests or examinations are there to access and diagnose if I do have a fertility problem?

- If I haven't been able to fall pregnant naturally, what medical procedures are available that could assist me to conceive?

- Are there things I can do to help prevent miscarriage?

- What kind of nutrients and foods are important to take that could help to improve conception and are beneficial during pregnancy?

- What can I expect to happen if I choose to go ahead with a specific treatment?

- What types of medical drugs do the doctors and IVF specialists use for infertility?

- If I have to use fertility drugs, what are the positive and negative effects of these medications?

- When I fall pregnant what can I do if I develop any other health problems?

All of these questions and many more will be answered throughout this book!
The way in which you use this guide may not necessarily be sequential; you may only want to know the basics to gain some general ideas about fertility or you may want more in-depth information for a greater understanding and clarity about fertility.
Depending upon your situation or what level of intervention that you may be contemplating, there are relevant sections suitable which should cover everyone's requirements. Whether you are just starting out on a fact-finding mission as a part of your preparation, or you are currently having medically assisted procedures, the information in this book may prove to be invaluable to you.

*Disclaimer* – Please note this book is not intended to replace advice from a qualified medical practitioner; however, by reading this book you will be more aware of the options available to you. For those people who combine both natural and orthodox medicine, it is very important to keep your practitioners aware of all medications and supplements that have been prescribed for you.

# Prologue

Virtually from childhood we start to rehearse for later life by role-playing mummies and daddies, with the expectation that we will become parents ourselves one day.

During our adolescent years when our sexual hormones kick in we become more aware of the fact that boys and girls are definitely made differently, and we become more concerned with the experimental act of reproduction (getting sex), rather than the consequence of the act (getting pregnant), let alone the issues of reproductive health.

As adults, we quickly need to find our feet to adapt to life with all the liberties and restrictions that go along with it. For most of us we will begin to formulate our plans for what we want and need in our future. We may wish to work on achieving that dream career in the hope of gaining financial security and personal satisfaction, get that nice house with all the mod-cons and trappings that go with it, or we may wish to travel to broaden our horizons and search for the elusive meaning of life and so on.

There may well come a time during our life's journey that we will all, at the very least, wrestle with the notion or idea that children may become part of our grand plan.

At some stage the body's maternal time clock will start to tick and it is extremely hard not to take notice when it does. For a large majority of women, and the occasional male, we may try to suppress these feelings, possibly for years, until we can't ignore them anymore and need to fill that void in our lives. Today the choice of whether to have children appears to be continually pushed further down the long list of life's priorities, until the day when we feel satisfied that the time is right. Now our perspective shifts from avoiding becoming pregnant just yet, to 'now it's time for action to start our family!'

Certainly we hear about other couples who haven't been able to have children for one reason or another, but until it strikes us personally we don't give it much thought. Many couples, when starting down the baby-making road, naturally expect a pregnancy to occur within a short time after they get serious about trying. But if too much time passes by, hope and expectation change to anxiety and doubt. If the problem continues we can begin to feel a sense of frustration, desperation and isolation.

The situation isn't helped by well-meaning friends and relatives with their less-than-subtle hints and reminders about time running out, or your body clock ticking away. Others may question why you would want to mess up your lifestyle by burdening yourselves with raising children, why not just enjoy the finer things in life, isn't having each other enough?

If that's not enough, everyone around you seems to be proving their fertility by getting pregnant and having babies, which just compounds your sense of inadequacy. Not to mention how difficult it is to keep on smiling, as the hot topic of conversation among your circle of friends revolves around their children.

There can be no doubt that infertility causes considerable emotional stress; however, we now know just how much of that very stress is in itself a <u>cause</u> of the infertility. Infertility can become an emotional, physical and financial roller-coaster ride. Failing to conceive a baby can be heartbreaking and devastating. Each monthly cycle becomes an agonising waiting game. With every disappointing attempt hopes and dreams feel like they are slipping through your fingers.

Infertility, when it directly affects you personally, can be intensely frustrating because it takes away your sense of control and forces you into a situation of dependency on others for help and support. Just when you thought you were getting your act together, the universe appears to single you out and throws a huge spanner in the works and disrupts your well-laid plans.

When one aspect of your life becomes negatively impacted it will naturally affect the others like a falling house if cards. People's confidence is crushed, decision-making becomes increasingly erratic and feelings of demoralisation and powerlessness are common among many couples.

Those who haven't suffered the anguish of involuntary childlessness cannot begin to comprehend how it can take over your lives. Stuck in limbo, desperate and disillusioned, feeling irrationally responsible for their affliction, blaming themselves for past decisions, lifestyles and health neglect, asking themselves 'what have we done to deserve this?'

During previous generations, conceiving a baby came easily to many couples. One would just have to look at their partner in that 'special way' and conception happened. But today, for some couples, climbing Mount Everest appears to be a less daunting task. Life is full of cruel ironies; for the couples that desperately want a family the road to parenthood seems frustratingly bumpy and difficult, while others who may not necessarily have pregnancy in mind, have a quick roll in the hay and fall pregnant.

There are many things that can be done, from both natural and orthodox medicine, to help ensure your best chances for success. There are many ways to treat reproductive problems. Natural pre-conception health-care can be very beneficial, not only for you and your partner, but can also greatly influence the odds of having a much happier and healthier baby.

Conceptual health-care does not just stop when a positive pregnancy has been diagnosed, but is encouraged to continue to support you throughout the pregnancy, labour and postnatal periods as well. If you are properly prepared, then you will feel more in control over your reproductive destiny!

## An Action Plan to Prepare Towards Pregnancy

### *The stages of a woman's reproductive life and what to expect*

Nowadays we are discovering more and more potential influences that may impact upon our reproductive health, and can prevent the delicate reproductive tissues from correctly functioning, thereby affecting our capacity to conceive. Because of all these compounding internal and external factors, it would seem sensible to take some active measures in the preparation for pregnancy. There are many things that can be done from both the prospective mother's and father's points of view to help in minimising potential problems from occurring that may hinder your fertility, or if reproductive problems do arise what positive steps you can take to rectify them.

Depending on your respective reproductive age and how long you have been trying to conceive, there are numerous issues to be aware of that may help you to gauge at what stages of your reproductive life you may require certain intervention, to assist with your planning towards a safe and trouble-free pregnancy.

This check-list can provide you with a basic guide that may help to clarify and assess if there is any reproductive problem that may require addressing and what you can do to optimise your preparation.

During the early stage of a woman's reproductive life, say from **puberty to the age of 20,** normally the follicle-stimulating hormone (FSH) and oestrogen hormones are within clinically acceptable ranges. After the onset of puberty the regular pattern of the menstrual cycle may take several years before it falls into place, usually 26 to 31 days between periods.

During this early stage it is not uncommon to experience some menstrual irregularities as the body's hormone feed-back system may not be strong enough to induce ovulation precisely every menstrual cycle. For this reason women who fall into this age group may not be quite as fertile (clinically speaking) as women in the following age group. As pre-conception issues are not as relevant to this group, medical investigations to determine fertility problems are less likely to take place during this stage.

The middle stages of a woman's reproductive life, you could say, are between the ages of **20 to 38 years**. Hormonally, oestrogen and FSH levels are usually more stable during this stage. A very small percentage of women experience menopause (or ovarian failure) before age 40; this may be indicated through blood tests that show the premature sustained elevation of FSH.

During this reproductive stage, the issues of preparing for conception become much more relevant, and this is the peak age group that woman may seek advice and undergo preliminary investigation, to assess their reproductive health.

The majority of woman during this time may have regular gynaecological examinations that include pap smears (high cervical swab), pelvic examinations, blood pressure, breast examinations, blood work to investigate full blood count, hormone function, thyroid function, rubella (German measles), hepatitis and HIV status, urine analysis for glucose and protein. Screenings to rule out sexually transmitted diseases (STDs) such as chlamydia, and other potential reproductive conditions that are more likely to occur during this stage such as: endometriosis, ovarian cysts, tubal blockages, and polycystic ovarian syndrome (PCOS).

Males should also have sperm tests and a physical examination to rule out potential problems that may contribute to infertility such as varicoses (all these conditions and many more will be discussed in-depth in following chapters). The times between 20 to 27 are recognised as the peak female fertile years. From 28 to 35 it is believed to begin to decline slightly, and from 35 onwards fertility starts to drop away more rapidly.

The later end of the reproductive stage is around the **38 to 42 age group**. This is not to imply you cannot carry a successful pregnancy to term after this age, though statistically speaking the odds are declining more so after this stage. Some women's FSH levels may have increased marginally at this age and may fluctuate somewhat from month to month.

With the increase in FSH, the ovary follicles become less responsible and the viable egg reserves begin to rapidly decline. Oestrogen levels may become slightly more erratic, though not necessarily enough to greatly affect ovulation and menstrual periods, which are usually still fairly accurate. Some women may begin to notice an increase in thrush and bladder infections as the fluctuations of hormones, particularly oestrogen, affect the acidity and elasticity the reproductive tissue.

The vaginal area may also become dryer and less lubricated. Because of the slight changes in hormone levels, you may find that you could experience some mood swings and period discomfort. Conditions such as fibroids, breast cysts, altered menstrual bleeding, and increased damage to the eggs can raise the potential incidence of birth defects.

This is the most common age group of the couples that I see at my clinic who come for reproductive counselling, most of whom have already been through numerous tests and examinations. If any medical conditions have been identified or diagnosed that may be impeding their fertility and potential to conceive, formal treatment protocols may be recommended (this will be covered in other chapters).

If couples have already undertaken medically assisted reproductive procedures such as IVF or ICSI, there is an endless resource of alternative/natural therapies that can be employed to increase the couple's preconceptual health care to optimise their chances of successful conception, either naturally or supportively, with the various medically assisted approaches. Most of us know of the important role of nutrients such as folic acid in conceptual care. Folic acid indeed has its vital place, but it is only one of many important nutrients required to maximise reproductive and foetal health.

The essential information presented throughout the following sections will educate and enlighten you to the importance of finding balance in your nutrition, lifestyle and environment.

Between the ages of **42 to 50** can be classified as the (Climactic) Peri-Menopausal stage. During this time a woman's FSH levels may dramatically rise and the oestrogen levels dramatically fluctuate and fall. Follicle quantity and quality may also be lowered. The further a woman transitions towards menopause, the less oestrogen and progesterone is released by the follicle. Ovulation during this stage may become increasingly hit-and-miss as hormonal feed-back signalling is less responsive. With the decline in the release of these hormones the uterine lining is lessened also. Because the uterus preparation has diminished it is not uncommon to notice the shortening of the length of time between periods, say, between 24 to 27 days instead of 28 to 31 days. Medically assisted reproductive intervention to pregnancy increases greatly during this stage; progesterone supplementation may be commonly recommended by your doctor to help enhance the uterine lining quality.

Other issues that arise during this stage may include: aging eggs that can become increasingly harder to penetrate by the sperm; and adhesion problems to the uterine lining, which also tend to increase. When the eggs reach this point in aging, the embryo quality many not be as good (in comparison with younger eggs) and the incidences of miscarriage may also greatly increase. Other health-related conditions are also more common during pregnancies during this stage. These may include: gestational diabetes; Caesarean births; and elevated blood pressure problems. Genetic counselling with a specialist in the field may help to clarify any concerns you may have regarding genetic or chromosome disorders. Most IVF centres offer PGD or similar testing to identify if genetic problems are likely to be relevant.

Menopause and the post-menopause stages normally occur after the 50-plus years. The FSH levels have peaked and stay elevated during these stages. The adrenal glands may still produce a small amount of sex hormones but the ovaries' production is very insignificant now. The clinical definition of menopause is when a woman has not had a true menstrual period for an entire year. The up-side to menopause is that if you previously suffered from endometriosis, fibroids, and ovarian cysts, they tend to greatly decrease and shrink during this stage.

At menopause most women may still have several hundred to thousands of eggs still remaining, but rarely are they viable to fertilise. The transition into menopause for some woman can be a traumatic experience: mood swings; hot flushes; sweating; and libido fluctuations are just some examples of symptoms that are commonly observed.

Menopause is not a disease and in the past, it was very much treated as such. There are numerous supportive treatments available through natural and orthodox medicine that can support you through these changes in symptoms so you don't have to suffer through this change-of-life phase.

## The Basics of Natural Conception

### The different roles of the man and the woman

Short of rehashing the story of the birds and the bees (hopefully that has been explained correctly to you by now), this section will help to set the scene of what is involved during the process of natural conception.

It's the reproductive system that sets the sexes apart. Male and female bodies are built differently, are powered by different hormones and complete vastly different functions. The female sex organs are stimulated to develop when a girl reaches puberty. The ovaries begin production of the hormones oestrogen and progesterone, breasts begin to grow, body hair forms and body shape changes.

During child-bearing years, the ovaries are smooth and firm, enabling them to produce the eggs, called ova, and the hormones that nourish a foetus. Every 28 days, hormones from the pituitary gland cause an ovum to leave the ovary and enter the fallopian tubes. If sperm are present, one may bind to the ovum to form a pronucleus.

The fallopian tubes are connected to the ovaries and lead to the uterus, a thick-walled pear-shaped organ. At the bottom of the uterus is the cervix, which opens into the vagina. At the opening of the vagina are the vulval region and the clitoris, an organ containing spongy erectile tissue and nerve endings. The male sex organs comprise the penis, two testes, the prostate gland and the intricate tube system that allows sperm produced in the testes to be ejaculated. During puberty (usually during a boy's early teens) the brain signals a secretion of hormones to stimulate development of the reproductive system.

The testes, walnut-shaped glands within the scrotum, release hormones called androgens, of which the most powerful is testosterone. Testosterone causes the sex organs to grow, and sexual characteristics develop, such as deepening of the voice and the growth of body hair.

Stimulated by thought or by touch, arteries in the penis become dilated and fill with blood, leading to an erection. The blood cannot drain away as veins at the base of the penis are closed off by surrounding tissue. When sexual stimulation becomes most intense, sperm and fluid created in the prostate gland and the delicate tube system is ejaculated through the urethra.

During sexual intercourse, when the erect penis is inside the vagina, ejaculated sperm swim upward to fertilise the female egg. After ejaculation, the veins in the penis reopen and the blood drains back into the body.

## Genesis – the Symphony of Life's Little Miracles

It's the moment when all new life beings are formed. Conception, when a male sperm fertilises a female egg, is usually the result of sexual intercourse between a man and a woman.

The exception to this is when science, through in-vitro fertilisation, helps couples who have trouble conceiving. From the time a male reaches puberty until he dies, a man is usually capable of producing sperm that can fertilise an egg. A man's testes produce millions of sperm daily and a healthy male can deposit 200 to 600 million sperm during one ejaculation.

Women are usually capable of conceiving a child from puberty to menopause. A woman is born with a lifetime supply of eggs. One egg or ovum is released each month by one of her two ovaries. Yet the chance of an egg being fertilised naturally by a sperm are many millions to one. Critical to the success of reproduction is the timing of sexual intercourse.

Women have an ovulatory or menstrual cycle, made up of complex physiological and biochemical changes. In the first phase of the menstrual cycle a follicle grows in the ovary, while the lining of the uterus builds up to receive a fertilised egg. At mid-cycle, when the egg is ready, the ovary releases the egg. This stage is called ovulation and is the best time to conceive.

The egg enters the fallopian tube, where it is caught up in the waving arms of the tiny filaments (fimbriae) that are at the end of the fallopian tube. The fallopian tube internally only has a width similar to that of a bristle of a hair brush. The egg has commenced its journey on its way towards the uterus. If the egg is not fertilised it is flushed from the body when the uterus sheds its lining and a new menstrual cycle begins.

As a couple engages in sexual intercourse, a man inserts his erect penis into the woman's vagina. During intercourse muscle contractions propel semen from the penis into the vagina. Once semen is deposited at the neck of the woman's uterus, the sperm begin the long journey to fertilisation. This must be completed within 48 hours, before the sperm die. The environment for the sperm in the woman's reproductive system is a hazardous place for them to survive long enough to complete their tasks to fertilise the egg.

Sperm move via a thrashing motion of their tails; this action propels them in a progressive movement hopefully toward their goal of reaching the egg. Sperm can potentially survive for 3 to 5 days after ejaculation, but due to the environment many are destroyed and the live sperm reduce by one-third each day. An average life span of a sperm is roughly 16 to 18 hours, so they need to get a wriggle on.

The sperm's journey may take about an hour to swim from the neck of the uterus called the cervix to the location in the fallopian tube called the ampulla, where if timing is right, the egg should be there waiting to be romanced by the swarm. The egg is only able to wait for her Mr Right sperm to show up for 12 to 24 hours. If by this time she has been stood up and the sperm hasn't arrived then the egg will give up and die.

But, while the egg is waiting for her white knight (the sperm) to save her, a substance that surrounds the egg is released that is believed to help attract and direct the sperm to assure they are swimming in the right direction. The sperm at this stage travel up the lining into the fallopian tube. Up to 1000 sperm surround the egg, but only one lucky winner can penetrate it due to the release of a special chemical. As soon as that happens, the cell membrane of the egg changes, preventing other sperm from entering.

The fertilised egg is now called a zygote. The zygote now comprises the complete 46 chromosomes (genetic material) from DNA of both the 23 chromosomes from the male's sperm and the 23 chromosomes from the woman's egg joined together to form the genesis of new human life. The zygote divides to form more cells, while being pushed along the fallopian tube. After 4 days the zygote has 100 cells and is called a blastocyst.

When the blastocyst reaches the uterine lining it floats for two days, implanting itself in the uterine wall by the sixth day after fertilisation. The blastocyst then secretes the hormone HCG, signalling a successful pregnancy. It is the level of HCG in the urine that is measured by a pregnancy test.

# Chapter 1

# *Facts of Fertility*

### *The stats of the matter*

Infertility is clinically diagnosed after a couple have been unsuccessful in their attempts to conceive after one year of trying to fall pregnant (after regular intercourse, sexual activity during the time of ovulation). It may also refer to the inability to carry a pregnancy to term. The condition may affect the male or female partner, or both. Of the 20 per cent of couples who experience infertility, the causal factor can be in found in 80 per cent of couples. Therefore, 20 per cent are medically defined as infertile due to unknown origin or **Idiopathic**.

First-degree infertility is the term used to describe those who have never had children. Second-degree infertility describes those who have had children but find themselves unable to conceive again at any point in their reproductive life.

The phenomenal decline in fertility and reproductive health may have various explanations but there are three main factors that stand out: One – couples are waiting until they are over 35 before trying to have children; Two – there is a marked increase in sexually transmitted diseases such as chlamydia; and Three – rapidly falling sperm counts and quality, largely suspected of having something to do with the last several generations of increased 'hormone-disruptive' chemicals that we, our parents and our parents' parents have become exposed to. The fertility problems that we are having today were possibly set in motion generations before we were even born.

Statisticians at the World Health Organisation (WHO) have estimated that the ability of a couple to conceive and to bear a living child affects some *80 million-plus* married couples around the world at any one time and is increasing. Estimates also suggest that infertility now impacts on more than *1 in every 6 Australian couples (over 3 million Australians)* and current trends are showing that this rate may continue to alarmingly increase and afflict more couples trying to have families in the foreseeable future.

Experts are predicting that infertility will affect a shocking *1 in 3* in just the next ten years. If we are currently up to generation 'Y' then we are seriously running out of letters in the alphabet.

**Late bloomers to parenthood – the elixir to the fountain of youth!**

Demographically, in society it appears that we are choosing to pursue parenthood much later in our reproductive lives. Many factors may be considered as to why this shift in reproducing is declining, although socio-economics and the changing attitudes to early parenting would have to play a major part of this current trend. This trend is not only prevalent throughout the general population; you only need to pick up a tabloid magazine to read about many of the Hollywood celebrities who are having children later in their reproductive years.

Cheryl Tiegs had twins at the age of 52, Elizabeth Edwards (wife of former US Senator and Vice President nominee – John Edwards) at 49 and 51, Beverley D'Angelo had twins at the age of 49, Holly Hunter fell pregnant with twins at 47, Geena Davies at 46 had her first bub and also had twins at 48, Susan Sarandon at 46, Christie Brinkley at 46, Jane Seymour had twins aged 45, naturally; Cherie Booth (wife of Tony Blair, former British prime minister) at 46; Jane Kaczmarek at 41, 43 and 46, Helen Fielding (Author of Bridget Jones' Diaries) at 43 & 48, Mimi Rogers at 45 and Marcia Cross (twins) at 44. Madonna had her second child at 41, Jerry Hall at 41, Annette Bening at 41, Halley Berry at 41, Nicole Kidman gave birth to Sunday Rose also at 41. All are members of the late bloomers club.

Some of the oldest celebrity fathers include: Julio Iglesias Sr. at 89, Saul Bellow at 84, Anthony Quinn at 81, Charlie Chaplin at 73, Rupert Murdoch at 72, Pablo Picasso at 68, Luciano Pavorotti had twins at 67, Larry King at 65 and 66, Warren Betty at 62, Paul McCartney at 61, Rod Stewart at 60, Eric Clapton at 59, Michael Douglas at 58 and Mick Jagger at 57. These guys were not shooting with blanks!

Some studies are estimating that the average age for females to conceive for the first time is approximately 30.2 years of age, in comparison to previous generations, which were approximately 24 years of age. Figures from the Australian Bureau of Statistics show over the last 25 years, the percentage of births in women over the age of 30 has doubled. Women aged between 35 and 39 are having more babies than women aged 20 to 24. In Australia in 2004, there were 53.4 births per 1000 women aged 20 to 24, compared to 57.4 births per 1000 women aged 35 to 39. Fifteen percent of couples medically investigated for infertility have been found to have more than one cause for their infertility. Male reproductive failure may now comprise 50 to 70 percent of infertility cases in western countries. During the past twenty years the birth rate for women under the age of 29 has almost halved. The highest birth rate with women is now between the 30 to 34 age group. Also during the past twenty years women aged between 35 and 39 have an increased birth percentage rate of around 65 percent in comparison to twenty years ago. The 'baby boom' period during modern times peaked during 1961, with an average of 3.5 babies per woman.

At the beginning of 2000, this number had declined to 1.75 babies per woman, a dramatic reduction by half in only forty years with trends reflecting that this will continue to worsen. Children from the 'baby boomer' era are now entering into the 'middle-aged' category of the population. This is now placing more of a strain on our fragile economies because there are not enough younger generations of future taxpayers to match and support this aging population.

Finding Mr or Mrs Right and committing to a long-term established secure relationship is a significant factor in the decline in conception rates in recent times; the modern trends in society towards remaining single during our twenties has rapidly increased during the last decade. Studies by Monash University over the past 15 years have observed a decline in marriage rates during this time. In 1986, 72 percent of women aged 30-34 and 65 percent of men aged 30 to 34 were married. By 2001, the comparable figures were 55 percent for women and just 47 percent for men. Marriage is occurring later in this current generation. In 1979 the median age of a woman marrying was 21 – in 2002 it was 29. This would be the equivalent of a woman aged 21 having over 1 million eggs dropping to some 250 thousand eggs on average at the age of 29. In 1976, 92 per cent of women had their first child under the age of 30 – in 2006 this had dropped to 27 per cent.

Infertility now affects tens of millions of couples worldwide at any one time, approximately *6.1 million* clinically recognised sub-fertile or infertile American couples alone are being medically 'treated' at any given time; this number does not account for people who haven't sought formal treatment. This data was published in 1995, therefore, considering present trends this number has possibly increased greatly since such time.

Recent research reported from the Mayo Clinic in the United States has indicated that an average healthy couple in their 20s has a 20 percent chance of successful conception during any given month. After the age of 30, fertility drops another 20 percent – a small decline; after the age of 35 a drop by 50 percent (10-15 percent chance) – a more significant decline, and a woman over 40 the odds drop to 95 percent or a 5 percent chance of conception.

Comparatively in the grand scale of matters a decrease from 20 to 5 percent between the ages of twenty to forty does not appear to be a very wide gap considering the pressure media reports put on older women attempting to have a baby. After the age of 45 the conception percentage is about 1 percent. This may be largely due to the increasing rate of chromosomally abnormal embryos that can occur during this stage of reproductive life. Even with these statistical odds, the number of births among women aged 45 to 49 today has increased a remarkable five hundred (500) per cent from only a decade ago.

The greatest chance of achieving successful conception is believed to occur in the 25-to-30-year-old age group.

Infertility can be a multi-faceted condition with potential causal influences coming from physiological, environmental, social as well as mental and emotional origins. Pinpointing the exact cause of the problem can sometimes be difficult. Ovulation, fertilisation, and the difficult journey of the fertilised ovum through the fallopian tube and finally into the uterus are highly intricate processes, and the struggle of life to find its way is fraught with many obstacles. Many scientists and environmentalists believe we are rapidly approaching a *'Fertility Crisis'*.

Recent evaluation of infertile couples revealed that male infertility or reproductive system problems (partially or wholly) affected between 40–50 percent of the cases. Of the 10 percent of couples that are unable to conceive, the male is found to be the cause in 60 percent of cases. The average male after the age of 24 has been identified to lose potency by 2 percent for every year thereafter.

# Chapter 2

# *Male Reproductive Overview*

## All about the Boys

There are many similar hormonal processes at work in men as in women. The hypothalamus gland releases gonadotrophin-releasing hormone (GnRH) every 60 to 90 minutes to trigger the pituitary gland to release follicle-stimulating hormone (FSH) and luteinising hormone (LH). What differs between men and women is that men normally produce these hormones at an even rate throughout the month, whereas women have various fluctuations of these hormones during the differing stages of the monthly menstrual cycle. The balance of these hormones is of essential importance to his fertility.

LH stimulates the Leydig cells in the testes that produce the hormone testosterone. Testosterone is required for numerous functions including: development of male characteristics; facial hair; penis enlargement at puberty; production of seminal fluids; sperm maturation; and sexual arousal. The testes are comparably about the same size as women's ovaries and are surrounded by the scrotal sac located outside the body. The testes are comprised of thousands of very tiny coiled tubes known as seminiferous tubules.

The process of spermatocytes is stimulated via FSH: primary sperm cells within the tubes divide and develop into spermatids which are tail-less young sperm. Normally, sperm is constantly being produced in the testes. A healthy male can produce over 50,000 sperm a minute, which is an incredible 72 to 120,000 million every day (up to 1,500 per second – an impressive production line).

These sperm travel to the epididymis where they are nourished by the Sertoli cells that line the tubules and form over a 72-day period, and then take another 20 to 30 days to mature completely. If the sperm are not ejaculated after this time they are broken down and are absorbed back into the body's system.

Every tiny sperm is made up of three parts, which are visible under a microscope:

- The head of the sperm contains the chromosomes and genetic information that are the male contribution to the child's heredity.
- The neck is the system of nerves that nourish the sperm, creating an energy supply aiding movement.

- The tail (flagellum) is the 'motor', which propels the sperm forward by lashing energetically from side to side, using stored Fructose (a form of sugar) as its 'fuel'.

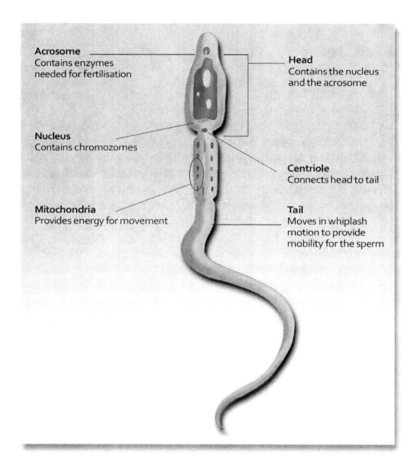

**Acrosome**
Contains enzymes
needed for fertilisation

**Head**
Contains the nucleus
and the acrosome

**Nucleus**
Contains chromozomes

**Centriole**
Connects head to tail

**Mitochondria**
Provides energy for movement

**Tail**
Moves in whiplash
motion to provide
mobility for the sperm

*Figure.1. A healthy sperm*

The sperm is forced out through the urethra by rhythmic contractions of the *epididymis*, sperm ducts and other muscles, giving enough thrust for the sperm to have the best chance of fusion with the egg (ovum). Sperm alone is not enough; for it to make the journey successfully and fuse with an egg, a rich fluid must nourish sperm.

The seminal fluid is protective, energising, and lubricating, and is also composed of three parts:

- An alkaline fluid produced by two seminal vesicles, or pouches, which protects the sperm from and acidity in the female vaginal fluid. This fluid accounts for about 70 per cent of semen volume, sperm cells account for about 20 per cent of the volume. Fibrinogen, a substance that holds or coagulates the seminal fluids together, and prostaglandins that help the sperm penetrate the cervix are also produced.

- A fluid containing a form of sugar called fructose is released by the prostate gland, which enables the sperm to move rapidly and sustain energy.

- A pre-ejaculatory fluid produced by the Cowper's gland at the end of the urethra, acts as a lubricant along the path taken by the ejaculate.

- Seminal fluid is composed of some 22 different substances such as: Vitamins B12, Vitamin C, Vitamin E, fructose sugar, potassium, sulphur, zinc, fatty acids, prostaglandins and also contains other antioxidant factors that protect the cells from damage. In sub-fertile males, this seminal fluid may not contain adequate amounts of these protective elements.

The semen cocktail contain some 83 identified proteins. These proteins play various crucial roles in conception. Some of these proteins are needed for the sperm to follow the chemical trail that leads them to the ovum; other proteins help to fight bacteria. A protein known as *PLCzeta* has a vital function at the end of a sperm's journey once the egg has been penetrated; its function is to trigger a calcium cascade that allows the egg to start growing. Faults in this protein could be a root cause of male infertility.

Another discovered peptide in semen called *TGF-beta* appears to have a very important function of reducing the woman's immune killer cells from destroying the sperm. Again faulty interaction of this protein within the female's body can be a significant cause behind immunological compatibility problems and a high sperm kill-off ratio.

When semen is ejaculated it is usually in a soft gel, viscous consistency (coagulum); this is possibly to protect the sperm during ejaculation. After approximately five to fifteen minutes of being inside the female's body the semen turns into a liquid consistency allowing the sperm to become mobile. Many people confuse sperm with semen. But men with no sperm can still have semen. This is because semen is a fluid that normally contains only 2 per cent sperm. These aforementioned fluids are to keep the sperm healthy and help to counteract vaginal acids that can destroy sperm.

The *vas deferens* and the seminal vesicles connect to the ejaculatory ducts in the prostate. The vas deferens tube is an incredible 6 metres (18ft) in length and is capable of storing enough sperm for about 30 ejaculations. These tubes in turn empty into the *urethra*, which carries the sperm outside the penis on ejaculation. Ejaculation (seminal release) is usually achieved via rapid muscular contractions from orgasm.

On average it is estimated that less than one in ten sperm will survive in the vagina before the arduous journey through the cervix and uterus up the fallopian tube to meet up with the egg. Some 'super-charged' sperm are able, after ejaculation, to potentially reach the entrance to a woman's fallopian tubes in as little as five minutes; other sperm may take much longer and can possibly survive up to five days after ejaculation. Fertilisation of the egg is still possible after five days if the environment is suitable to sustain sperm activity. Sperm is ejaculated for the male's body at an impressive force, approximately 16 kilometres per hour (10 mph). This may not sound very fast to you or me but when you consider how tiny the sperm cells are that speed would be equivalent to the G-forces experienced by an astronaut blasting off in a space rocket away from the earth's orbit.

Per average ejaculation a male produces about 3 to 6 ml of seminal fluids, which normally contains between 60 - 200 million sperm. If a male ejaculated 250 - 350 million sperm on average (approximately equivalent to the population of the United States of America); only 100 million would survive to make it to the cervix. Approximately 1 hour after ejaculation about 50 percent of the sperm lose their motility. Of the original 300 million sperm that started out on this journey, only 200 or so lucky fellows will get to the fallopian tube to have a chance at fertilising an egg.

Errors in the male's sperm production and replication are much more likely to occur than in the female's eggs. This is because the sperm go through an estimated 328 - 380 cell divisions before they reach the stage of an adult tadpole-shaped cell ready to be used to fertilise an egg. Each time a cell divides genetic copying (transcription) faults can occur. In comparison, the female's egg has much less opportunity for errors to arise as the egg undergoes only about 23 cell divisions making them less likely to develop copying errors.


**'Sperm ain't what it used to be'**

*Sick sperm syndrome – It's a tough life for a sperm*

In 1938, the average sperm count was 113 million per ml; by 1990 that value had dropped to 66 million, in 2003 the numbers have fallen further to 40 million per ml. Adding to this, the amount of semen fell almost 20 percent from 3.4 to 2.75 ml. Altogether, these changes mean that men are now supplying about 35 percent of the number of sperm ejaculate compared with 1938 levels.

Young adult males that possibly fought during the World War Two era were approximately three times more potent on average than the same aged males of today.

Now we are into the 21<sup>st</sup> century, going by progressive trends these amounts would be expected to be worsening. The gravity of these findings is not showing an encouraging outlook for the next 50 years. Not only are sperm counts generally declining, the motility and formation of the sperm that are being produced is also reducing. Overall sperm fitness is now proving to be a vital key to the success of male fertility. Indeed having adequate sperm numbers and motility (athletic potential) are vital criteria to the success of conception, as is the quality of the genetic load the sperm is carrying.

There are many other factors to male fertility that are simply overlooked or are still unknown. Statistically, *30 per cent* of men with perfectly adequate sperm (tested under current scientific standards) have trouble fertilising a healthy female's ovum to achieve conception. There must be other factors involved that are contributing to this men's infertility.

A look into the future: In 2006, biologist Professor Karim Nayernia was the first person to successfully 'grow' artificial mouse sperm from blank stem cells that fertilised a female mouse's eggs and produced life of seven mice offspring using ISCI technique. This major breakthrough in reproductive medicine may in the future be a significant stepping stone to curing numerous human male infertility conditions and offering fresh hope to the millions of couples blighted by infertility. By the year 2011, scientists believe that immature sperm cells removed from the testicles will be able to be grown in the lab to fully functional sperm that can then be put back into the man's body to then be able to fertilise a female's egg. This technique may potentially be able to create sperm free of inherited genetic flaws.

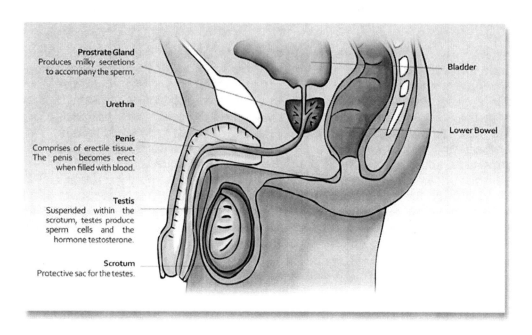

**Prostrate Gland**
Produces milky secretions to accompany the sperm.

**Urethra**

**Penis**
Comprises of erectile tissue. The penis becomes erect when filled with blood.

**Testis**
Suspended within the scrotum, testes produce sperm cells and the hormone testosterone.

**Scrotum**
Protective sac for the testes.

Bladder

Lower Bowel

*Figure.2. The Male Reproductive System (Cross Section)*

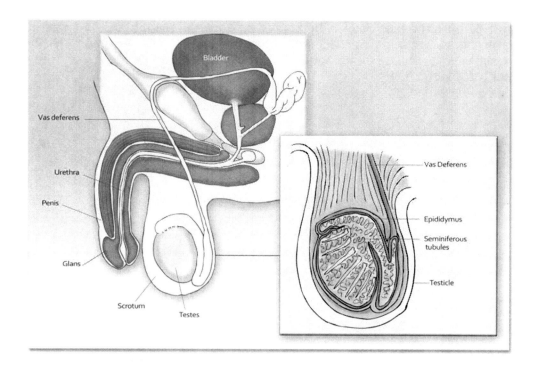

Bladder

Vas deferens

Urethra

Penis

Glans

Scrotum

Testes

Vas Deferens

Epididymus

Seminiferous tubules

Testicle

*Figure.3. Internal Cross Section of Testis*

30

# Fertility Tests

There are a number of tests – for women and men – that may be performed if conception does not occur within a twelve-month period or longer. It is both easier and more cost-effective to test the male partner first before going on to the more invasive techniques needed to test the female partner.

Even if the male's test results return with passing marks from your pathologist, there are many other factors that need to be considered from the male's point of view before he is ruled out diagnostically.

# Tests Performed on Men

*Endocrine test*: Blood tests are done to determine levels of follicle-stimulating hormone (FSH); if the levels of FSH are low to normal then treatments are available, though, if the levels are abnormally high, the man is considered permanently sterile. This is not necessarily my personal view; I believe that there are many natural medicine treatments worth trying first!

*Luteinising hormone (LH), and Thyroid hormones (T)*: LH levels are usually only tested if thyroid hormone levels are abnormal. Free testosterone, aldosterone and even prolactin hormones may be investigated to rule out if they are the cause of the problem!

*Postcoital Test (PCT)*: The partners have sexual intercourse during the middle stage of the female cycle (around day 14) and the ejaculate is tested for surviving sperm approximately 12 to 14 hours thereafter. A vaginal swab is retrieved to analyse the interaction of the sperm and mucus to predict any problems. Doesn't that sound like great fun to have done?

*Kremer test*: Many specialists now prefer to use the Kremer test as opposed to the postcoital test. This examination involves analysing the sperm's capacity to penetrate or swim through the mucus secreted in the women's vagina around the time of ovulation.

A sperm sample is supplied by the male and a mucus vaginal swab at mid-cycle is retrieved from the female. The sperm and mucus are placed together and examined under a microscope to observe penetration and anti-sperm antibody reactions. Donor sperm is also used to analyse a controlled comparison. This is a particularly useful test for evaluating the presence of any significant antibodies that may be contributing to cause of infertility.

The majority of pathology and physical examinations that are mentioned will require a doctor's referral to a pathology lab or IVF speciality centre.

# Semen Analysis

A sample of semen is examined no longer than one or two hours after ejaculation. The male sperm analysis should be one of the first procedures carried out before other examinations take place as it is one of the easiest and cheapest tests to perform. Not forgetting that males account for 40 to 50 per cent of the causes of infertility, problems associated with conception is not an exclusive condition only limited to females.

### Fertility is a couple's issue, not a women's issue

*'It takes two to tango'* and from my experience a large majority of the time the males can be overlooked as part of the fertility process until quite late in the investigative stages. When I am consulting on fertility it is usually only the female partner that initially attends. The earlier the males can be encouraged to get involved and be investigated, the better, as it can save a lot of trouble further down the track. Particularly if it is eventually diagnosed that it is the male partner contributing to the fertility problem, a lot of time and effort can be avoided. I know that rearranging work commitments is not an easy thing to do, but for a matter as *important* as this, you would expect to see a united partnership commitment. The guys are also contributing half the genetics necessary to make a baby and should not be forgotten.

A semen analysis is a very useful procedure to help determine if there is anything going wrong from the male's side of things and can assist in narrowing down the field of possible causes that may be hindering conception. Depending on the clinic performing the analysis, the sperm sample may be preferred to be produced or collected on site at the clinic facility. The process of normal sperm collection does not require a degree in rocket science from the male participant, though the basic laws of propulsion do apply! Next to having a physical prostate exam, giving a sperm sample is possibly number 2 on a male's list of fear factors.

In a nutshell – the male is required to take himself into a private room where he needs to masturbate (the 'wank-a-torium' I've heard it described) so the ejaculate of semen is fully collected into a sterile container, so it can be either processed for the purpose of the analysis or if you are at the stage of attempting a medically assisted conception procedure, then the sperm may be specially stored awaiting its use for the fertilisation stage. Most men may find that having to masturbate on cue is somewhat awkward and embarrassing as part of their contribution to the conception process, though when you consider what procedures the lady may have to go through and the other alternatives there are for extracting the essential sperm, this is a relatively painless and simple activity. The initial anxiousness surrounding the whole event is quickly forgotten. Keep your mind on the goal; this procedure may be a very important stepping stone along the road to you and your partner having a baby.

Some males may really not feel comfortable about producing the sample at the clinic, so arrangements may be made to produce the sample at home, if correct storage and transport guidelines are strictly adhered to, such as getting the sample to the laboratory within a 2-hour period and storing it in a warm area like the pocket of your jacket (make sure it's securely sealed in the sterile container or that could be messy!). The sterile surroundings of an IVF clinic or pathology centre may not be very conducive to getting a male aroused enough to achieve ejaculation. Some centres provide some inspirational material such as magazines or videos to help take his mind off the embarrassing aspects of what they need to do and focus on the job at hand (forgive the pun!).

A percentage of males may not or do not masturbate for whatever personal reasons. Therefore, a special type of condom may be provided by the clinic so the sperm sample can be obtained through intercourse. This may not be the preferred method by some clinics but using this type of condom (not the ones you may normally use) can minimise unwanted contaminates. It is important to bear in mind that all the ejaculate should to be collected for the accuracy of the analysis; the first part of the ejaculate is especially required as it usually contains the highest amount of sperm concentration.

The results are correlated and the specialist or doctor reviews the results. This information will assist in ruling out certain issues and may help to shed light on what future plan of attack is warranted. If for some reason, the sperm results are not looking too favourable (e.g. many abnormalities or low numbers, etc) after the first attempt, a future follow-up sample may be needed in approximately 2 months to rule out any false-negative results, as there are many influencing factors that can temporarily affect a sperm result.

The sperm may require going through a **wash** procedure; this is normally done prior to egg fertilisation in IVF, ICSI or AIH procedures. The sperm is washed particularly if foreign matter (debris) or sperm antibodies are seen to be present. Debris in the semen can also be an indicator of possible infection or prostate health issues. Washing the sperm increases the chances of correct fertilisation to occur and minimise immune reactions against the sperm. In some situations where sperm is known to be produced but is unable to be ejaculated, the sperm may require extraction via medical intervention to be retrieved through an **aspiration technique**. This procedure may be recommended in conditions that involve absence or blockage of ducts and when the sperm production may be extremely low.

Sperm can be retrieved by several techniques. The most common is via testicular biopsy with local anaesthetic (when you're awake) or general anaesthetic (when you're asleep). The aspiration of the sperm is performed using a needle that is directly inserted through the scrotum skin and into the testicle or epididymis and the fluid containing the sperm is then sucked out via the needle. That sounds like having as much fun as a kick in the head, though the swelling and discomfort usually stop within a few days after the procedure is completed. It's not as bad as it sounds, guys!

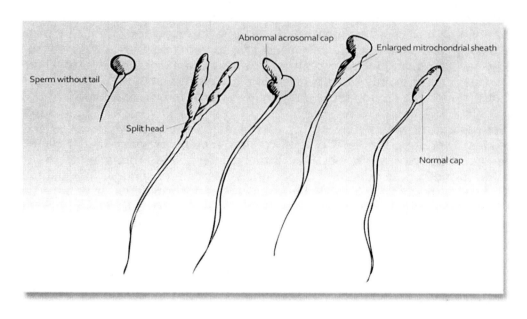

*Figure.4. Various types of sperm abnormalities*

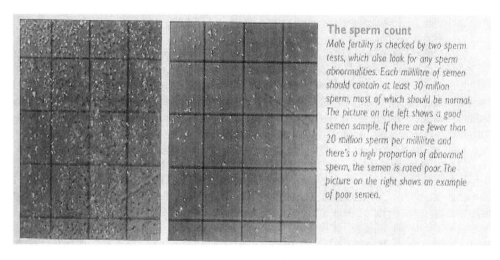

## The sperm count

Male fertility is checked by two sperm tests, which also look for any sperm abnormalities. Each millilitre of semen should contain at least 30 million sperm, most of which should be normal. The picture on the left shows a good semen sample. If there are fewer than 20 million sperm per millilitre and there's a high proportion of abnormal sperm, the semen is rated poor. The picture on the right shows an example of poor semen.

*Microscope grid used to examine sperm for count and abnormalities*

# Tests for Male Fertility

- **Sperm motility**. The percentage of sperm swimming should be more than 60 per cent.

- **Concentration**. The number of sperm (both alive and dead) that are in the ejaculate. The normal amount is 20 million sperm per millilitre or more, or a total greater than 40 million per ejaculate.

- **Morphology**. The percentage that is normally shaped should be more than 30 per cent normal.

- **Semen volume**. The total amount of ejaculate produced should be 1.5 to 5ml, or approximately a teaspoon.

- **Semen colour**. Semen is normally cream in colour; white-coloured semen may indicate an infection; clear-coloured semen may indicate low sperm content, red colour in semen may indicate blood due to possible kidney damage, testicular injury, or prostate gland damage.

- **Viscosity/density, time of last ejaculation, sperm count**. Usually reaches its highest levels after two (2) to three (3) days of abstinence from any sexual activity (including masturbation – no choking the chicken, spanking the monkey, or jerkin the gherkin)! Sperm that remains in a man's body for longer than a month is less effective at fertilising an egg (ovum). Depending on which pathology organisation is performing the test (SCALES MAY VARY!), it is preferable to see numbers over the 40 million range with better than 50+% motility and morphology.

- **Agglutination**. Where sperm stick to each other – may also be observed to see if the sperm is 'clumping' together appropriately. Also 80 per cent of sperm should still be active an hour after ejaculation.

- **Forward progression**. Is a rating on a scale of 1 to 4, at least 2 plus means a good number of sperm are moving forward.

- **Acrosome reaction test**. The tip of the sperm is the acrosome. It contains enzymes that allow the sperm to penetrate the egg. If the proper enzymes aren't present, the sperm can't get through the egg zona (outer layer - shell).

- **Hypo-osmotic swelling (HOS)**. Greater than 50 per cent of the sperm tails should swell when exposed to a hypo-osmotic solution; this swelling is a sign of normal functioning.

- **The Ph – (Acid/Alkaline level)**. The Ph level should be in the alkaline (7.2 – 8.0) to protect sperm from the acidic environment of the vagina. White blood cells: Should be no more than 0 to 5 per high-power field; more can be an indication of infection. Levels should be fewer than 1 million per ml.

- **Hyperviscosity**. The semen should gel promptly but liquefy within 30 - 60 minutes after ejaculation.

- **Velocity**. The average speed at which the sperm travels; the normal speed is 30 microns per second or more.

- **Low Sperm Count (Oligospermia)**. Men with counts of less than 20 million/ml may be contributing to the infertility. An average male ejaculate should contain nearly 200 million sperm; however, because of the natural barriers in the female reproductive tract only about 40 million sperm will ever reach the vicinity of the egg (ovum).

  Oligospermia/Oligozoospermia could suggest anatomic disorders from toxin exposure, trauma, stress, and nutrient deficiency such as protein; endocrine disorders, varicocele, sperm immaturity, congenital abnormality of the vas deferens, cystic fibrosis and general ill health.

- **Oligoteratozoospermia - (OATS)**. The sperm count is less than 20 million per ml. with motility less than 50 per cent.

- **Aspermia**. Aspermia means that there's no ejaculate with orgasm, usually indicating malfunction of the glands that provide the seminal fluid, the prostate and the seminal vesicles.

- **No sperm in the semen (Azoospermia)**. The most common causes of Azoospermia can be due to an obstruction or failure of the testes to produce sperm.

- **Poor sperm motility (Asthenozoospermia/Asthenospermia)**. The sperm do not swim in a good progressive manner and therefore lack the ability to make their way to the egg (ovum) to fertilise it. Less than 40 per cent of the sperm are motile and they are poorly formed.

  Various causes of this condition could include: Varicocele, poor nutrition such as zinc status being low, infection and the use of certain drugs. Other factors could also involve the semen specimen being tested too late or not stored in ideal conditions, which could return a false negative pathology. If the results return with suspect or poor levels, a follow-up test with another sample or different pathology lab may help to verify if the report is correct. An average sperm's motility rate is propelled at 18cm per hour.

The World Health Organisation recommended that sperm parameters should be more than 20 million sperm/ml with equal to or greater than 85 per cent normal levels of viable sperm. If the sperm are assessed as being normal but the count is low or the sperm are sluggish in motility, a medical drug similar to caffeine called Pentoxifylline may be prescribed to improve the liveliness of the sperm.

- **Poor Sperm Morphology (Teratospermia).** The shape of most of the sperm is abnormal, a factor we know to be associated with inability to penetrate and fertilise an egg (ovum). There are many contributing factors that could cause sperm abnormalities.

  Some of these may include an infection or low-grade infection (e.g. flu) during the last 72 days, toxin exposures, stress, excess acidity (review acid food/beverages in diet), chronic illness, pancreatic dysfunction, drug use, varicocele, congenital abnormalities and nutritional deficiencies. Teratospermia indicates that more than 70 per cent of the sperm have forms of abnormalities.

- **Necrospermia** - all sperm are dead.

- **Pyospermia/Leucospermia** - white blood cells are present implying infection.

- **Aggregation** - dead and live sperm are clumped together with debris.

- **Agglutination** - antibodies are clumped with live sperm.

- **Morphology** - the sperm structure (head, mid-piece and tail).

- **Polyspermia**. Polyspermia refers to having less than 25 million sperm in the sample. Factors contributing to this condition may include dehydration (poor water intake), excess alcohol consumption, abstinence for ejaculation may be too long, metabolic or endocrine imbalances, inadequate prostate secretions or enzymes deficiencies which are needed to nourish the sperm.

- **Spermatogenesis**. Spermatogenesis is the complete production line of sperm development, from dividing stem cells in the tubules of the testis (the spermatogonia), through the phase of meiosis, namely spermatocytes and the spermatid, to mature, released sperm cells, or spermatozoa. Its duration is about two months.

- **Spermiogenesis**. Is the last section of the spermatogenesis, the remodelling process that turns a round spermatid, already haploid, into an elongated swimming machine, the spermatozoon that takes about two weeks?

- **Sperm Penetration Test**. Sperm is tested to see if it has the ability to penetrate hamster egg cells. This indicates the sperm's ability to penetrate the partner's egg (ovum).

- **Testicular biopsy**. A sample of testicular tissue is examined under a microscope to determine the condition of the sperm, or to determine if sperm are being made.

- **Sperm Aspiration**. Sperm can be aspirated from either epididymis, which sits on top of the tests, or from the testes themselves.

- **MESA – microsurgical epididymal sperm**. This procedure can be done for obstructive azoospermia, because men with non-obstructive azoospermia rarely have sperm in the epididymis. A small incision is made in the scrotum, and then a dilated tubule in the epididymis is cut open and examined through a lighted microscope.

  Fluid is collected from the tubule and examined for sperm. This procedure can be done in the doctor's surgery. Men may be given a spermatic cord block and sedation during the procedure. You can generally return to work the next day.

- **PESA – percutaneous epididymal sperm aspiration**. A blind needle stuck into the epididymis is used to extract sperm. Local anaesthesia and sedation may be given.

- **TESE – testicular sperm extraction**. A small incision is made, and a piece of testicular tissue is removed. Testicular sperm doesn't freeze (Cryostorage) or thaw as well as epididymal sperm but may be the only sperm found in men with non-obstructive azoospermia.

- **TESA – testicular sperm aspiration**. This procedure also involves aspiration from the testes using a blind needle. All techniques involved in aspiration can cause bleeding and hematomas (a collection of blood that can be mildly painful and form bruising).

- **X-Ray**. This test is done to check for damage to the ducts in the male responsible for transporting the sperm to the penis. Though a useful diagnostic test, exposure to certain x-ray radiation may also cause problems.

- **Osmosis sugar test**. This is a simple test that is used to determine if sperm are dead or extremely lazy. Live tissue will soak up fluid, while dead tissue will not. Sperm are soaked in a sugar water solution; the sperm that are alive will swell up, while the dead sperm will not.

## Blood tests to investigate for male fertility

**FSH and LH**: If these hormone levels drop to low or are imbalanced, sperm development can be deficient. FSH and LH are the same hormones produced by the brain that control female egg production. Low FSH may be a cause of infertility; high levels of FSH may be caused by testicular failure or disease that can cause problems with sperm production.

Testing inhibin B is useful where no sperm are found in the semen (e.g. azoospermia). Normal levels of inhibin B in males are measured at 300pg/mL. Inhibin B levels that are over 80 pg/mL is a good indicator that viable sperm can be found, testicular biopsy may be required. Levels below 80 are a gauge of poor fertility and if viable sperm are to be found, a PESA procedure may be required. If relevant, having inhibin B testing may be recommended before considering having vasectomy reservals; if inhibin B is low, success is less likely.

Low LH may be a cause of infertility, or hypogonadism (underactive testes). High levels of LH can cause premature puberty in children. FSH levels in adult males should range between 1 – 5 IU/L. LH levels in adult males should range between 2 – 9 IU/L. Note: ranges may vary between pathology laboratories.

**Testosterone**: If testosterone levels are low this may indicate that the testicles are not functioning correctly or that there may be other imbalances of biochemical factors that require investigating. The normal amount of testosterone present in the blood of an adult male can be measured between *2 – 34 nmol/L*. Before puberty levels may range between *0.4 – 0.7 nmol/L*.

Low testosterone hormone levels may occur in hypogonadism, pan-hypopituitarism (underactive pituitary gland), andropause, delayed puberty, Addison's disease (underactive adrenal glands) and other causal factors of sterility. Excessively high levels may be indicative of an adrenal tumour. Blood tests for testosterone should be done in the early morning when testosterone levels should be at their highest.

**T3, T4 and TSH thyroid function tests**: If thyroid function is imbalanced such as in hypothyroidism sperm production may be compromised. Appropriate thyroid medication may be recommended to balance thyroid hormone levels.

**Prolactin**: Prolactin is more commonly recognised as a female hormone that promotes breast milk production. But prolactin is also produced in males. If prolactin is too low or too high this may cause imbalances in FSH and LH, thus affecting sperm production.

# Medical drugs that may help to increase sperm production

**Aromatase inhibitors**: These types of drugs are used to block the conversion of testosterone to oestrogen, the role of testosterone in part is to stimulate the testes to produce sperm.

**Clomiphene citrate**: This drug can help to kick-start the pituitary gland into increasing the production of FSH and LH to stimulate sperm production. The drugs used in males can be taken on a daily or day-on-day-off regime. Dosage of clomiphene citrate medications such as Clomid may range from 25 to 50mg in table or capsule form daily. Clomid is usually taken from days 2 to 6 of the menstrual cycle.

**HCG**: Is given via injection twice weekly to stimulate the testes cells to produce testosterone, therefore stimulating sperm production.

**Metrodin or Pergonal**: Used to stimulate FSH and LH production, used over a 3 – 6 month period has shown to improve severe sperm production problems.

**Indomethacin**: Is a drug that inhibits prostaglandins, which are produced in the body in response to inflammation. The 'BAD' prostaglandins can produce inflammation which can affect sperm motility and count levels.

**Parlodel**: Is used to reduce prolactin levels in conditions such as hyperprolactinemia. By normalising prolactin production, testosterone can than stimulate sperm production.

# Factors Impeding Male Fertility

This section is a basic summary of the potential causal factors that may impede or be implicated as a cause of male infertility. The majority of these factors will be discussed in-depth throughout the following chapters.

- **Poor sperm production – (Oligospermia)**. Sperm factors such as low sperm count or abnormalities contribute approximately 30 to 40 per cent of the detectable cause of infertility. Some of the causes for poor sperm production are: infection of the testes (orchitis); germinal aplasia – failure of sperm producing cells in testes to develop; cryptorchidism – small testes developed from birth; endocrine disorders – pituitary or thyroid defects; excess heat; drugs; poor nutrition; radiation exposure; mumps; surgery; testicular dysgenesis syndrome (TDS) and Y chromosome abnormalities.

- *Impaired sperm motility or agglutination*.

- *Testicular varicoceles*. Enlarged varicose veins that may be twisted or taut; hernia operations may also contribute to this problem. Varicoceles can cause overheating of the testes, therefore affecting the condition of the sperm. A varicocele is believed to cause more that 37 per cent of cases of sub-fertility in males.

- **Seminal tract obstructions**. Prostatitis, orchitis, epididymitis, vasectomy reversals, scar tissue, testicular atrophy, hydrocele, hypospadias, epispadias, phimosis, excessively small or large penis, bent penis, testicular torsion and undescended testes (cryptorchidism) can all potentially affect sperm production and/or ejaculation.

More men and women have had either a vasectomy or a tubal ligation at a young age and then decided to have another child. Needless to say, they may immediately face fertility issues due to their previous procedures. If a sperm analysis shows the presence of erythrocytes or haemoglobin (haematospermia – blood in with sperm), this can indicate injury to the penis or prostate gland, use of blood-thinning medication e.g. Warfarin, kidney damage or genital cancer.

- **Poor nutritional status**. Imbalances of nutrients such as: zinc, Vitamin C, Vitamin B12, arginine, taurine, carnitine, selenium, lysine, Vitamin E, Vitamin A, essential fatty acids (omega 3 and 6), co enzyme Q10, octacosanol, DMG, sulphur amino acids (methionine, cysteine), carnosine, and histidine can contribute to infertility problems in men.

Coeliac disease is also implicated in infertility as it can cause malabsorption of multiple nutrients and immunology problems; a strict gluten-free food diet may be recommended in this condition.

- **Heavy metal toxicity**. There is a large amount of documented information that implicates heavy metal exposure to reproductive dysfunctions. Some of these may include: aluminium, arsenic, cadmium, excessive copper overload, lead and mercury.

Cadmium for example is linked to the destruction of cells of the testes. It is found in tobacco, refined flour, some water supplies and is used in manufacturing batteries, fertilisers, paint and TV sets.

A Hair Tissue Mineral Analysis may be a useful diagnostic tool to consider if further investigation is warranted. Naturopaths and some medical practitioners will be able to advise you how to go about having this analysis done. People working with chemicals or in an industrial trade such as builders or mechanics would be particularly at risk.

- **Various drug and chemical exposures**. All chemical groups are potentially dangerous and everyone is exposed to them. We breathe them, eat them, and drink them. There are nearly 50,000 different pesticides alone based on some 600 or so active ingredients, and combinations of two or three compounds at low levels can be 1,600 times more toxic than any one individual compound.

There are countless numbers of chemicals that may need to be investigated when considering their impact on fertility.

Some of these may include:
- Ulcer medications such as Cimetidine (Tagamet) and Ranitidine (Zantac), which may decrease sperm count and even produce impotence;
- Marijuana and cocaine use can also lower sperm count and may affect motility;
- Sulfasalazine used to treat colitis and bowel conditions is known to reduce the sperm count sometimes to azoospermia;
- Dioxin, an infamous component of the defoliant known as Agent Orange, used for removing vegetation in the Vietnam War, has been implicated in oligospermia; Dioxin is also linked as a causation of endometriosis for women. The US environmental protection agency investigations have found that Dioxin was three thousand times more carcinogenic than DDT;
- Working with items such as certain glues and oven cleaners has been found to cause an approximate 230 per cent rise in miscarriage rates;
- Aflatoxin is a naturally occurring mycotoxin produced by two types of mould particularly found in grains and hulls of peanuts. A study of 50 infertile men, and 50 tested normal men, showed the infertile men had higher afatoxin in their semen and showed a 50 per cent higher level of sperm abnormality than in the fertile male group. Therefore, diets high in poor quality grown grains may be a possible link;
- MSG (Monosodium Glutamine) is a commonly used food flavour enhancer that is linked to multiple health issues; studies have shown that it may greatly reduce pregnancy success; and
- Chlorine and Aspartame (NutraSweet) are also linked to many conditions that may affect fertility.

- *Xenoestrogenisation (foreign hormones)*. Diethylstilboestrol (DES) exposure in-utero can possibly be associated with lowered sperm counts in males. High rates of vaginal, breast and cervical cancers, spontaneous abortions, ectopic pregnancies and infertility are all linked to DES.

- *Chronic Disease and Auto-Immune Disease.*
  - Sperm antibodies; mumps; gonorrhoea; syphilis; HIV; arthritis; heart attack (myocardial infarction); leukaemia; liver cirrhosis; renal failure; sickle-cell anaemia; and thyroid disorders are all conditions that have been associated with affecting male fertility.
  - Lupus (S.L.E.) can be indicated by lowered testosterone and raised prolactin hormones.
  - Diabetes – 40 per cent of diabetic males may have retrograde ejaculation, a condition in which sperm back up into the bladder.

- **Radiation exposure**. Frequent plane travel, computer monitors, electro-magnetic fields, electric blankets, heated waterbeds, and ionised x-rays are linked to causing infertility.

  Studies have proven that x-ray exposure is directly linked to damage caused to chromosomal material and an estimated increase in infertility of 450 per cent, and can have prolonged effects of up to 3 years for both sexes after initial exposure; chemotherapy and testicular cancer can cause problems with the sperm.

- **Prolonged fevers**. Regularly coming down with the 'flu', infections, or chronic allergy reactions can affect sperm quality. An elevated level of leucocytes in a sperm analysis is commonly indicative of infection and/or inflammation affecting the reproductive system.

- **Overheating of testes**. Sperm do not thrive very well under conditions that cause excessive fluctuations in temperature. The sperm can tolerate a change of only a couple of degrees. Extreme temperatures changes can cause sperm damage.

  Cooler bathing or showers would be greatly beneficial; avoid heated spa baths and saunas; wear loose non-restrictive clothing. Sitting for long hours could be a problem for people in occupations such as truck drivers, cabbies, and computer terminal workers. Male athletes may also be susceptible to this problem.

- **Chromosomal genetic defects**. Genetic defects of the Y chromosome. A number of genes that are needed for sperm to form normally are located on the Y-chromosome.

  - Klinefelter's syndrome (Sertoli-cell-only) is a rare condition where the man's chromosomes contain at least one extra X (female) chromosome (47, XXY), leading to low testosterone levels and usually a total absence of sperm production.
  - Young's syndrome potentially can cause very low sperm production.
  - Frohlich syndrome is a pituitary tumour that can cause a lack of sexual development.

  A group of genetic causes on the Y–chromosome, however, can be detected with DNA and PCR tests. Men with CBAVD (congenital bilateral absence of the vasa deferential) can be carriers of one or more genes for cystic fibrosis.

  PGD (pre-implantation genetic diagnosis) tests and Sperm Chromatin Structure Integrity Assays (SCSA) can be performed via advanced pathology centres and most IVF clinics using sophisticated machines such as a fluorescent activated cell sorter to help identify various genetic and congenital defects. A higher level of DNA fragmentation is sperm appears to also increase with the male's age.

About 1000 genes are needed to work well for spermatozoa to form in the normal numbers. What is currently known is that the genes involved in decreasing male fertility are not the same genes involved in decreasing female fertility.

Small deletions of genetic material from the Y-chromosome that remove or disable one or more genes required for the manufacture of sperm are called micro-deletions that will transmit to all male offspring. Karyotypes have shown to have a higher risk among children born from medically assisted procedures (IVF, ICSI) than from natural conception.

- **Obesity (High Body Mass Index)**. Conditions involving atherosclerosis, blood pressure fluctuations, diabetes, cardio-vascular or circulation diseases, and excessive fat tissue surrounding the scrotum can raise testicular temperature and impair sperm production. Conversely, males who have low body weight or have rapidly lost weight can have decreased sperm function and count.

- **Impotence**. Impotence can be defined as having problems with ejaculation or the ability to sustain an erection. Ten percent of men between the ages of 18 and 59 have experienced erectile problems in the last year and 10 per cent of men between the ages of 40 and 70 have complete erectile failure.

Factors that contribute to male impotence may include:

Low testosterone levels; low seminal prostaglandin levels; excessive prolactin levels; imbalances in nitric oxide (NO) levels; drugs such as anti-depressants; neuroleptic; anti-histamine; anti-hypertensive; blood pressure medications like beta blockers; digoxin; narcotics; sedatives; phenothiazine; anti-neoplastic agents; stomach acid inhibitors; and steroids (if abused). A prolactin-producing tumour, less common in men than in women, generally produces profound impotence as the sperm count falls.

- **Surgery**. Surgeries that may cause erectile or ejaculation issues: Abdominal perineal resection, proctocolectomy, radical prostatectomy, spinal cord injuries, and transurethral resection of prostate.

- **Excessive intake of pharmaceutical and recreational drugs**. Alcohol, caffeine, and cigarettes are only a few examples of external substances that can impede reproductive health.

- **Emotional and hormonal problems**. In about one in 200 cases of male infertility, the testes are inactive because of a deficiency of FSH (Follicle stimulating hormone) and LH (Luteinising hormone) from the pituitary gland. As well as inhibiting the maturing of sperm, such a deficiency causes the other main tissue in the testes – the Leydig cells, which produce the male sex hormone testosterone – to be inactive, which means the male sex characters are stopped from forming or from being maintained.

A deficiency of FSH and LH in men, as in women, may in turn be because of a deficiency of the gonadotropin releasing hormone (GnRH), produced by the hypothalamus to drive the pituitary gland.

Emotional and physiological stress can affect the body's delicate balance of the endocrine system function, thus unbalancing hormones and affecting correct sperm production.

- **Immotile cilia syndrome**. This is a rare group of disorders characterised by defects in the structure of the microscopic hair (cilia) that line tissue ducts and tubes, e.g., Fallopian tubes and Vas deferens. These syndromes can cause immotility or poor motility of spermatozoa tie (Kartagener's Syndrome). In males, testicular biopsy is normal and the sperm count is usually adequate but sperm motility is either markedly reduced or absent.

- **Associated effects of the environment**. Environmental influences such as global warming may contribute to reproductive problems and the decline in male sperm counts.

# Chapter 3

# *Female Reproductive Overview*

## All about the Girls

### *The Vagina*

The Vagina is the opening between the rectum (the opening from the bowel) and the urethra (the opening from the bladder). It is the structure via which the uterine secretions are shed during menstruation and conveyed to the outside. Vaginal tissue, being primarily muscular, serves as a passageway, first for the penis to deliver sperm up near the opening of the uterus. The vagina contains glands that secrete fluid during sexual arousal that makes it easier for the penis to enter the vagina. The vagina can also stretch to many times its normal size during the birth of a baby and then return to normal.

The *hymen* is a non-functional piece of circular tissue found at the entrance to the vagina. The bleeding many women have the first time they have intercourse comes from the tearing of the hymen. An *imperforated hymen* is one that has no holes and can cause blood to back up behind the small opening; this blood can be forced back up into the fallopian tubes and can lead to a higher incidence of endometriosis.

The external genitalia of a woman are known as the *vulva*. This is a collective term that incorporates the other structures including the *labia majora* – large fleshy skin folds that encompass the inner structure of the vulva, *labia minora* (clitoris hood, prepuce), joined together at the front to form the covering for the clitoris, and is lined with mucous membranes. The *vaginal* and *urethral openings* – within the folds of the labia minora, the *clitoris* and the *Bartholin's glands* – are glands that secrete mucus to lubricate the vagina during intercourse or sexual arousal.

### *The Cervix*

The Cervix is the lower part of the uterus. The lower third of the uterus is the tubular cervix, about half of which protrudes down into the vagina; the other half of the cervix is above the vagina attachment. The cervix has also been referred to as 'the neck of the womb'. The cervix is an important reproductive area that women need to monitor as it is prone to become infected, inflamed and the tissue may develop cancerous changes. Pap smear tests should be performed regularly during reproductive years to avoid these problems.

The opening of the cervix is usually tightly closed except during childbirth, menstruation to allow an outward passage for menses fluids, and during the peak fertility stage (ovulation) to allow sperm to enter.

During a woman's fertile phase of the cycle the cervix when physically examined feels softer and less firm when touched gently with your finger. It may also feel slippery with fertile mucus and its *dimple (os)* opens a little until it is big enough to put the tip of your finger into gently. The position of the cervix during this stage of the cycle may have moved across slightly so it is right in the middle of the topmost part of the vagina, rather than to one side.

During pregnancy, the cervix serves to help keep the baby maintained in the uterus and helps guard against infection from the mucous secretions that form a barrier between the vagina and the inside of the uterus.

An *incompetent cervix* is a term that means that the cervix doesn't stay tight and closed during pregnancy. This condition can be corrected usually by having a suture called a *cerclage* performed to prevent the loss of the baby due to the increasing weight as it grows.

### *The Uterus*

The Uterus (or Womb) is a flattened pear-shaped muscular organ and is one of the strongest muscles in the body. The uterine muscle is called the *myometrium* and is designed to stretch, hold and nourish a developing foetus and during childbirth rhythmically contracts.

The lining of the uterus, called the *endometrium,* thickens every month in preparation to embed and nourish an embryo. If a conception has **not** occurred, then the endometrial lining breaks down and sheds away as menstrual fluid; regular shedding of this endometrium is known as a *period*.

The endometrium develops due to the influence of the ovarian hormones oestrogen and progesterone. During the first stage of the menstrual cycle just after the period, the endometrium is at its thinnest and the lining is caused to change and develop via the influence of oestrogen.

At ovulation, progesterone is produced in increasing amounts and the endometrium not only thickens but its structure changes to become *glandular.* The average amount of blood loss during a normal menstrual cycle is about four tablespoons or 50ml; a heavy period is classified as anything over 80ml of blood loss.

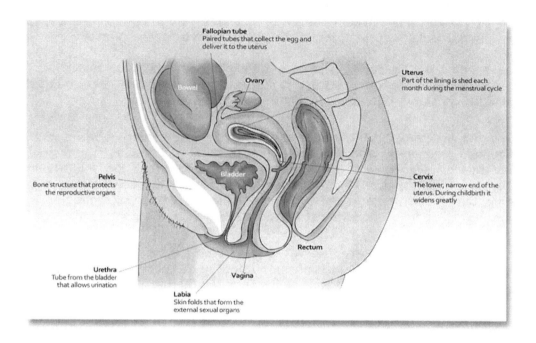

*Figure.5.   Female reproductive system - cross section internal view*

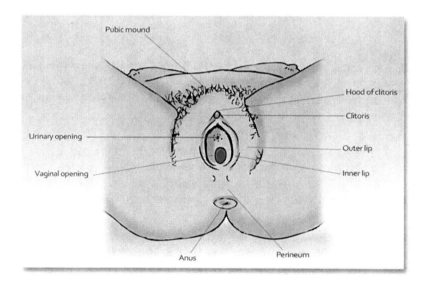

*Figure.6.   Female reproductive system - external genitalia*

About 2 or 3 per cent of women may have shape abnormalities of the uterus. The most common of these is a *septate uterus*, meaning that there is a partial or complete divide inside of the uterus. Approximately 20 per cent of women also have a *retroverted* or tipped uterus. *(These and other conditions that affect the uterus such as *polyps* and *fibroids* are discussed in other chapters). During pregnancy the uterus increases in size and shape; an enlarged uterus may be medically referred to as 'bulky'.

## The Fallopian Tubes

Normally, there are two fallopian tubes that connect the two ovaries to the uterus, also referred to as oviducts or egg ducts. The fallopian tubes are cylindrical (funnel) shaped muscles, internally lined with microscopic hairs called *cilia* that propel in a continual wave-like motion. When ovulation occurs this tubes rhythmically contract to convey the ovum (egg) into the uterus and assist the transport of sperm towards the ovum. This contraction motion of the tubes is also believed to partially prevent the backflow of menstrual blood known as *retrograde menstruation* and may help to keep infection from getting to the pelvic cavity that may cause *peritonitis*.

The average length of a fallopian tube is about 10 cm in length and at the ends are small finger-like projections called *fimbriae* that sweep the ovum into the fallopian tube. Damage to the fimbriae and infections such as chlamydia, endometriosis and adhesions can adversely affect the tubes that can cause infertility and increase the chances of ectopic pregnancies occurring.

## The Ovaries

There are normally two ovaries that are oval in shape similar in size to a flattened hen's egg. The ovaries are not actually attached to the fallopian tubes but to the uterus by ligaments. The ovaries are complex structures that carry literally hundreds of thousands of eggs (ova), of which many are used during an ovulatory cycle and are necessary for conception. Conditions that can affect the ovaries may include: endometriosis, 'chocolate cysts', polycystic ovaries, ovarian cancer and other various ovarian-type cysts. *(These conditions will be discussed in other chapters).

A newborn baby girl at birth already contains about 1 million eggs (ova), and that is only after a loss of 2.5 million eggs in the last three months before she is born. Every day throughout a female's reproductive life-span, many eggs are lost via *atresia*, which means that they die off because they're not being stimulated to mature.

By puberty, only 300,000 to 400,000 eggs remain, and every month, 500 to 1,000 are lost, along with the one or possibly two eggs that make it to maturity and are released each month. On average a female will have approximately 400 menstrual cycles during her reproductive life.
By age 50, only approximately 1,000 or so eggs remain. It is possible that at this stage of reproductive life, many of the remaining eggs have abnormalities, because the majority of 'good' eggs get used up first. Food for thought, when

you think that it is not only the one ovulated egg that gets used each month of the cycle. A woman's ovarian egg reserves may be estimated by having a full hormone function blood test and abdominal and/or internal ultrasound to assess if egg reserves are good or are failing. On average 1 in 10 women will have premature ovarian failure; ovarian egg loss is believed to accelerate almost by double after the age of 37!

The ovary is quite adaptive; if one of the ovaries is damaged or has been removed by surgery, such as from ovarian cancer or an ectopic pregnancy, depending on ovarian reserves, and even though they have now basically been halved in number with the loss of one ovary, the single remaining ovary can increase its existing workload to compensate and continue to produce eggs each ovulatory cycle. Similar to when one kidney fails or is removed, the other adapts and increases its work load to compensate – the body has a back-up plan by providing us with two. Therefore, fertility does not really decline as much as you may think with the loss of an ovary as long as the remaining ovary is functioning well, preferably with no fallopian tube blockages.

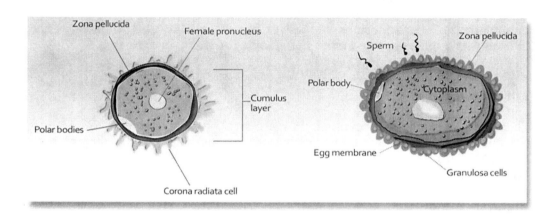

*Figure.7. A normal mature human egg*

## The Egg Enigma - Mother Nature vs Father Time

Recent studies conducted at Harvard Medical School and Massachusetts General Hospital in Boston (USA) have demonstrated in mice and primates that female germ line stem cells could give rise to ovary follicular renewal, that may potentially extend and enhance ongoing egg (oocytes) production.

If these findings are also found to be true in humans then all previous theories about female reproductive system aging will need to be revised. This breakthrough in research (even though at its infant stages) could possibly rewrite the textbooks of the half a century-old doctrine that females are born with a fixed lifetime supply of eggs with a limited reproductive lifespan. If similar *stem cells* are to be found in human females this could lead to future treatments that may ultimately postpone menopause, delay ovarian failure, extend childbearing years and restore fertility to women.

Regardless if females are born with a set number of eggs, germ cells are continually regenerating. Correct follicle development (folliculogenesis) is what largely dictates the future health or quality of the egg. This intricate process starts some four (4) months prior to the domain follicle releasing the mature egg. Fundamental to the success of this growth phase, good blood flow and nutrient supply to the target reproductive tissue is of vital importance and the balanced regulation of hormone feedback messaging is necessary for correct protein synthesis, hormone utilisation, and growth factors required to control the communication signalling for normal follicle development and egg maturation to occur.

There are numerous female animals that are known to be capable of bearing offspring throughout their entire adult life. This same reality may also be proven of humans. Researchers have stated that the aging process of the body is only caused by about 35 per cent genetic factors and remaining 65 percent is caused by various environmental influences. The body makes an incredible 300 billion copies of your DNA every day, and regenerates 100 trillion cells. If 65 per cent of our aging process can be influenced by environment, then even the subtlest of changes must have a ripple effect on our overall health and wellbeing, therefore impacting on our reproductive potential, for better or worse.

### Just for the record - 'Age had no Boundary'

Omkari Panwar from Uttar Pradesh, North India, is believed to be the world's oldest mother, who at the age of 70 gave birth to twins (a boy and a girl) after an IVF treatment with her husband, Charan Singh Panwar, aged 77. The twins were born at 34 weeks by emergency caesarean section at a hospital in the nearest town of Muzarffarnagar on the 27th June, 2008. The elderly couple already have two daughters in their thirties and five grandchildren.

The world's previous oldest mothers were a Spanish woman, Carmela Bousada from Cadiz, Spain, who at the age of 66 years and 358 days, gave birth to twin boys at St. Pau Hospital in Barcelona, in December 2006. Romanian Woman, Adriana Iliescu, who at the age of 66 and 320 days, gave birth to a daughter, Eliza-Maria, in January 2005, after nine years of fertility treatment.

In March 2007, an unnamed Austrian woman aged 66 gave birth to her third child, at the age of 61 her 2nd child was born in December 2002; her oldest is

30 years old. This could be the first and only known case in the world of two pregnancies and births over the age of 60.

Indian woman, Satyabhama Mayapatra, from Natagarh in Orissa, at the age of 65 gave birth to a baby boy in April 2003. Husband Veenarani Mahapatra was the sperm provider after being married for 50 years.

In 2006, 62-year-old American great-grandmother Janise Wulf gave birth to her twelfth child.

Britain's oldest mother is 62 years old. Dr Patricia Rashbrook (aka Patti Farrant) who received donor IVF treatment in Russia (as the unofficial age limit in Britain to be a candidate for IVF was 50) from Italian IVF specialist Dr Severino Antinori. Mrs Rashbrook already had three older children, aged 17, 22 and 26, from a previous marriage.

Dawn Brooks is believed to be the oldest natural conception mother in Britain. She gave birth at the age of 59, with her 64-year-old husband Raymond.
Australia's oldest known mum is believed to be aged 56; giving birth in 2007 via IVF, *Wendy Kenyon* (Australia) gave birth to IVF triplets in 1998 aged 54.

Obviously many ethical debates have risen regarding having children at such an age, but it has proven that pregnancy is possible later in life and is encouraging to women who may also be in their later reproductive years and who are trying to have a child, that age barriers can be broken and women can indeed stay fertile longer.

The world's oldest known father was an Australian mineworker Les Colley, who was 92 years and 10 months old when he fathered a son, Oswald in 1992.
Indian farmer, Nan Ram Jogi fathered his 21st child at the age of 90, to his fourth wife (who was one of his son's wives with whom he married after his son passed away). Mr. Jogi has 12 sons and 9 daughters. His first daughter was born in 1943 and his last daughter (so far), Girija Raj Kumari, born in August 2007 - 64 years apart. Mr. Jogi has stated that he didn't want to stop and plans to continue producing children until he is 100.

For interest, the world's youngest mother is believed to be five (5) years eight (8) month-old Peruvian girl, *Lina Medina,* from Andean Village of Ticrapo (Peru). Lina gave birth to a six-pound baby boy *Gerardo* on 14th May 1939 at Lima Hospital, Pisco, Peru. Lina's parents thought their daughter had a large abdominal tumour; doctors discovered otherwise. Lina was said to have started menstruating from the age of eight months old; her father stated that she was having regular periods from the age of three. Lina was tested and found to have the ovaries of a fully mature woman. It is believed that Lina had an extra ordinary pituitary gland disorder. Menstruation had stopped some seven and a half months prior to visiting hospital.

Birth of the baby was via caesarean section and Lina's father was arrested for suspected incest but was released from jail due to lack of evidence, believe it or not!

## The Glands and their Functions

### The Adrenals
The adrenals are small glands that are located on top of the kidneys. The adrenals produce *glucocorticoids*, which affect carbohydrate and protein metabolism, *mineralocorticoids*, which play a role in regulating sex hormones, stress hormones, and body fluid concentration. These hormones are released into the bloodstream daily.

### The Hypothalamus
The hypothalamus gland (the 'mission-control' part of the brain) is located at the base of the brain, and is connected by nerves to the brain and spinal cord. The function of the hypothalamus acts as a link between the endocrine and nervous system via receiving information from sensors in the brain.

The hypothalamus plays a vital role in regulating numerous body functions such as: controlling appetite, thirst, sex drive, pleasure sensation, temperature, aspects of stress response (e.g. fight and flight), and the menstrual cycle.

### The Thyroid
The thyroid gland is located just below the larynx in the neck. This gland is comprised of two sections called the *lateral lobes,* which are positioned on each side of the voice box and are connected via a bridge called the *isthmus*.

The main functions of the thyroid are to monitor metabolism, build nerve and brain tissue, relay messages signalled from the pituitary gland, and regulate growth patterns. The thyroid and adrenal glands have a close symbiotic relationship in regulating numerous metabolic functions. *Triiodothyronine (T3)* and *Thyroxine (T4)* are produced by the thyroid to increase the metabolic rate. They are stored and released into the bloodstream, which transports them to their respective target areas. These hormones are regulated by thyroid-stimulating hormone (TSH) that is secreted from the anterior pituitary gland in response when the levels of T3 and T4 become too low. Symptoms of underactive thyroid may include: hair loss, weakness, memory loss, mood swings, sensitivity to cold, weight gain or loss, heavy or irregular periods.

An under-active thyroid can cause lowering of SHBG (Sex Hormone Binding Globulin), which eventually increases the availability of oestrogen in women. An over-active thyroid leads to a greater conversion of androgens to oestrogen. Both situations can lead to amenorrhoea due to ovarian failure;

menstruation usually recommences with appropriate treatment. Medical treatment for underactive thyroid is daily doses of thyroxine (synthetic or bovine) ranging from 50 to 200 mg.

## The Pancreas
This gland is situated above the stomach in the upper abdomen. It is approximately 15cm in length and regulates two main functions in the body:

1. Eighty per cent of the pancreas' function is to produce digestive juices involved in the assimilation of foods.
2. The pancreas contains microscopic cellular units called the *islets of Langerhans* which secrete hormones: *Secretin* to stimulate a bicarbonate and water solution to maintain the pH (acid-alkaline) balance, and *Cholecystokinin* that activates the acinar cells within the pancreas to produce the essential enzymes.

   The islets of Langerhans are divided into four parts:
   A – alpha: secrete the hormone *Glycogen*
   B – beta: produce *Insulin*
   D – delta: contain *Somatostatin* which suppresses insulin and glycogen
   PP –pancreatic cells are present in both the exocrine and endocrine sections of the gland. Their secretions pass directly into the pancreas veins and into the bloodstream. All the islets work closely with the liver.

Malfunction of the pancreas can lead to conditions such as: coeliac disease (gluten intolerance), lactose intolerance (sugar found in milk), poor body fat metabolism, autism (has been linked to *secretin* malfunction), and diabetes mellitus (blood sugar imbalances).

## The Parathyroids
These glands are located behind the thyroid. There function is to maintain blood calcium levels. When blood calcium levels are low parathyroid hormone (PTH), is produced to raise calcium blood levels.

## The Pituitary
This gland comprises two parts called the anterior pituitary and posterior pituitary. The pituitary is recognised as the master gland. It is connected to the base of the brain stalk and is about the size of a pea with a mushroom-like appearance.

The function of **the anterior pituitary** is to produce: adrenocorticotrophic hormone (ACTH), growth hormone (GH), follicle stimulation hormone (FSH), luteinising hormone (LH), thyroid-stimulating hormone (TSH) and prolactin (PRL).

FSH and LH are called *gonadotrophins* because they target the primary sexual organs – the ovaries and the testes. These protein hormones are constantly being produced and are released about every 60 to 90 minutes. These hormones' main function is to promote ovulation in females and sperm in males.

Prolactin (PRL) stimulates milk production to the breasts during lactation.
Just prior to ovulation the dominant follicles reach full size (around days 12-13), the hypothalamus pulses the release of GH that sensitises the pituitary to make it release the LH. This surge of LH, and other interactions with the follicle, regulates the growth of the follicle and its release. Within 24-36 hours after the LH surge reaches the follicle, it bursts out of the ovary with a fluid that carries it to the uterus, and this is ovulation.

**The posterior pituitary** produces *oxytocin,* which helps to induce labour and milk release, as well as producing *antidiuretic hormone (ADH),* which promotes water retention by the kidneys.

## The Normal Female Cycle

A normal female cycle is 28 days from the start of one menstrual period to the start of the next. Ovulation, the release of the ripe, but unfertilised egg (oocyte) from the ovary, occurs usually on days 13-14. A fertile woman can notice changes in her cervical mucus as the days of the cycle progress. Starting with the first day of menstrual bleeding as day one, bleeding will usually occur for 5-7 days. On about day nine, the cervical mucus will be noticeable but fairly thick in texture.

By day twelve and for approximately the next four days the mucous will be thin and the woman will feel moist. Her underpants will often be quite wet during this period of the month.

As well as being aware of the wetness, a woman will feel fullness in the pelvic area and a strong desire for sex. If she happens to be around any male dogs at this stage, they may become embarrassingly interested.

*This is confirmation of the fertile stage*.

At the time of ovulation, a pain may be felt in one side of the abdomen. The side of pain may alternate from month to month as the unfertilised eggs are released alternately from the right and left ovaries. Often the sensitivity to the pain is greater on one side where there is a problem. Sometimes this pain can be quite sharp. A temperature chart is an old method of identifying the day of ovulation and it is an easy personal check to see that everything is normal. The basal temperature should be taken before getting up in the morning.

Because mouth breathing can alter the oral temperature, and most of us do a bit of mouth breathing (even snoring) at night, it is best to take the vaginal temperature. Make sure that you use a thermometer that is designed for this purpose. At the start of the menstrual cycle the basal temperature will be about *36.6°C* (the average internal human body temperature) and will remain there until about day 12. On day 12 or 13, there will be a dip in the temperature of about *0.2°C*, which reduces the temperature to about *36.2°C*. Each time there is a drop in hormone production there is a drop in the temperature, and it is this dropping of the hormone production that is actually being recorded on a basal temperature chart.

This drop in temperature is also conducive for the survivability of the sperm. Sperm are normally stored at a temperature of 36.2 degrees and the transference of sperm to the female during this ovulation temperature dip phase also helps to minimises any interruption to their environment.

The temperature dip does not usually last 24 hours so it may not always be detected. The dip coincides with a surge of the hormone oestrogen that precedes the next hormonal surge of luteinising (ovulating) hormone (LH), which induces the ovulation event.

Ovulation is also accompanied by many other biochemical changes. One of these is a drop in the body levels of a body regulator call *X1-anti-trypsin*. The function of this chemical is to act as an antagonist to the enzyme *trypsin*, which is important in breaking down protein.

By lowering X1-anti-trypsin, trypsin can be active in the ovulation process. A woman who is studying her cycle may make two other observations. One is that she might feel slightly unwell or nauseous on the day of her oestrogen surge. The other is that she might experience sinus-like symptoms on the day of ovulation. The temperature dip does not usually last 24 hours so it may not always be detected.
Following the dip, the temperature rises over the next two days to 37°C. It will remain at 37°C until about three days before the next menstrual bleed. Then it will gradually move back to the basal level. If pregnancy has occurred the temperature will remain at 37°C and menstruation will not occur.

During the fertility phase, check the vaginal mucus, and the female's temperature, and make love on days 10, 12, 14 and 16.

Make sure the man saves up his sperm during the days between to ensure that there is a higher volume of sperm on the days you make love. Multiple ejaculations on these days (10, 12, 14, and 16) will only result in less ejaculate being available each time.

There are several methods behind the madness for this day on, day off regime:

1. To increase the male's sperm pooling effect (improve sperm numbers); and
2. To decrease the female's immune defences from developing allergies or antibodies against the sperm, as it is falsely recognised as a foreign invader and needs to be dealt with extreme prejudice!

For women who have shorter cycles, try days 9, 11 and 13. If you are having a long cycle, e.g. 30 to 32 days, then try during days 14, 16 and 18. Attempting natural conception at the peak of the lunar cycle may also warrant consideration.

Males' hormones usually peak in the morning as do sperm counts, so it may be worth changing your routine around and try having intercourse in the morning rather than at night to see if that may yield a better result. Ovulation is controlled by body chemistry and your internal body time clock; due to hormonal changes throughout the different times of the day the most likely time for a woman to ovulate is at *midnight*. Contradictory to this, other studies have monitored ovulation patterns and found that *4pm* may be the time when women mostly ovulate. If this is true, then having sexual intercourse or making love around this time may be worth trying.

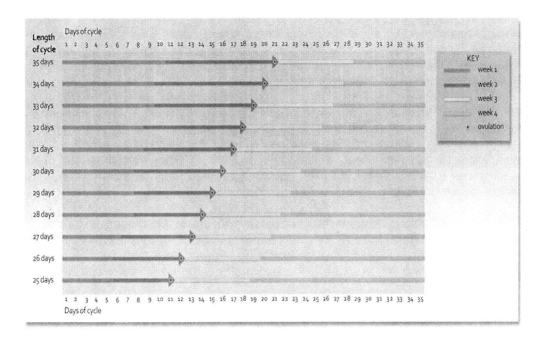

*Chart for calculating timed intercourse for variable ovulation times*

## Timing of Intercourse

Timing of intercourse for conception is best to coincide with the day before ovulation (usually mucus peak) to allow the first swarm of healthy sperm to reach the egg just as it is released. This accounts for and ensures fertilisation takes place before the less healthy or slower sperm catch up.

Sperm normally live *3–5 days*, but are less viable after 3 and enough will die to lower sperm count below viable levels. Several days of abstinence (3–5) before conception will ensure high count and fertilisation by fresh sperm. The life span of a viable ovum (egg) is normally between *12–24 hours*. Fresh sperm and eggs are less likely to result in miscarriage.

At the end of the menses cycle, simultaneous low levels of oestrogen and progesterone (due to degeneration of the corpus luteum) 'give the green light' for gonadotropin-releasing hormone (from the hypothalamus gland) to stimulate the anterior pituitary gland to release follicle-stimulating hormone (FSH). This occurs at about day 25 (new ovarian cycle begins). Low oestrogen and progesterone also cause spiral arterioles (which develop with the thickening endometrium) to constrict. Bleeding starts at day 1 of the new uterine cycle.

With the release of follicle-stimulating hormone (start of ovarian cycle), growth of primary follicles in the ovaries is stimulated. The primary follicles contain the female eggs (primary oocytes at this stage). The growing follicles start to produce oestrogen. By producing oestrogen, they govern their own growth and the need for follicle-stimulating hormone decreases. On approximately day 6 of the uterine (menstrual) cycle (menstrual cycle is usually completed at day 4 or 5), one follicle begins to outgrow all the others.

The increased level of oestrogen produced inhibits (blocks) follicle-stimulating hormone and less developed follicles undergo atresia. The strongest follicle becomes self-sufficient with its own oestrogen. The oestrogen produced also stimulates the growth and thickening (repair) of the endometrium. New endometrial glands develop, and spiral arterioles coil and lengthen. The endometrium doubles to 4–6mm thick (stratum functionalis).

Near the mid-point of the uterine cycle, high levels of oestrogen produced by the growing follicle, promotes secretion of both gonadotropin-releasing hormone (GnRh) and luteinising hormone (LH). GnRh in turn increases luteinising hormone (LH) further and also causes a 'bump' in follicle-stimulating hormone production.

The surge in luteinising hormone (LH) peaks at about day 13. Luteinising hormone causes the follicle to secrete even more oestrogen and grow bigger. It ruptures on day 14 and expels the egg (secondary oocyte). The ruptured follicle collapses, then grows and forms the corpus luteum (yellow body) under the influence of luteinising hormone. The corpus luteum, stimulated by luteinising hormone (and leuteotropic hormone) secretes oestrogen and progesterone.

The second half or postovulatory stage of the uterine cycle thus begins, the luteal phase of the ovarian cycle i.e. pertaining to the corpus luteum. Oestrogen levels drop off when the follicle ruptures but oestrogen and progesterone are produced by the corpus luteum and steadily increase. Progesterone continues to stimulate growth of endometrium and the glands to secrete glycogen, thus preparing the endometrium for the arrival of the egg;

this takes up to 7 days. (A day or two before ovulation, *fimbriae* become active by peristaltic action and 'fan in' the egg into the fallopian tube; cilia within the tube also help to create currents).

If fertilisation of the oocyte does not occur, simultaneous rising levels of oestrogen and progesterone inhibit both gonadotropin-releasing hormone and luteinising hormone. As luteinising hormone drops, the corpus luteum begins to degenerate. Ironically, this causes a falling of oestrogen and progesterone as the corpus luteum degenerates.

Rising oestrogen and progesterone levels together cause their own demise. The simultaneous falling levels subsequently give gonadotropin releasing (and thus follicle-stimulating hormone) the green light again.

If the oocyte (ova-egg) is fertilised, the embryo produces human chorionic gonadotropin (HCG), which maintains the corpus luteum, despite rising oestrogen, and progesterone it produces. The chorion of the embryo later develops into the placenta. HCG is the gonadotropic hormone produced by the chorionic villi of the placenta in response to the implantation of a fertilised ovum. This hormone is the basis of most pregnancy tests.

The placenta eventually takes over the corpus luteum and its production of oestrogen and progesterone. Oestrogen supports pregnancy and progesterone both supports and develops breasts for lactation. The role of the corpus luteum then becomes minor.

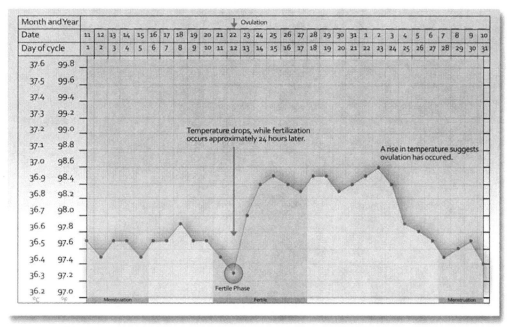

**Figure.8. Basal Body Temperature (BBT) Chart showing normal cycle**

# In a Nutshell – What Makes an Egg Develop and Mature?

- Follicle-stimulating hormone (FSH) is released from the pituitary gland.

- In the ovary, 10 to 15 eggs begin to grow. The tissue surrounding each egg forms a follicle, a fluid-filled sac. Each follicle contains one egg.

- Luteinising hormone (LH) is released from the pituitary gland. The follicle begins to produce oestrogen.

- One follicle becomes dominant, growing faster than the other.

- As the dominant follicle grows, it produces more oestrogen. The amount of FSH released decreases, and the smaller follicles stop growing.

- A large amount of LH is released as the oestrogen rises. This makes the egg inside the dominant follicle mature.
- The follicle bursts, and the egg is released.
- The leftover part of the follicle, now called the corpus luteum, produces progesterone to help an embryo implant.

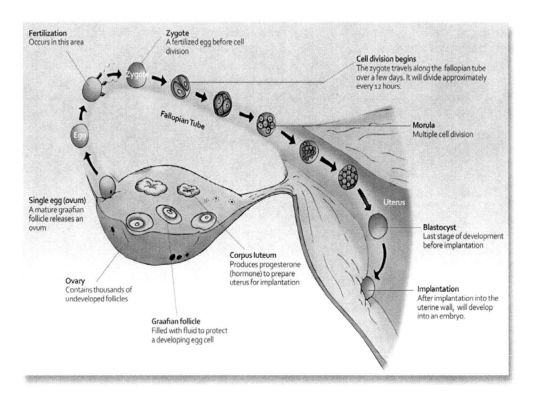

*Figure.9. The normal female hormone cycle (the process of fertilisation)*

# Ovarian Hormones and their Function

These hormones are the ones released by the ovaries and are the major female sex hormones. These are the ones most familiar to women.

## *Functions of Oestrogen*

The oestrogen hormone is responsible for all kinds of physiological effects including the development of female characteristics at puberty and during the menstrual cycle. Oestrogen causes the cervix to soften and rise, and its opening the *os* to widen, thus facilitating the entry of sperm.

- Oestrogen stimulates mucus secretions in the cervical crypts to change in quantity and quality and becomes fertile, thus ensuring survival and transportation of the sperm.
- The endometrium (lining of the uterus) proliferates (grows), and thickens to prepare to receive the fertilised egg (if there is one).
- Oestrogen stimulates the pituitary gland to release a sudden surge of luteinising hormone (LH) and modulates vaginal activity, (ph3.5-4.5).
- Oestrogen is involved in secondary sex characteristics (feminine body proportion).

The oestrogen is measured usually 1-2 days before ovulation is due, when it should be peaking. Low levels of oestrogen can be caused by pituitary dysfunction and low follicle-stimulating hormone may be a factor, but it is more commonly a result of ovarian problems. Symptoms of low oestrogen can include delayed ovulation (which can also be a result of excessive oestrogen levels), and inadequate amounts of fertile cervical mucus, which will be obvious to anyone observing their mucus changes. Both oestrogen and progesterone work to develop the endometrium and increase mucous secretions mid-cycle.

Traditionally, oestrogen levels have been evaluated by measurement of serum oestrogen (E2). It has become clear, however, that improper oestrogen metabolism can also be a substantial contributor to oestrogen activity. As a first step, oestrogen is metabolised via enzymes belonging to the cytochrome P450 family into 2-hydroxy (OH) or 16-hydroxy oestrone. 2OH oestrone possesses mild oestrogen activity relating to E2, while 16-hydroxy oestrone retains much of the activity of E2. Therefore, the ratio of 2OH to 16OH oestrone that is produced is an important determinant of overall oestrogenic activity. A ratio of 2OH:16OH greater than 2 is considered to be protective against oestrogenic activity.

- Oestradiol (Estradiol in the USA) is measured in the blood as 17-beta-oestradiol. The normal test range is: female before ovulation: 180 – 1500 pmol/L (50-400 ng/L)
- Female after ovulation: 400 – 800 pmol/L (120-200 ng/L)
- Female post menopause: less than 200 pmol/L (less than 55 ng/L)

### Functions of Progesterone

This hormone is secreted by the corpus luteum, (the crater left after the follicle has released the egg). It transports from the ovaries to the endometrium in increasing quantities post ovulation and production peaks between days 21 to 23 of a normal 28 day cycle. The level of progesterone then falls to trigger menstruation if conception has not occurred.

### Progesterone:

- Adds to, and modifies oestrogen effects.
- Helps alter cervical mucus. (Mid-cycle becomes more viscous and tacky increasing to mucous hostility to sperm and infertile).
- Is required during secretory phase (second half of cycle) for endometrium development.
- Deposition of subcutaneous fat (helps use fat for energy).
- Stimulates uterus lining to thicken more, so that within 5-7 days it is ready to receive the egg.
- Raises basal body temperature (body at rest).
- Assists the cervix to lower, harden and close, Decreases uterine contraction.
- Stimulates the ovary to cease egg releasing.
- Increases skin sebum secretion, e.g. acne.
- Inhibits prolactin and normalises blood clotting.
- Decreases peripheral blood flow (internally heating).
- Acts as an anticonvulsant, diuretic, and vasoconstrictor.
- Helps balance the glucose tolerance levels; aids immune system and reduces CIN 1 and CIN 2 cervical dysplasia.
- Aids in the synthesis of corticosteroids in the adrenal cortex.
- Helps maintain pregnancy and is necessary for the survival of the embryo and foetus throughout gestation.
- Protects from fibrocystic breasts, breast cancer and endometrial cancer.
- Restores sex drive, and helps normalise blood sugar levels.
- Has a thermogenic (temperature-raising) effect and is a cortisone precursor.
- Has functions as a natural anti-depressant and protects from osteoporosis.
- Helps thyroid hormone action and restores proper cell oxygen levels.

### Excessive oestrogen dominance may contribute to:

- Premenstrual Syndrome (PMS).
- Mid-cycle spotting (break-through bleeding).
- Endometriosis, uterine fibroids, fibrocystic breasts, and uterine cancer.
- Infertility, miscarriage, depression and fatigue.
- Breasts tenderness, premenopausal bone density loss, accelerated aging.
- Bloating, irritability, foggy thinking, headaches, water retention, mimics hypothyroidism, hypoglycemia, increases blood clotting (increasing stroke risk) and gallbladder disease.

- Excessive nervous system stimulation, producing irritability and possible histamine release, which may produce skin and allergy problems and anxiety. Increased contraction and cramping of uterine smooth muscles.
- Menorrhagia – heavy menstrual bleeding.
- Irregular menstrual flow/cycle.
- Prolonged or excessive production of cervical fluid.
- Chloasma (brown pigmentation on the face).
- Delayed ovulation.
- Nausea, dizziness, leg cramps, elevated blood pressure, bilateral headaches, weight gain (particularly around abdominal area), low libido, sweet cravings, varicose veins, insomnia, period pain, mood swings and cystic ovaries.

Progesterone is usually measured approximately 1 week after ovulation (day 21), when it should be peaking. Low levels will be reflected in a shortened post-ovulatory phase (luteal phase), inadequate or sluggish temperature rise and various PMS symptoms such as sore breasts, fluid retention, and PMT.

### Excess progesterone may contribute to:
- Decreased Libido (sex drive).
- Depression / mood swings.
- Fatigue / extreme tiredness.
- Muscle weakness.
- Drowsiness.
- Increased appetite.
- Hyperinsulinaemia (high insulin blood levels).
- Oily skin.
- Breast tenderness.
- Thrush.

### Prolactin
Prolactin is another hormone released by the pituitary gland.

### Elevated prolactin may cause:
- Milky discharge from the breasts.
- Irregular or absent ovulation and menstruation.
- Shortened post-ovulatory phase (luteal phase). This can be due to increased prolactin levels interfering with release of gonadotropin releasing hormone.

Decreased follicle-stimulating hormone (FSH) stimulation results in a decrease in the number of gonadotropin-releasing hormone receptors and a subsequent response in progesterone synthesis.

Excessive elevated prolactin is also called hyperprolactinemia. Prolactin can be measured at any stage of the cycle, though some women may only have elevated levels during the night, which can mislead conclusive testing methods.

Excessive oestrogen may contribute to increase prolactin, which can produce depression and dysphoria, breast tenderness, water retention and corpus luteon function.

Imbalances in prolactin level may be caused by disease of the pituitary, tumour or growth on the gland (not necessarily malignant), and decreased hyper thalamus or thyroid function. A CAT scan may be required to rule out possible pituitary growths.

Polycystic Ovarian Syndrome and various drugs can also be causal factors of excessive prolactin. When prolactin levels are too high symptoms may include: amenorrhoea, breast tenderness, depression and PMT.

The medical treatment for hyperprolactinemia commonly focuses on the use of the Dopamine Agonist, *Bromocriptine*, correction of hypothyroidism and hyper thalamus stalk lesions. Macro adenomas (tumours) are usually treated first by a trial of drug therapy and only surgical interruption is instigated when drug therapy is unresponsive.

Natural medicines: such as the amino acids *DL-Phenylalanine (DLPA)* and *Tyrosine* are precursors for dopamine synthesis in the brain, capable of enhancing dopamine levels. *Vitamin B6, Vitamin C* and *Zinc* are capable of enhancing enzymes involved in the production of dopamine. The Chinese herbal formulas *Rehamannia eight (Hachimijiogan)* and *Paeonia and Licorice combination* have also been successful in treating hyperprolactinemia.

Herbal medicines such as *Vitex-agnus castus* may also be effective at lowering prolactin levels and has shown in studies to mimic the action of dopamine. Vitex used in divided doses given through the day has shown to be more effective than when given in single doses. Excessive stress, beer consumption and numerous recreational drugs can also adversely affect prolactin levels.

Acupuncture points that may be used to lower elevated prolactin may include: Yintang, LI 4, Lv 2, Lv 3, UB 2, UB 62 and SI 3.

### Oxytocin
This hormone produced by the pituitary gland causes the contraction of the smooth muscle fibres and is responsible for making the uterus contract powerfully during labour. Low levels of this hormone may potentially compromise fertility by affecting the muscle fibres in fallopian tube walls, and in the walls of the blood vessels supplying the uterus lining. *Syntocinon* is a synthetic form of natural oxytocin hormone. It is usually administered intravenously via drip to induce labour and stimulate contractions. Syntocinon is usually given in situations where synthetic prostaglandins (applied in gel form vaginally, in pessary or oral tablet) are unsuccessful at inducing labour.

### Females and Testosterone

Women also produce small quantities of male androgen hormones such as testosterone. This hormone is greatly responsible for regulating the sex drive in men and women. Conditions such as hirsutism, which causes excessive hair growth in women, are due predominantly to excessive or hyper-androgen states. Specific drugs, such as phenytoin, minoxidil and steroids can also cause hirsutism as can malnutrition (anorexia) or rare genetic disorders.

Clinical hirsutism is generally associated with acne, temporal balding, increased muscle strength, altering of the libido and in virilisation in women (masculine), clitoral enlargement and deepening of the voice. Generally there is defeminisation with amenorrhoea and a decrease in breast size. Two main causes of hirsutism are idiopathic hirsutism (which means the cause is not fully known), and polycystic ovarian disease, which is rarely linked with virilisation or deepening of the voice.

Hair growth is usually first noted in the peri-pubertal period and tends to stabilise after progressing for a few years. Adrenal and ovarian gland tumours will generally be present in adults. Most ovarian tumours are palpable on physical examinations. Most cases of overt virilisation are caused by androgen-secreting ovarian tumours. Adrenal tumours usually have weaker androgen secretion and are rarely the cause of this problem. Excess testosterone output in females can also cause increased aggression, undue competitiveness, weight gain, skin problems and anovulation. It is uncommon in cases of idiopathic hirsutism or polycystic ovarian syndrome to find increased levels of plasma testosterone, but ovarian tumours are often indicated to cause significant testosterone elevations.

Adrenal lesions, congenital adrenal hyperplasia or malignant tumours will have high plasma DHEA sulphate levels. Medically, treatment protocol for benign, congenital adrenal hyperplasia may include dexamethasone. DHEA sulphate should be suppressed after 3 days on treatment. Patients with tumours, however, will not have DHEA sulphate. High testosterone levels associated with polycystic ovarian syndrome can be medically tested via an oestrogen-progesterone pill; herbs such as Vitex, Peonia and Licorice may also be useful.

Testosterone should be suppressed with polycystic ovarian syndrome but patients with ovarian tumours will have a lack of suppression in contrast. Ovarian and adrenal tumours are treated through surgical intervention. Congenital adrenal hyperplasia is suppressed with glucocorticoid replacement. Idiopathic hirsutism and polycystic ovarian syndrome are treated with contraceptives, glucocorticoid or anti-androgens, the most commonly used being *Cyproterone*. Normal adult female testosterone blood levels range between: *0.4 – 3.6 nmol/L.*

### Luteinising Hormone (LH) and Follicle Stimulating Hormone (FSH)

These hormones are usually measured at the mid-cycle peak, a few days before ovulation. Luteinising hormone is often high, when polycystic ovarian syndrome is present, as the pituitary sends out increasing amounts of this hormone to try to stimulate the release of an egg from the unresponsive ovaries (this also happens at menopause). Raised levels of both pituitary hormones can be caused by *resistant* ovaries, or by the presence of auto-immune diseases.

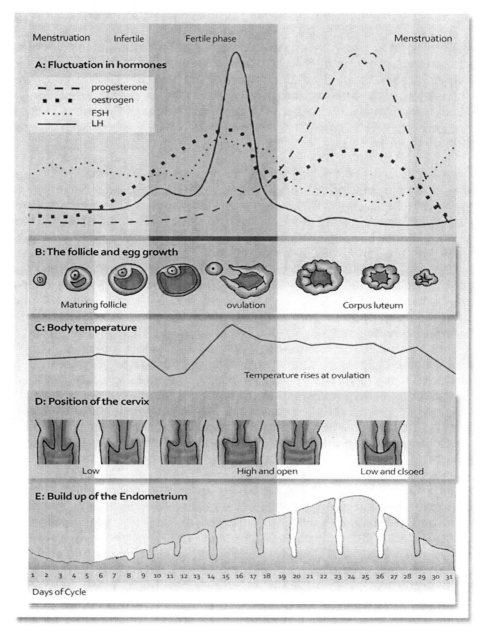

*Figure.10. Females hormone changes during 28-day cycle*

66

# Tests for female fertility

### Endometrial biopsy
A tiny sample of the endometrium (the lining of the uterus) is taken in the later part of the menstrual cycle and tested in order to see if there is enough progesterone in the lining as it matures. If not, the condition is called *Luteal Phase Defect*. It can be treated with hormone and/or natural medicine therapies. The current thickness of the endometrial lining can be an important indicator in determining if a pregnancy is likely to carry to full term.

### FSH test
A blood sample is taken on day three of the menstrual cycle and tested for follicle-stimulating hormone (FSH). FSH levels increase as a woman reaches menopause. If there is a high FSH level, pregnancy is unlikely. Prolactin (the forgotten hormone) is usually released after childbirth to assist with the production of breast milk.

If prolactin levels rise higher than approximately 20 per cent above normal, this will lead to temporary infertility while these levels remain elevated. Stress, drinks containing caffeine, such as soft drinks (soda), coffee and tea can contribute to elevated levels. Polycystic Ovarian Syndrome is also a condition that may have high prolactin output.

### Sonohysterogram
A sonohysterogram or HyCoSy (Hystero-contrast Sonography) is similar to a hysterosalingogram (HSG), except that a saline solution, rather than a dye, is injected, and ultrasound, rather than an X-ray, is used to show uterine abnormalities such as polyps (small growths), fibroids, blockages, and obstructions.

### Hystero-salpingo-gram (HSG)
Dye is inserted through the cervix into the fallopian tubes and uterus, and an x-ray is taken to determine whether the tubes are open and if the uterus is a normal shape. The fallopian tube has the approximate diameter of a hairbrush bristle, though the dye flush again is a useful diagnostic tool.

The dye can flatten out the villi that line the mucous membranes in the tube, which are vital to assist how the sperm and ovum are washed towards each other. The villi require some months to rejuvenate their proper function, which may delay conception for some couples.

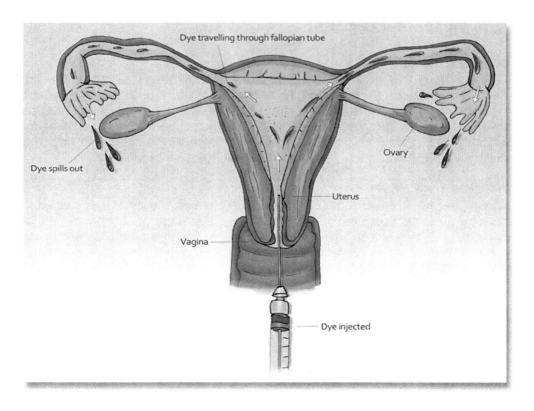

Dye travelling through fallopian tube

Dye spills out

Ovary

Uterus

Vagina

Dye injected

*Figure.11. Hysterosalpingogram*

### Laparoscopy

A laparoscopy is a surgical procedure in which a physician (medical doctor) examines the reproductive organs by means of a tiny scope. If scar tissue or endometrial build up is found, it can be removed by means of the scope as well.

This test/procedure is very useful where large areas of *endometriosis* and/or adhesions require de-bulking, though the benefits may only be temporary because the endometriosis and scar tissue usually grow back, and sadly, it can become much worse the more times this procedure is performed. With conditions such as endometriosis for example, lymphatic system drainage and regulation of excessive oestrogen clearance should be considered! Laparoscopy is the most commonly used endoscopy and it is also utilised for other procedures such as:

*   Evaluation of ovarian disease and pelvic inflammatory disease (PID).
*   Diagnosis tool for cysts, fibroid tumours, and tubal patience.
*   Removal of ovarian adhesions, cysts, ectopic pregnancies, and fibroids.
*   Used to perform biopsies of the tubes, ovaries and uterus.
*   Used to repair various types of damage to fallopian tubes.

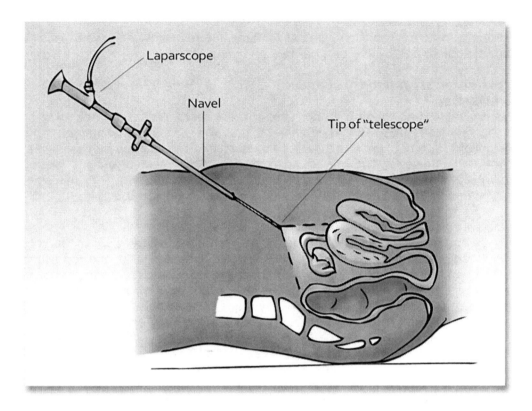

*Figure.12. Laparoscopy*

### Some of the symptoms of laparoscopy procedures may include:

Post-operatively after a laparoscopy procedure many women may experience varying degrees of discomfort, that can possibly cause general unwell feelings for a week or so afterwards.

- Pains in the abdomen, the neck and shoulders. This can be very intense. It is caused by the gas which has been blown into the abdomen. It has nowhere to escape to.
- Sore throat as an after-effect of the anaesthesia.
- Staining from vaginal secretions which are expelling the dye used in the tubal testing.
- Vaginal bleeding.

One of the latest advance techniques is called *Ovarian Diathermy*. This involves laser or what is called *Monopolar electro-cautery* and simultaneously destroys parts of the ovary and repairs it.

### Postcoital Test (PCT, Sims-Huhner Test)

The partners have intercourse 2-8 hours before this test. A sample of cervical mucus and tissue is removed and examined to determine whether the mucus or the cervix is prohibiting fertilisation. Undergoing a PCT is said to be much the same as having a Pap smear. *Refer to test performed on males section.

### Transvaginal Ultrasound

A probe is inserted into the vagina to look for fibroids or ovarian cysts. This can also be done to track early pregnancies.

### Trans-cervical Balloon Tuboplasty (TBT) & Selective Fallopian Tube Canalisation

This procedure has roughly 90 per cent success rates in removing obstructions of the fallopian tube. TBT is similar to the artery-clearing technique called angioplasty. A tiny balloon is inflated and stretched to clear the blocked section of the tube. However, there is an approximate 20 per cent chance of the tube blocking again, therefore, further procedures may be advised. (Chronic stress and chlamydia should be investigated with blocked fallopian tubes)!

### Dilation and Curettage (D&C)

This procedure is routinely performed and commonly ordered with the other mentioned procedures. Its method involves the scraping out of the top section of the endometrial lining. Dilation and curettage may be used during instances when menstruation is delayed due to the endometrium not coming away properly. A D&C may be required in early stage miscarriages when the placenta has not come away properly, thus potentially leading to infections.

### The Clomiphene Citrate Challenge Test – (CCCT)

A measurement of estradiol and FSH is taken on day 2 or 3 of the period and then measured again after taking the medication *Clomiphene citrate* for five days. This drug is used to stimulate egg production. The estradiol and FSH are re-checked. The estradiol levels should rise by the 5th day, but if the FSH level is elevated on either day two or after five days, then the result may be send to be a failed CCCT.

This result may mean that the ovaries have depleted reserves that may decrease chances of conceiving with your own eggs. Further investigations would be warranted to verify results.

### Follicular glycoprotein inhibit-B and Insulin growth factor binding protein-3 (IGFBP-3)

These are a few of the new screening tests to help predict pregnancy success. The protein substances are directly produced by the ovaries and help to produce healthy eggs. The measuring of these proteins may assist in assessing with more accuracy if conception is more viable.

### Exogenous follicle-stimulating hormone (EFORT) and GRH agonists

These substances may be useful diagnostic measures that can help to assess the ovaries response to hormone stimulation, therefore indicating whether ovarian function is working and receptive to hormone messaging; at present EFORT and GRH agonist are used as a fertility 'marker'.

* Additional information of these diagnostic tests may also be addressed in the medical-assisted reproduction techniques section.

# Factors impeding female fertility

This section is a basic summary of the major causal factors that can potentially impede or be implicated in female fertility. The majority of these factors will be discussed in-depth throughout the following chapters.

## *Tubal or peritoneal factors*
Account for approximately *25 to 30 per cent* of the cause behind female infertility. In the United Kingdom reports indicate tubal factors account for *15 per cent* of primary infertility and *40 per cent* of secondary infertility problems for women.

## *Endometriosis / endometritis*
Endometriosis is believed to be the number one gynaecological cause behind female infertility. Endometriosis accounts for *10 per cent* of primary infertility and *5 per cent* secondary infertility.

## *Ovulatory failure / anovulation / endometrial polyps / peri menopause*
Ovulatory dysfunctions including hormone imbalances account for approximately *20 per cent* of the causes of primary infertility and *15 per cent* of secondary infertility.

## Tubular obstructions/Incompetence
Rokitansky-Kuster-Hauser-Mayer syndrome (born without a vagina), and Incompetent cervix are two examples of conditions that will require surgical intervention to restore fertility.

## *Uterine fibroids / prolapse*
Cervical or uterine factors account for approximately *10 per cent* of the causes of female infertility. All of these conditions or structural abnormalities can affect fertility:

Sub mucous, intramural, subserous fibroids – adhesions; scar tissue (in uterine cavity may be caused by Asherman's syndrome); adenomyosis; Mullerian duct defect; imperforated hymen; absent uterus and vaginal; septate uterus; sub septate uterus; bicornuate uterus; double uterus; double vagina; and longitudinal vaginal septum.

Meigs syndrome (Demons-Meigs syndrome) is an ovarian fibrous growth that can cause abdominal swelling and sex hormone abnormalities that can contribute to infertility.

## *Poly cystic ovarian syndrome/disease (PCOS/D)*
PCOS is becoming one of the most complicated and increasingly diagnosed endocrine related disorders that affect female fertility.

### Immunological problems
Immunological factors account for approximately *5 per cent* of the cause of female infertility. For example, the body may develop antibodies in defence to attack against the sperm and/or embryo. Hughes syndrome is an anti-phosholipid syndrome that affects blood clotting that can cause infertility and miscarriage.

### Chronic infection and auto-immune disease
Measles, mumps (paramyxovirus), rubella, chicken-pox, (T-helper lymphocytes Th1 and Th2) imbalances, chronic allergies, chronic tissue-specific inflammatory damage, anti-cardiolipin antibodies – specific for miscarriage, also lupus anticoagulant, anti-phospholipid syndrome – causes clotting disorders and affects placental development, immunoglobulin M & IGG (can cross the placenta), thyroid disease such as hashimotos and liver disease such as Hepatitis should also be investigated.

### Pelvic inflammatory disease (PID)
The incidences of sexually transmitted diseases that contribute to conditions such as cervicitis and hydrosalpinx are increasing. Hydrosalpinx is a condition that involves having chronically infected and/or inflamed fallopian tube/s that may affect the passage of the egg through the fallopian tube and can possibly affect an embryo's survival due to infective matter draining down into the uterus. If both tubes are dilated, the condition is known as hydro-salpinges. These conditions may require surgical removal of that affected tube.

### Genito-urinary tract infections
There are large number micro-organisms that have been studied and implicated in affecting reproductive health.

These may include: Chlamydia trachomatis (Fitz-Hugh-Curtis syndrome); ureaplasma; systemic candida albicans; gardnerella; gonorrhoea; genital herpes simplex virus; mycoplasma; ureaplasma; enterococcus; B.strep; staph auteus; Haem influenza and Haem strep; E.coli; klebsiella; toxoplasmosis; cytomegalovirus (CMV); parvovirus; rubella; HIV, syphilis and hepatitis.

Chlamydia is said to affect more than 4 million American's a year and is a major cause of infertility and tubal dysfunction.

### Antibody incompatibilities and Genetics
An example of a genetic condition that can affect female fertility is Turner's syndrome. This condition is caused when a baby girl has only one of the normal pair of X chromosomes. Turner's syndrome can result in very few or no eggs (ova) and occasionally, no ovaries.

### Cervical mucus abnormalities
Excess acidity (hostile mucus). The use of certain artificial lubricants and even saliva may affect fertility.

### Endocrine/hormone imbalances

Early ovarian failure, luteal phase defect, oligomenorrhea (infrequent periods), periods exceeding six days, menstrual cycles shorter than 24 days or more than 35 days apart; imbalances or fluctuations of reproductive system hormones such as Follicle Stimulating Hormone (FSH), Luteinising Hormone (LH), oestrogen, progesterone and prolactin. Some endocrine disorders that may contribute to infertility include: diabetes, hypothyroidism, and Addison's disease (adrenocortical insufficiency).

### Luteal phase defects

The term describes inadequate transformation of the endometrium during the secretary (luteal phase) of the cycle that can cause infertility. Luteal phase defects are estimated to affect *3-4 per cent* of women who have unexplained infertility and up to *63 per cent of women who repeatedly miscarry*.

It has also been shown that *6-10 per cent* of women who are infertile have an inadequate luteal phase. Luteal phase defects can be associated with inadequate or deficient progesterone production relative to oestrogen (also known as corpus luteum insufficiency) or normal levels of progesterone that do not adequately stimulate the endometrium. Abnormally low cholesterol levels can also affect progesterone production and cause luteal phase defects.

### Chronic stress and psychological issues

Psychogenic/nutritional or metabolic factors may account for approximately *5 percent* of the causes of infertility. These are a few examples of potential psychological issues that may contribute to infertility.
 Having a baby to some may seem like searching for the 'Holy Grail'; the harder one tries to reach out for it, the further away it appears to be. Past issues such as sexual abuse, history of abortion/s, recurrent miscarriages, previous emotional trauma, handicapped siblings, guilt, fear of parenthood, fear of added responsibility, trying to have a baby as a means to saving a strained relationship, and actually trying too hard to conceive.

Stress has a significant effect on hormone control, often contributing to related conditions. The principal effect of stress is the depletion of the 'mother' of hormones DHEA that is produced via the adrenal gland. Stress increases cortisol production at the expense of DHEA and subsequent sex hormones. Stress can greatly influence the intricate balance of the hypothalamus / pituitary / adrenal axis, which regulates over multiple bodily functions.

Excessive stress may be both a direct or indirect contributor to infertility. The stress of infertility alone may also be a major factor of why conception may not be occurring. Pseudocyesis is a psychotic delusional state when a woman believes that she is truly pregnant when in reality she is not. This condition can be contributed to by intense stress.

### Outside body fat percentage ranges
If a female is carrying less that *15 percent* body fat or over *35 percent* body fat, this can potentially affect her fertility.

Fat is used by the female body to convert androgens to oestrogens, and affects the biological effectiveness of those oestrogens. Obesity can affect the correct utilisation of body hormones and other chemical reactions; therefore, ovulation failure is more likely to occur. Studies published by the *British Journal of Medicine* and *Journal of Reproductive Fertility Development* have reported that women with a high waist-to-hip ratio (an 'apple' shape) had far more difficulty conceiving that those with low waist-to-hip ratio (a 'pear' shape).

### Effects of contraceptive pill
The intake of contraceptive medications is known to deregulate the natural menstrual cycle and depletes a large number of nutrients with ongoing use.

### Pollution and radiation exposure
Excessive exposure to X-rays, TV screens, mobile phones, microwaves, computer screens, photocopiers, main-cables, electrical appliances, fluorescent lighting, and power outlets, are all known to potentially affect fertility.

Radiation can greatly affect people in occupations such as VDU operators, pilots, and flight attendants. Studies have stated that every one high-altitude flight (over 30,000 feet) of 4 - 5 hours duration gives the equivalent exposure to cosmic radiation as a full-body x-ray. Polar areas involve increased exposure; frequent flyers, dentists, and radiographers require compensatory treatments.

### Excess alcohol and caffeine intake
Caffeine stimulates the production of the neuron-transmitter dopamine, which has an inhibitory (blocking) effect on prolactin production. Deficiency or excesses of prolactin can promote infertility. Studies have reported that even one (1) caffeinated soft drink a day has been associated with a temporary 50 percent reduction in conception.

Excessive alcohol ingestion in women may provoke hyperprolactinemia (excess prolactin), and also prevent proper adhesion of the embryo to the uterine wall, hence causing infertility.

### Other biological contaminates of our air, food and water quality
Toxic chemicals: Approximately 70,000 manufactured chemicals are in use worldwide and not all of them have been tested for toxic effects on human reproduction. There are more than 300 new fertility-robbing chemicals used today that didn't exist 50 years ago. It is also estimated that some 60,000 different chemicals may be contaminating our water supplies today. Some examples may include: solvents; glues; many paints; carbon monoxide; anaesthetics; pesticides; agrochemical fertilisers; vinyl chloride; household

cleaners; insect sprays; aromatic hydrocarbons; some food additives; PCBs; xenoestrogens; and formaldehydes.

Many chemicals commonly found in the environment have the capacity to interfere with hormonal balance, via disruption of enzyme activity or directly binding to oestrogen receptors. These chemicals are known as 'endocrine disruptures' and have become an important drive for both male and female reproductive pathology. These chemicals can cause disruption via epigenetic changes to the genes sequence without necessarily mutating the gene. These epigenetic changes have been shown be passed on through several future generations of offspring. Breakdowns in the effective detoxifications processes within the body increase our risk of exposure to these chemicals.

### Nutritional Deficiencies
There are numerous nutrients that are vitally important for maintaining correct bio-chemical function of the body's various systems.

Some of the following nutrients are particularly important for female reproductive health: Vitamin A (moderate amounts); folic acid; Vitamin B12; zinc; selenium; Vitamin B complex, esp. Vitamin B6, Vitamin B5, Vitamin B2; PABA; iron; Vitamin C; Vitamin E; magnesium; calcium; potassium; manganese; and essential fatty acids.

**Amenorrhea** (absence of menses), **Menorrhagia**, (excessive menses), **Polyps**, and excessive vaginal dryness can affect fertility.

### Excessive physical exercise
Can cause a condition called 'Marathoner's amenorrhea' that can affect fertility; mild exercise though may actually be beneficial to reproductive health.

### Low cholesterol levels and poor protein intakes in diet
Cholesterol and proteins are required for the proper production of reproductive and other body hormones' enzymes, and the integrity of cellular membranes. It is particularly important in strict vegetarian diets to assure that enough primary proteins are being consumed by combining various foods.

### Dehydration
At least 70 per cent of the constitution of our body is water. The amount of water is critical to the regulation of the concentration of the various minerals and organic chemicals found in the cells. Cells are extremely sensitive to the concentration of their contents and normal cell function depends on this being strictly controlled. Dehydrated cells will not divide properly and chromosome errors are likely to result. Dehydration can be a cause of both infertility and foetal abnormality.

**Unexplained infertility** (infertility of unknown medical cause)
Unexplained infertility accounts for approximately *20 to 30 percent* of infertility cases. Factors that may be involved include mind-body issues and undocumented miscarriages.


# Ovulation – timing (self-testing)

If you wish to become pregnant, there are a number of tests available over the counter that can help you determine the best time to attempt to conceive. These tests predict the time of ovulation by detecting the release of Luteinising Hormone (LH), which in turn triggers the release of the egg (ovum). You may have heard of women who have conceived outside their predicted ovulation time. Studies have revealed that women can also spontaneously ovulate due to other factors such as changes in the lunar moon cycles, from orgasms and even with the onset of menstruation.

**Ovulation test kits (OPK)**
A chemically treated dipstick detects the luteinising hormone (LH) in urine sample. If the hormone has been released, the stick changes colour. It can take 8 to 12 hours for LH to filter from the bloodstream to the urine. After a positive result, ovulation takes place within twelve (12) to thirty-six (36) hours. Testing for LH in the urine tends to be most accurate when the urine sample is taken between 11am and 3 pm. Remember, however, that no test is 100 per cent accurate.
 To improve the accuracy of the test, the urine is best to be reasonably concentrated. Don't drink fluids two hours prior to obtaining the urine sample.
Storage of the test kit is best in a neutral weather environment; extreme hot and cold conditions may affect the test's accuracy.

If the menstrual cycle is shorter than 26 days and the test is performed too late, or the menstrual cycle is longer than 35 days and the test is performed too early then the results may be inaccurate. Some examples of ovulation test kits include: *BioSelf* – electronic basal body temperature fertility indicator, *Baby-Comp* – basal temperature monitor. *Persona* and *Clear-Plan* are LH urine test strip monitors. BBT charts are usually provided with the various ovulation test kits.

Note: Women with polycystic ovarian syndrome and hyperthyroidism may produce a relatively high level of LH, for this reason a false negative result may occur during testing.

**Saliva Tests** such as the *Maybe Baby* scope can also be useful to determine that you're coming into a fertile phase by observing fern-like pattern changes to the saliva scope, which may indicate mucus changes at the time of peak fertility. During the non-fertile period, the scope may show a series of tight, dot-like patterns. Usually 2 to 3 days before the woman starts the fertile phase, the ferning pattern then appears. This can remain until 3 to 4 days after the peak fertile time has passed.

There are now **electronic saliva tests** available such as *OvaCue II* (by Zetek) although this version is not quite as portable as the manual types. This electronic saliva test also comes with both an oral and vaginal probe. It comes with a spoon-sized sensor that can be placed on the tongue for eight seconds in the morning for greater accuracy. Clinical trials have shown this method of fertility time diagnosis to be 25 per cent more accurate than the basal body temperature and cervical mucus viscosity methods.

Both **Basal temperature (BBT) charting** and **The Billings (rhythm) Method** are self-help techniques that may assist in isolating your ideal time to fall pregnant. To get a more accurate reading from your BBT it is best to take the temperature vaginally rather than orally, as many individuals may be mouth breathings during sleep and this may affect the accuracy of the readings.

**The symptom-thermal method (STM)** is an approach that observes more than one fertility indicator, most commonly BBT and cervical mucus; the position of the cervix is another (Dr Weschler's fertility awareness method).

**The lunar cycle (or lunar phase) –'synchronising with the stars'**
We know that the affects of the lunar changes influence our planet in many ways. These same changes can also influence the body's physiology and bio-rhythmic cycle of fertility depending on the various phase of the orbiting moon when it travels around the earth.

A female's peak fertility is greatest when mid-cycle ovulation is synchronised or coincides with her lunar fertility phase. This peak fertility phase can be predicted in advance. This requires accurate calculation of what is known as your personal 'natal angle' during the lunar cycle from your time of birth. Not only can these lunar cycles enhance fertility peaks, the child's sex selection may also be influenced during the various zodiac times.

Male (positive) signs (fire and air) - Aries (fire), Gemini (air), Leo (fire), Libra (air), Sagittarius (air), Aquarius (air).

Female (negative) signs (water and earth) – Taurus (earth), Cancer (water), Virgo (earth), Scorpio (water), Capricorn (earth), Pisces (water).

Approximately every 2.5 days the moon travels from one sign to the other. If this method of fertility prediction is used it is best to time the respective zodiac phase to coincide with your lunar fertility peak. Many women are known to ovulate on the full moon and have their periods on the new moon. A method called 'lunaception' involves sleeping in complete darkness (no illumination or electrical applicances near by) until three (3) days before the full moon; then the blinds and curtains are opened to allow the moon light to flood in.

This is said to help promote ovulation and trying to conceive at this time would be worth giving it a go!

If you would like further information in regards to this method, Author Francesca Naish has several books on this subject: *The Lunar Cycle (a guide to natural and astrological fertility control)* and *Natural Fertility.*

# Chapter 4

# *Plan A: Timed Intercourse*

## *'Making babies the old fashioned way – the ups and downs'*

There are three basic stages that will be discussed throughout this book that identify the various stages of intervention that may be required to achieve conception. The first stage or **Plan A** involves using *timed intercourse* around predicted ovulation. Stage two or **Plan B** may involve incorporating the use of *alternative/natural therapies* to enhance reproductive health to improve your chances of conception. Stage three or **Plan C** involves having to utilise *medical assisted intervention* in the hope of successfully falling pregnant. All of these various stages can have both pros and cons. Plan A is an example of what many couples have experienced and what you could expect if you are going into this unprepared.

Timed intercourse can potentially be a great strain on you as a couple. Sex can lose its spontaneity, women feel desperately anxious to 'hit the right moment', and men can feel they have to 'perform on cue'. These factors can contribute to other possible problems: for the males, impotence, loss of libido, frustration, and if time goes by without a positive outcome he may feel a sense of personal failure and worthlessness as his ego becomes bruised, due to his inability to perform his manly duty and impregnate his partner.

Women are under equally, if not more, stress, due to charting her temperature changes, or measuring her hormone levels, in order to know the day, possibly even the hour, that she may be ovulating, in an attempt to predict the best time/s to have intercourse.

A single episode of intercourse, once in mid-cycle, is a bit hit-and-miss. Alternatively, being too enthusiastic can also have a down side, using up too much of the good viable sperm and possibly contributing to immune reactions against the sperm as well. Predicting the timed release of the egg is rather like trying to hit a moving target. So to cover all bases, timing intercourse around the event of ovulation gives you much better odds of success. The time around ovulation really needs to be 'peppered' with intercourse!

This regimented cycle of planned intercourse can potentially raise problems, if as a couple, you let them. For example (one possible scenario – to some this may sound familiar), let's say that the lady may feel 'tonight's the night' because the basal temperature has fallen and it's day 12 to 14 of the menstrual cycle. It's now time to have nooky (intercourse). Your partner may not appreciate the blunt nature of your plan (in his perception) and may feel that tonight he would rather watch the footy on TV.

After trying all the persuasive threats, tears, and eventually having to pull out all stops by giving him the 'come-hither' moves (irresistible to all warm-blooded mortal men) your now-willing sex machine (bewitched by your feminine charms) and torn between the choice of sex or football (possibly his two most favourite things in the world), turns off the TV and grumbles all the way to the bedroom.

As even the most virile of men with seemingly endless sex drive can have a difficult time performing when having to prove their manhood, communicating each person's intentions before the event can avoid much unnecessary distress and make the experience more pleasurable than painful.

This routine is then repeated several times during this time of the month, keeping your fingers crossed, anxiously hoping that your temperature rises and does not come down. Almost two weeks have gone by of nervous waiting, but depressingly the menstrual period does show up once again, meaning you have to go through the whole process again the next month.

Another hurdle that may plague some couples when attempting timed intercourse is the difficulty of actually getting both partners together in the same place at the same time to attempt this method. Some partners may have to travel for their work or are involved with shift work schedules that can potentially hinder accurate timing to coincide with the female partner's ovulation cycle.

As time goes by, the pleasure and joy of love-making is replaced with the chore of baby-making (sex-for-reproduction). As more time elapses, the tension continues to build and intercourse may be replaced with yelling and screaming at one another that may even threaten your very relationship. The compounding stress for many couples is immense and you both need to distinguish when the stress is impacting on you too much, so you can take a bit of time out from this rigid routine, to replenish your energy and refocus on each other before trying again.

If natural conception has *not* occurred after a full year of attempting to fall pregnant using timed unprotected intercourse, consider moving forward to investigating *Plan B* and/or *Plan C* methods under the advisement from a qualified practitioner in the appropriate field. *These methods will be discussed in other chapters.

## Sexual Positions and Conception

There is much debate about whether certain sexual positions are better than others for improving the chances of conception. Some individuals may have mastered the art of Tantric sex and others may be able to contort themselves to do every possible position of the Karma Sutra, but do any of them really enhance your odds of falling pregnant?

For the purpose of baby-making the consensus is the 'oldie but goldie' technique of the standard 'missionary position' (which is when the woman lies on her back and the man is on top).

Because of the way the female reproductive system is designed, the semen/sperm tend to run down the vagina and into the cervix when a woman is on her back. The depth of penetration by the male penis into the vagina may benefit the delivery of the sperm at ejaculation, by placing it higher in the vaginal tract closer to the cervix. This may also give the sperm a good chance of avoiding many of the vaginal defences such as hostile mucus that can destroy a very large quantity of the sperm before it gets a chance to make it to the next stage.

Placing an object such as a pillow in the small of the women's back to elevate the hips can help, to not only allow greater penetration, but with the added benefit of gravity to assist the correct down flow of the sperm. Another favoured position is the classically known 'doggie style' or spooning technique. For this manoeuvre the male needs to enter the woman's vagina from behind while the woman is kneeling on her hands and knees. I promise that this position was not just conjured for the male's benefit; there is reasonable scientific validation to warrant giving it a try.

## 'G' marks the Spot not the 'X'

Does having an orgasm affect your chances of conception? We know that if a male doesn't ejaculate then there is no sperm to fertilise the egg if you are trying to fall pregnant the old fashioned way and the male orgasm usually goes hand in hand with this process. Though, the type of orgasm the female has may have some bearing on the outcome. It has been suggested that orgasms via the G-spot, or Graftenberg spot, stimulation are more likely to result in conception than orgasms via clitoral stimulation, although this has not been conclusively proven.

The theory is that when there's G-spot stimulation, the uterus pushed downward into the vagina and the cervix dips into the pool of sperm. This may explain why studies have observed the presence of sperm entering the fallopian tubes with hours after intercourse, rather than much later for those who did not experience the same type of orgasm. During clitoral stimulation the uterus has been shown to pull up.

The G-spot is the highly sensitive area of tissue and nerve endings on the upper wall of the vagina, just a short distance back from the opening towards the cervix. The clitoris is located under the soft lips of the labia minora that surround the vagina and the opening of the urethra. It has been said that men can read street directions better than women, but when it comes to finding a woman's G-spot some instructive coaching may be required for some men. The guys may also need to be reminded that the word 'foreplay' doesn't mean the lead-up sports talk that goes on before a footy game.

# Influencing the sex of the baby

*'Life is like a box of chocolates, you never know what you're gonna get'*

### *Gender Selection methods*
The cells of the body are normally comprised of 23 pairs of chromosomes, our genetic blueprint, a nucleus that is the control centre of the cell and cytoplasm the fluid material that is contained within the cell. The 23 pairs of chromosomes are the ones that depict the sex characteristics. The female has two similar XX chromosomes and the male has two dissimilar XY chromosomes. The male's chromosomes are the ones that will select the sex characteristics of the offspring: combining either the father's X chromosome with the mother's X chromosome for a girl baby or the father's Y chromosome with the mother's X chromosome for a boy baby.

Two types of sperm are believed to be produced, one with the X chromosome and the other the Y chromosome, which predict the final sex characteristics of the child (male or female).

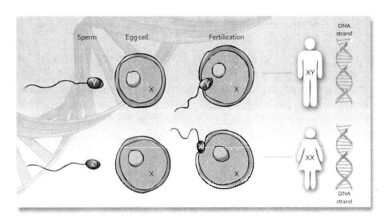

The male sperm (Y-carrying) is said to be much smaller in size to the female sperm (X-carrying) type, much more agile and faster swimmers (the sprinters of the sperm world). The Y chromosome-carrying sperm, also referred to as *Androsperm,* have a much rounder head than the female X or *Gynosperm* counterpart.

The female-type sperm (the endurance swimmers) are believed to be much hardier than the male type, and therefore are said to be more resistant to being destroyed by the defences of the women's reproductive system. The gynosperm may also have a longer life span, are more oval-headed in shape, but are produced in lower numbers in comparison to its androsperm (the sprinters) counterpart.

The sperm's obstacle course to the ovum is not unlike the children's story of the Tortoise and the Hare race. The male sperm (the hare) are the quick ones out of the starting blocks, but run out of puff halfway through the race and need a rest. The female sperm (the tortoise) takes it slow and steady, although they have a habit of pipping the stamina-deprived male sperm at the post on many occasions. The race to the egg is a contest of *endurance versus speed.* For every 100 girl babies born there are about 105-6 boys babies, a very close race in the number of the sexes.

The Billing's (rhythm) method of timing female reproductive fertility states the closer intercourse is to the peak ovulation time, the better chances of conceiving a *male child* and the further away from ovulation (within viable sperm life span, two to four days) the better chances of a *female child*. Studies that have examined this method have reported very high success rates of conceiving with that particular sex baby!

Some men only produce one type of sperm, which restricts their offspring to one sex. Similarly, the Ph (Acid/Alkaline) balance of the women's vagina and uterine secretions are more favourable to one sex.

Female chromosome-carrying sperm appear to be more resistant to hostile environments like excess acid in the vagina, but male sperm make up for this through strength in numbers, which are usually in excess of the female sperm. This is where specific dietary intake could be useful in potentially tipping mother nature's scales, by slightly adopting either an alkaline or acidic type of diet.

A study claimed two French scientists had reported a 95 per cent success rate for sex selection by placing the prospective mother on a particular diet for a month prior to her conception. Following are examples of the various foods that may be particularly beneficial to try. When my wife and I were thinking about trying for our third child, we came across these foods that may help for the different sex types. We did try it and we did have the same sex baby we were trying for. Many other people that I have discussed this topic with, have also said that they were successful – worth a thought?

**For a BOY**

*'What are little boys made of? Snips and snails, and puppy dog tails, that's what little boys are made of!'*

This ole early 19th century Mother Goose nursery rhyme may not be all that far from the truth!

*Foods to eliminate from the diet:*
No milk or dairy products, including sauces made from milk or cheese; chocolate; cocoa; mustard; nuts; pizza; all whole grains, wholemeal breads, and breakfast cereals and biscuits made from these foods; shellfish; molluscs; spinach and green leafy vegetables including cabbage, cauliflower.

*Include these foods:*
Meat, fish, (except shellfish and prawns); all fruit and fruit juices; pasta with egg base; white bread products – providing they are not calcium enriched; vegetables (those not on eliminated list) including lentils, beans, parsley, peas, artichokes; mushrooms; all fruit, both fresh and dried; sugar is allowed but not chocolate; tea, coffee, cola and soda drinks; pastries; refined grains such as cornflakes; white rice; and pasta.

*Increase sodium and potassium-based foods and minerals.*


**For a GIRL**

*'What are little girls made of? Sugar and spice and all things nice, that's what little girls are made of!'*

*Foods to Eliminate:*
Meat; smoked fish; all pre-cooked bacon; ham; salted products (including crisps); hard cheese; oranges; cherries; peaches; plums; pineapples; dried fruits; red apricots; melons; popcorn; parsley; spinach; cabbage; cauliflower; mushrooms; sweet corn; zucchini; avocado; raw tomatoes; dried peas and beans (except soybeans); lentils; alcohol; fruit juices; tea or coffee; chocolate and sweets; preserves; mayonnaise; pickles; shellfish; cakes; biscuits; bicarbonate soda; olives; vinegar; frozen and tinned meals; tea; coffee; and alcohol.

*Include these foods:*
Milk; fish; eggs; yoghurt; unsalted cheese; soft cheese; veal; lamb; chicken; crispbreads especially unsalted breads; potatoes; carrots; celery; peas; green beans; cucumber; onions; leeks; capsicums; cooked tomato; eggplant; potatoes; green salads; soybeans; nuts; sugar; honey and any sauces; apples; pears, strawberries.

***Increase calcium and magnesium-based foods and minerals.***
The theory is that sodium and potassium attract to the male-bearing androsperm (Y). Calcium and magnesium attract female-bearing gynosperm (X). The idea of the sex selection diets and nutrients is to alter the chemical composition of the egg so that it attracts the desired sperm type, similar to that of a magnet.

**Another method that may have some benefit in gender selection**

**To assist with selecting a BOY**

***Douching*** - the use of a mildly alkaline douche prior to intercourse may help. Dissolve 5 grams of baking soda or bicarbonate soda in half a litre (about 2 pints) of water and wash the vaginal area with it.

***Orgasm*** - The alkaline secretion that is released during a female orgasm is favourable to the male type sperm (Y or androsperm). Therefore females that experience orgasm in synchronisation (just prior or with) the male orgasm may assist in improving the chances of a male child.

***Intercourse positions*** – Deep vaginal penetration from the rear or the classically known 'doggy style' position may help to avoid many of the male sperm from being destroyed as the cervical entrance is more alkaline than the more acidic environment of the vaginal area. The deep penetration at the time of the male's ejaculation allows the Y chromosome sperm to be deposited further in the female reproductive tract giving the male type sperm a better chance. This position may also allow for the cervix to open wider.

***Abstinence from intercourse*** for several days prior to the 'ideal' conception time may increase the sperm-pooling effect and therefore increase the percentage of possible male Y-carrying sperm. Intercourse should be timed to synchronise as close to the female's ovulation as possible (preferably on the day).

Cooler testicular temperature may influence the male-type sperm, therefore increasing the odds of a male child. Cold showers, wearing loose-fitting clothing and underwear such as boxer shorts may be beneficial.

**To assist with selecting a GIRL**

***Douching*** - the use of a mildly acidic douche prior to intercourse may help. Add 20ml of white vinegar in half a litre (about 2 pints) of water and wash the vaginal area with it.

***Orgasm*** - for increasing the odds of having a female-gender baby it is believed that the female should not orgasm on the 'ideal' conception day/s. This may avoid making the vaginal environment too alkaline, which can favour the male sperm chances. This is definitely not as much fun for the ladies as the boy method!

*Intercourse positions* - Shallow penetration may be better in the 'missionary' position or face-to-face technique, where the male penetrates the vagina on top of the female. The male is required to ejaculate as he is withdrawing from the vagina closer to the entrance. The vaginal entrance is usually more acidic than near the cervix; this may assist the female X (gynosperm) type as they are more resistant to the hostile environment that the male Y type are.

Another theory to assist selection for a girl is to have intercourse during the mid-afternoon as the male's testosterone is normally low during this time and is believed to help influence the chances for a girl.

Also studies have shown that having intercourse at the time of a full moon shows a very high conception rate of female babies. The science behind some of these theories is not completely understood but eclectic research into these methods holds some validity.

*Abstinence from intercourse* – It is believed that when attempting to conceive a female baby *no abstinence* is required as lower sperm counts of your male partner may actual increase your odds of a female child due to the fact that the male-type sperm is usually produced in higher numbers to make up for their lack of resilience.

Increased intercourse at the beginning of the cycle may help to lower the male type of sperm therefore increasing the odds of a girl child. Increase in testicular heat such as from wearing tight clothing may also lower the male type sperm numbers also!

### Did you know these facts?

- The first-born are more often boy babies.
- Older couples are more likely to have girls.
- Males who are highly stressed are more likely to have girls. A reason for this could be that stress can temporarily reduce a male's sperm counts via increased prolactin output and reduced testosterone production.
- Women treated with ovulation-enhancing drug such as Clomid are more likely to have girls.
- Throughout history there have been many old wives' tales regarding ways to influence the sex of babies. One of these beauties worth mentioning was proposed by Hippocrates, who is regarded as the 'father of modern medicine'. Hippocrates believed that the man's right testicle produced boys and the left produced girls. This led men to tie string around one testicle during intercourse to prevent the 'undesired' sperm from leaving their body. Also during the eighteenth century numerous male aristocrats had their left testicle removed by a doctor in the belief that it would ensure them of fathering a male heir! Thank goodness that practice has fallen out of favour.
- Aristotle stated that when a warm wind blows it will be a boy; during a cold wind it will be a girl. This statement may actually hold some validity given the different environmental factors that andro-sperm and gyno-sperm best thrive in.

# Medical procedures that may assist with the gender selection process

**The Percoll method**: This method is used to separate the female (XX) sperm from the male (XY) sperm. In the lab the sperm are laid on to a media in a sterile container. The female sperm are heavier than the male sperm as they contain approximately 2.8 percent more DNA material and are generally slower swimmers as well. The female-type sperm tend to sink faster than the males and settle on the bottom layer ready for retrieval. Though not perfect it is reported that this method has a 75 percent success rate in conceiving a girl.

**The swim-up method**: Essentially the same as the Percoll method but performed basically in reverse. Because the male sperm are faster and lighter the sperm is placed in the bottom of a sterile container first and the media is placed over the top of them. More sperm are believed to reach the top layer before the female sperm and are used in the insemination procedure. It is reported that this method has a 65 per cent success rate in conceiving a boy.

**Microsort**: This newer method also uses the fact that female sperm contain more DNA and are larger in size. A fluorescent dye is used to stain and bind to the DNA material. An instrument called a flow cytometre is used to sort out the sample. The female sperm may be observed to appear a reddish-pink colour, whereas the male sperm appear more greenish in colour. This method is said to have slightly better results though is still quite expense and only a few IVF clinics still perform this procedure.

**The SELNAS Method**: A computer data program developed from gender selection. Personal information details are collected and entered into the computer program. A personalised year gender selection calendar is correlated to predict when ovulation is most likely to occur, for example, five days prior to try for a girl and the day of ovulation if you are trying for a boy. Studies of couples using this method have reported an accuracy of between 96 to 98 percent success rate. This program was largely based on the studies conducted by European physician Dr Josep Stolkowski and European biologist Schoun.

**Pre-implantation genetic diagnosis (PGD)**: This technique involves removing a single cell from the embryo to identify the presence of genetic disease. PGD can also be utilised from gender selection as the isolated cell can reveal what sex the embryo will develop into. This can allow the geneticist to pre-select which embryos to transfer, depending if a particular sex child has been advised by the prospective parents.

In the future, a technique called *microarray analysis* may be available to examine embryo genetic make-up before implantation. Microarray analysis may also be utilised for sex selection, and to assist in indentifying the best quality eggs that can be used for fertilisation.

These are some things that can help Mother Nature, but remember, while she appreciates our efforts to help her in any way, for those who try to force or change her designs, she can also be ruthlessly savage.

# Cervical Mucus Changes

The cervix produces different types of mucus from little pockets that open into the cervical canal called *crypts*. There are approximately 100 of these crypts in the neck of womb and are controlled by changes in hormones during certain stages of the menstrual cycle.

At the beginning and end of the menstrual cycle, the oestrogen levels should be low; this results in the production of minute or scanty amounts of sticky, tacky-type mucus which is normally opaque in colour and texture. This is infertile mucus. As oestrogen levels rise closer to the ovulation phase, the mucus becomes clearer, more profuse, thinner, and moister. Just prior to impending ovulation, the oestrogen levels have peaked and the mucus then becomes more jelly-like, and is still quite moist. The mucus now becomes stretchy and may resemble a substance likened to raw egg white. This effect is known as *spinnbarkeit* or *spinn*. This is fertile mucus.

Changes in this cervical mucus are the only physical symptom that is observable and reliable in predicting impending ovulation and fertility. There are 4 known types of mucus: the G-type, L-type, S-type and P-type, and all have differing functions. Some are needed to repel sperm during the infertile phases of the cycle, others filter out the defective sperm and invading microbes, and other types of mucus actually nourish, channel and guide the sperm through the cervix and uterus just prior the ovulation. This type of mucus also makes the environment more alkaline and is more favourable to the sperm's survival.

The vagina is normally an acidic environment; acidity immobilises sperm. During the fertile phase of the cycle, this mucus provides a buffer of protection for the sperm from the acidity. During the infertile phase of the cycles, this mucus provides little if any protection and the armada of sperm is usually quickly destroyed in this hostile environment.

The life span of sperm can be viable up to three days, though live sperm can live up to 5 days, but the numbers are usually too low to effect a conception. Each day approximately one-third of sperm are destroyed. The average life expectancy of sperm is about 16 to 18 hours; the more favourable the environment it needs to work in the better chances of extending their life span and improving the number of sperm able to reach the site of the ovum (egg). The more sperm around the ovum, the better the chances that one will take up the challenge and breach the egg's shell to achieve fertilisation.

Testing cervical Ph (acid/alkaline) status should be one of the earlier investigations to rule out the level of mucus hostility.

The use of *Tes Tape* (from your pharmacy or drug store) is an old but favourite way of testing cervical mucus and for predicting ovulation. Hold a portion of the tape to the cervix for a few seconds. Remove and observe whether the colour of the paper changes. A few days prior to ovulation the paper should turn an olive colour; just before ovulation it should turn dark green or blue when the cervical mucus is alkaline. If vaginal dryness is a problem during the fertile stage of your cycle a 'sperm-friendly' lubricant called *Pre-Seed* ™ by INGfertility may be worth considering. When applied it may improve the sperm's viability and reduce uncomfortable friction soreness during intercourse.

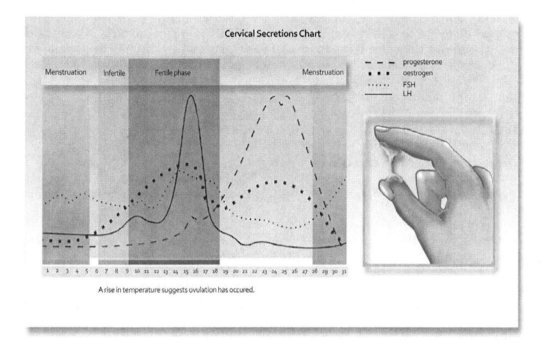

*Figure.13. The various types of cervical mucus*

### Natural treatments to increase fertile mucus production
Herbal medicines to balance hormones may include: False unicorn root; dong quai; black cohosh; peonia; saw palmetto; and other oestrogenic herbs and foods taken prior and during the pre-ovulation stage.

Tonic herbs for the mucus membranes: golden seal and bayberry.

Nutrients such as: calcium; magnesium; zinc; and potassium chloride.

### Increase consumption of Alkaline-forming foods in the diet:
Avocados; buttermilk; corn; dates; fresh coconut; fresh fruits; cherries; vegetables; goat's milk; honey; maple syrup; molasses; nuts (almonds, hazelnuts); raisins; cider vinegar; alfalfa; red clover; sea vegetables; seeds; soy products; whey; and yogurt.

***Avoid or decrease Acid-forming food in diet; these are some examples:***
Meat; fish; eggs; all animal products; sugars; coffee; tea; alcohol; artichokes; asparagus tips; aspirin; beans; beer; cakes; cheese; cocoa; cranberries; custard; doughnuts; eggs; flour products; milk; mustard; noodles; jams; pasta; pastries; peanuts; pepper; poultry; sauerkraut; shellfish; spaghetti; and white rice.

To maintain good health the human diet should comprise a ratio of 70 per cent alkaline foods to 30 per cent acids. The human body normally has a Ph (acid/alkaline ratio) of between 6.0 and 6.8 (that is mildly acidic). If this value rises above 6.8 then the body is too alkaline and can contribute to imbalances in homeostasis and cause numerous health problems from alkalosis. Similarly, if the Ph value of the body is under 6.3 then this can cause acidosis and also many health disturbances as well.

## Ovarian reserves

### *'There may be life in the old girl yet'*

Several tests are available that can help in assessing a female's fertility potential:

- Ultrasound of the ovaries during the first half of the cycles to examine the size and number of small (antral) follicles (developing eggs).

- Blood test to measure for *Anti-mullerian hormone* (AMH). AMH is made in the ovaries and is important for the production of oestrogen and assists in egg maturation each month. AMH is considered a marker of ovarian function; the levels of AMH can help to indicate both the quality and quantity of the remaining egg store. This test may also be used prior to undertaking IVF procedures. If the AMH levels are low than the ovaries may not response as favourably to drug stimulation.

  Women with Polycystic Ovarian Syndrome (PCOS), however, may have very high AMH levels due to the increased number of ovarian follicles. This hormone test may be useful tool in also identifying PCOS. AMH is presently considered the preferred gold-standard assessment test for predicting ovarian reserves.

- Another blood test is to measure for FSH (follicle-stimulating hormone), the hormone that stimulates the follicles to grow on the surface of the ovary. If FSH is high during the first half of the cycle, this may indicate that the ovaries are requiring more stimulation to grow follicles for ovulation. In effect the body has to work much harder in order to achieve ovulation; lower ovarian reserves are a likely cause.

# Chapter 5

# *Chemicals and Pollutants that can affect Fertility*

## We all have our own poisons ...

There are potentially hundreds of thousands of external influences that can affect the proper functioning of the body's reproductive processes, possibly leading to sub-fertility or infertility problems as well as hindering sperm, egg and foetal development. Approximately 800 new industrial agents are manufactured every month adding to the massive overload of current chemical pollutants that we are exposed to on daily basis. Exposure to environmental toxins such as heavy metal, drugs, poisons, radiation and electromagnetic fields, have all been linked to fertility problems. The following substances that will be discussed throughout this chapter have been extensively researched and studied in regards to their effects on reproductive health.

It goes without saying that avoidance or minimisation of exposure to these substances is vitally important to help maintain and protect your overall health and wellbeing. Having stated this we cannot live our lives in a sterile bubble in the hope of avoiding exposure to these chemicals, drugs and pollutants.

When you consider how external influences can impair our fertility, almost everything we come in contact with can have some form of impact. Many people work in particular careers and environments that expose them to these things. All I can say is, just be aware of your surroundings and take a commonsense approach to the avoidance of the toxins.

## Alcohol – 'A sobering thought'
Alcohol has long been known to have many harmful effects on the developing brain, nerves, heart cells, skeletal and urinary tract systems. It has been implicated in approximately 5 out of every 200 congenital malformations, particularly mental health retardation in children. Birth defects from alcohol abuse are, unfortunately, only identified after the birth of the child, so it is safer to abstain or restrict consumption to a very moderate intake. Alcohol may reduce absorption of folic acid and therefore affects the development of DNA.

Heavy alcohol consumption may reduce testicle size and decrease testosterone production leading to fewer mature sperm and more abnormalities. Alcohol can cause impotence, lowered libido, shrinkage or atrophy of the seminiferous tubules, increase sperm abnormalities and loss of sperm cells. Not to mention the detrimental effects on the cardiovascular and nervous system of the body. Continuing to consume high amounts of alcohol during pregnancy not only increases the chances for miscarriage, but can also cause foetal alcohol syndrome (FAS). FAS babies may have learning and behavioural problems and typically have small heads, a flat midface, small eye slits and a low nasal ridge.

Having mentioned all this about the evils of the drink, small amounts of alcoholic consumption such as quality red wine may have modest benefits by providing some antioxidant protection. As the old saying goes 'everything in moderation, know your limits and don't exceed them especially when it comes to alcohol consumption'.

### Cocaine
Cocaine or 'Crack' causes poor sperm development, damages sperm cells and can impair testosterone production. Cocaine use can cause constriction of the blood vessels, which can result in early miscarriage, pre-term delivery, and problems such as bleeding from the placenta. Menstrual irregularities can be caused by cocaine use, making pregnancy harder to occur. This drug can also have profound physical effects on the user and offspring. Babies born to regular cocaine-using mothers may also have withdrawal symptoms after birth.

### Anabolic drugs
Anabolics have been linked to testicular atrophy (shrinkage), and can lower levels of both follicle stimulating hormone (FSH) and luteinising hormone (LH), which lead to lowered sperm count levels. Testosterone-related steroids can shut down the pituitary gland and the testicles' production of hormones, though after stopping such drugs their effects are usually reversible. Anabolic steroids are normally used to enhance body and muscle mass and have been known to be abused among some body builders and sporting individuals who later have difficulties in conceiving children.

### Coffee and cola drinks – 'Calling all java junkies'
Caffeine can potentially impair blood flow and blood vessels leading to impotence. Studies have indicated that heavy coffee drinkers were shown to take an average 17% -30% longer to conceive than non-coffee drinkers. Cola drinks also contain high levels of both caffeine and phosphoric acid, which are linked to multiple health-deteriorating conditions. Several studies have shown that drinking several cups of coffee a day may increase the risk of developing endometriosis. Limiting coffee and tea intake to under 3 cups per day would be advisable, if not cut out completely.

Caffeine is a diuretic and can cause dehydration (water lose) which can lead to cellular damage (alters DNA repair and metabolism) and accelerated ageing; caffeine also leaches vital nutrients out of the body due to its high acidity; it can lower the production of the master steroid DHEA (dehydroepiandrosterone) and elevate stress hormones.

### Tobacco smoking – 'No ifs, ands or Butts'

There are at least 4,000 compounds in tobacco smoke and some of these compounds are known mutagens that cause genetic damage. Smoking can deplete Vitamin B12 levels, which can lead to a wide variety of problems including birth defects, miscarriages and sickly underweight babies. Smoking has been linked to diminishing sperm cell development causing poor sperm count motility. Nicotine can contribute to tubule obstructions and blockages such as varicoceles.

The cadmium content in smoke can accumulate in blockage and affect zinc status, which can cause additional obstruction due to seminal/plasma thickening.

Tobacco can decrease testosterone and lead to a decline in sperm quality and approximately 20 per cent decline in sperm motility. Various studies show the number of children born with a malformation rises directly with the number of cigarettes smoked by the father per day.

The ova (eggs) studied from smokers are prone to polyspermy, where two or more sperm enter an egg. The embryos that result are chromosomally abnormal and will not grow. The incidence of ectopic pregnancies has been observed to be two to four times higher in smokers in comparison to non-smokers. It may increase the risk of congenital abnormalities, miscarriage rate, cot death, meningococcal disease and lowered egg-binding capacity.

Smoking during pregnancy has been directly linked to multiple problems including: placenta abrupta (a placenta which separates prematurely); blood pressure fluctuations; placenta praevia (a placenta located dangerously low in the uterus); low birth rate; miscarriage; increased newborn deaths; SIDS (sudden infant death syndrome); behavioural and intellectual problems. Foetal heartbeat monitors that have been studied on pregnant women who smoke have shown that the baby's heart rate increased quickly and continued to rise abnormally for up to 15 minutes after the mother has had a cigarette.

The effects of smoking have also been shown to affect dopamine transport mechanisms; this can potentially link to child behavioural problems such as ADHD, impulsivity, opposition behaviour and addictive habits such as gambling (possibly when they're much older, hopefully not during childhood!).

The efficiency of the placenta and respiratory function was also notably affected. In the uterus of a pregnant woman, the blood vessels of the placenta contract with cigarette smoking; less nutrients and oxygen are available to the baby. Studies have shown that up to 500mg of Vitamin C levels can be depleted from smoking just one cigarette and that serum Vitamin C levels in smokers in comparison with non-smokers were 40 per cent lower in many cases.

(N.B. Refer to the nutrition section on Vitamin C to gain additional understanding of how detrimental this addictive habit is to your health).

To assist in throwing away the cigs (cancer sticks), associations such as QUIT are well worth contacting. Try some natural remedies such as sipping water with a teaspoon of bicarbonate soda (between meals), which helps to minimise withdrawal symptoms, as do nutrients such as tyrosine, which help with the stress and substitute for the nicotine fix when coming off the smokes.

### Marijuana – 'Don't be a dope'
Marijuana (also known as cannabis, grass, pot, hashish, ganja, wacky baccy, loco weed, and the devil's lettuce among its may other street names) may inhibit the ability of sperm to penetrate the ovum (egg); sperm quality and count decrease; abnormalities to eggs and sperm are high. The long-term use of marijuana has shown the reduction of testosterone levels and that luteinising hormone (LH) levels increased, therefore contributing to impotency and decreased libido.

Studies have indicated a higher percentage of female babies were conceived to heavier male marijuana smokers; this may be due to the female geno-type sperm that is believed to be more resilient than its male counterpart.

Marijuana is believed to have a direct negative effect on the menstrual cycle and ovulation. The regular user of marijuana has been shown to have shorter menstrual cycles, particularly the luteal phase or second half of the cycle. This can result in changes to the ability of a fertilised egg to implant in the uterus wall. The active compound in marijuana is *Tetrahydrocannabinol (THC),* which has a similar structure to hormones found in the adrenal gland. THC has been shown to accumulate in the ovaries and testes contributing to infertility, miscarriage, anovulation and weakened immune function. Offspring that survive are at greater risk of chromosomal and behavioural problems.

### Heroin – 'Playing Russian roulette'
Heroin can cause atrophy (shrinkage) of the testes and reduces testosterone production causing decreased fertility and possible stillbirths.

Other narcotic-type drugs that also include Methadone can possibly inhibit the brain hormone dopamine, which can increase the production of the hormone prolactin. This hormone can greatly affect both male and female fertility and disturbs the ovulation process.

The use of these drugs can have major effects on your general wellbeing causing increased infection risk, poor nutrition utilisation and excessive weight loss. All can indirectly affect reproductive capacity. Substitution drugs that are used to assist withdrawal from heroin include Methadone and Naltraxone to help flush the more addictive drug out of the body and reduce the 'cold turkey' symptoms and desire to resume taking heroin.

### Anaesthetic
Anaesthetic has been found to lower sperm count and may increase potential congenital abnormalities and is linked to miscarriages.

### Methylated chlorine
Methylated chlorine is used to extract caffeine from coffee and is a solvent in paint strippers. It may contribute to lowered sperm count and testicle atrophy.

### Dimethyl formamide
Dimethyl formamide has been linked to testicular cancer. It is used in the manufacture of pesticides, drugs, paints, artificial fibres and leather dyes.

### Phenol
Phenol is used as a food preservative, disinfectant, pesticide and is in some medications. The manufacturing industries also use phenol in cosmetics, dyes, paints and perfume, and in the lining of tin cans. Phenols are among the most common substances that cause allergic reactions.

### Phthalate
Phthalate is used in many day-to-day household items including: perfume; cosmetics; shampoo; nail polish; hand lotion; paint; vinyl flooring; plastic; teething rings; dummies (soothers); and food wrappings. This chemical has been shown to be toxic to the reproductive system.

Reports have claimed that even some types of female perfumes may affect the male sperm count. These substances have been found to be disrupters of the endocrine, nervous and immune systems as well.

### Paint fumes
A condition known as 'painter's syndrome' involving professional painters has been shown to have higher than normal sperm abnormalities and poor sperm numbers.

### Vinyl chlorine
Vinyl chlorine has been linked to higher neural tubal defects and miscarriage in babies from fathers exposed to this chemical. Correct nutritional status is necessary to detoxify this substance from the body. Vinyl chlorine can lead to other chemical intolerances. It may also cause problems of impotence and declining libido. It is commonly used in plastic goods.

### Carbon Disulfide, Dimethyl Sulphate, Boron, Ethylene Oxide and Bromide (EBD)
These chemicals may cause sperm abnormalities, impotence and loss of libido. Commonly used by electricians, fumigation agents, and leaded petrol manufacturing, clothing and textile industries.

### Organo chlorines; Dichlorodiphenyltrichloroethane (DDT)

DDT is one of the best known and most controversial of all pesticides. These substances have an action of mimicking oestrogens. It has been linked to causing damage to the immune and endocrine systems, as well as affecting DNA (Deoxyribonucleic Acid). Many health-related conditions have been associated with this substance such as cancer, convulsions, liver disease, and muscle disease, nausea and memory loss.

### Organo Phosphates: Diethylstibestrol (DES)

DES has been particularly indicated in affecting the embryo (in utero) due to exposure via the mother. It has been shown to be especially detrimental to the male reproductive system. These chemicals are linked to a wide range of symptoms and have suppressive activity on the immune and neuropsychological functions.

### Various steroids and antihistamines

Steroids and anti-histamines used on a regular basis can cause shrinkage of the mucosa and fine blood vessels. This action will reduce the production of mucus, therefore leading to the drying up of testicular, ovarian and vaginal secretions, which can prevent the numerous hormones and enzymes from reaching their target glands.

When the body is under stress it produces steroid hormones called glycosteroids, in much larger than normal quantities. The hormones are necessary to suppress the inflammatory reactions within the body.

Synthetically manufactured versions of these hormones are medically prescribed in conditions such as asthma and arthritis to reduce the symptoms of pain and allergy reactions. Ongoing use of these synthetically introduced medications may interfere and suppress the body' own glandular regulation of these responses. This can affect the pituitary activity in sending the correct chemical messages to the reproductive system, therefore, leading to potential fertility problems.


## Heavy Metal Toxicity that can affect fertility

### Heavy metal – 'Leave it to the head bangers'!

### Aluminium (Al)

Aluminium can be found in products such as aluminium cans; antacids; anti-diarrhoea medications; anti-perspirants; baking powder; buffered analgesics; aluminium cooking ware; cigarette filters; fabric softeners; foil wrapping; food additives; some milk substitutes; nasal sprays; softened water; tea (from aluminium tea pots); table salt; 'tetra' or 'popper' packs; some aspirin compounds; vaccines; toothpaste; and vaginal douches.

The effects of aluminium on the body can interfere with the metabolism of nutrients such as calcium, vitamin D, fluoride and phosphorus, which will contribute to mineral loss or leaching for the bones. Aluminium has also been linked to causing fatigue, gastrointestinal dysfunction, skin conditions, and lung and kidney problems. This heavy metal also can alter iron, zinc and copper metabolism; it can bind to DNA and displace magnesium and malic acid.

Aluminium can also interfere with the transport of other nutrients such as choline, which is needed by the nervous system to make acetylcholine which has shown to be low in neurological conditions such as Alzheimer's disease. This heavy metal tends to accumulate is tissue such as the brain, liver, lungs, and thyroid. Due to its wide effects on various nutrients status throughout the body, aluminium can indirectly cause problems with reproduction function.

### Arsenic (As)
Arsenic may be found in products such as some cereals; breads; drinking water; fish; meats; and pesticides. It has also been used in rat and insect poisons and in the production of beer, table salt, glass, pottery, and timber preservatives. This heavy metal can increase bleeding time and alter methionine metabolism in the body. Toxicity signs may include flu-like aches and pains; headaches; muscle spasms; and skin problems; gastric upsets; and fatigue.

### Cadmium (Cd)
Cadmium can be present in air pollution; cigarette smoke; contaminated seafood; soft water; pesticides; phosphate fertilisers; galvanised pipes; rubber tyres; solders; oysters; and urban sewerage sludge. It is also used in the manufacturing of some paints, batteries, and electrical appliances.

Excessive absorption of cadmium is caused by deficiencies in nutrients such as Vitamin D, copper, iron, calcium, zinc. Cadmium impairs calcium and phosphorus balance in the body and can compete with zinc for binding sites in various enzymes and proteins. This heavy metal may accumulate in organs such as the brain, liver and placenta and is linked to disruption of foetal development and growth that may lead to congenital abnormalities and miscarriages.

### Lead (Pb)
Lead toxicity has been reported to affect sperm counts and motility and increase the incidence of sperm abnormality. Lead is a neurotoxin that can cause damage to brain and nervous system. Long-term exposure to lead has been linked to conditions such as gout; fatigue; high blood pressure; dyslexia; mental retardation; renal dysfunction; epilepsy; convulsions; digestive upsets; delinquency and anti-social behaviour; learning problems; lowered IQ levels; and poor hand-eye co-ordination.

High lead levels in either partner have been shown to be a contributing factor to birth congenital abnormalities, miscarriages and stillbirths. Women who were reported to have excessive lead levels in the body had a higher incidence of antibodies against their partner's sperm and their cervical mucus was also more *hostile*; these conditions were greatly improved when the lead burden was decreased.

Studies have shown that the lead burden on the body is up to one thousand times higher in the average person than it was back before the industrial era. Over the years several products that had a high lead content, including many paints, have been banned, but there may be still exposure to these old products particularly when doing building or home renovations on older properties that were built prior to the 1960s. Lead toxicity can severely affect your body's haemoglobin formation as lead can cause iron deficiencies.

One good thing that has come of the research into lead is that lead-based petrols are not as widely available as they use to be, though even with all the damning evidence against the use of lead, it is still widely used in many products and industries that may include: lead smelters; coal burning; metal polishes; lead solder in the plumbing industry; petroleum products; batteries; lead water piping; some inks; black hair dyes; some ceramic ware; and pesticides. The regular intake of cigarette smoke, coffee, and alcohol have shown elevated blood levels of lead.

### Mercury (Hg)

Mercury has been shown to accumulate in the pituitary gland; any disruption of its usual function will affect our endocrine system, therefore contributing to reproductive dysfunction and possible infertility. Exposure to mercury (particularly in vapour form) may also cause long-term problems with sperm motility and loss of libido. A character in the story of *Alice in Wonderland* is the Mad Hatter. The Mad Hatter's madness may have been caused by the mercury that was once largely used in the millinery industry to line the hats, hence the phrase 'mad as a hatter'.

Mercury toxicity can contribute to miscarriage, birth defects and nerve damage. This heavy metal can easily pass through the placenta and into the foetal blood supply. Some of the signs and symptoms of mercury toxicity may include: Chronic fatigue; depression; mood swings; loss of memory and coordination; joint aches; skin rashes; hair loss; insomnia; nervousness; speech problems; and excessive salivation. Mercury can interfere with metabolism of selenium and zinc and can induce hypothyroidism. The heavy metals mercury, cadmium and lead all have the ability the concentrate in the placenta and cause serious damage to foetal development.

Avoid consumption of large fish that are high on the food chain, e.g. swordfish, blue fin tuna, shark (flake), deep sea perch, orange roughie etc (there's something fishy about the fish)! Identify the source of this fish and be wary of fish caught in estuaries. Smaller fish at the lower end of the food chain may be less likely to yield high heavy metal toxicity. Other areas that increase your exposure to mercury may include: some body talc powders; cosmetics; fabric softeners; dental amalgam fillings; incineration of industrial waste; cement and chlorine production. Fungicides and insecticides can also be sources.

### Nickel

Nickel is known to influence the production of the hormones prolactin, adrenaline, noradrenaline, and aldosterone. Nickel can bind to chromosomes and ion channels therefore potentiating oxidative damage of tissue. Nickel can antagonise the essential nutrients such as calcium, iron, magnesium and zinc. Nickel excess can contribute to poor growth rate, dermatitis, asthma, and altered blood pressure. It can also weaken immune function and affects glucose regulation. Foods that may contain nickel include oatmeal, dried beans, peas, nuts and chocolate.

## Drugs that can affect fertility

When you are undergoing certain treatments for various ailments, it may not be the disease that could be impacting on your capacity to conceive but the actual treatment itself. Consult with your doctor and go through your medicine cabinet to check out what medication could be a potential problem. Even common medications used to treat everything from acne to ulcers can contribute to fertility issues for both you and your partner.

*Disclaimer:* There are potentially hundreds of medications on the market that could affect the health of the reproductive functions in some negative way or another. It should not be assumed that the medications and drugs named in the relevant sections of this book will actually cause any or all of the problems mentioned. They have been included for example purposes only.

Listed below are just some of the many drugs to keep a look out for:

### Antibiotics

Certain antibiotics can lessen the effect of the contraceptive pill; other medications can influence hormone production and throw ovulation out of rhythm.

Some antibiotics may alter cervical mucus patterns, imbalance intestinal and vaginal flora contributing to thrush (Candida excess) and leave your body more vulnerable to urinary tract infection. Some antibiotics can also adulterate blood results of important nutrients such as folic acid and vitamin B12. High doses of various antibiotics may also affect sperm development and motility.

Medications may include: Tetracyclines, Gentamicin and Erythromycin.

### Antacids

Antacid medications have been linked to lowering libido, impotency, imbalancing intestinal flora and therefore, leading to conditions such as thrush, affecting the absorption of nutrients such as iron, and is reported to contribute to a condition known as gynecomastia (when the breasts are enlarged uni- or bi-laterally in men and women). By excessively lowering the alkalinity (Ph) of the body it can affect the normal health of the sperm and other necessary biochemical reactions that need to take place. The sperm health and survival is best in a relatively neutral environment of a Ph 7.2 to 7.8 - alkalinity. The sperm doesn't like fluctuations very much outside this range.

Medications may include: Cimetidine in Tagament, Losec, Tazac, Zantant and Zotone.

### Analgesics
Analgesics may: inhibit spermatogenesis; reduce serum testosterone; lower libido; cause testicular atrophy; affect ejaculation ability; contribute to gynecomastia; and generally give organs such as the liver a hard time. Drugs may include Codeine phosphate, Morphine and Pethidine.

### Anti-depressants
Some types of anti-depressant medications have been reported to potentially increase the risk of birth defects. These medications have been linked to: causing impotency; lowering libido levels; disrupting menstrual cycles; temporarily suppressing fertility; inhibiting ejaculation; and have caused swelling of the testicles.

Some types of antidepressant medications have been shown to excessively elevate prolactin hormone production.

Drugs may include: Monoamine oxidase (MAO); Phenelzine (Nardil); Tranylcypromine; Typtonal; Allegron; Aropax; Cipramil; Efexor; Luvox; Zoloft; and Prozac. Some anti-anxiety medications such as alprazolam (Zanac) and diazepam (Valium) may also cause similar problems.

### Cold and Flu Medications (including anti-histamines)
Many are used to dry up over-active mucous membranes, though their effects may not necessarily limit their action to the site for which they were intended, such as the nose and throat. This type of medicine can occasionally cause thickening and/or drying up cervical mucus, which will greatly hinder the sperm's ability to swim its way to the egg. Expectorant medications on the other hand can possibly assist the sperm's progression by thinning out the cervical mucus.

Anti-histamines can also contribute to ejaculation problems in men and orgasm problems in women, as well as lowering libido, affecting urination, causing gynecomastia, and actually weakening the body's natural immune function. Anti-histamines may include Dilosyn.

### Anti-convulsants
Some medications have been reported to contribute to Peyronie's disease, a condition where the tissue of the penis develops fibrous thickening inhibiting full erection and causing pain. Anti-convulsants may also increase prolactin levels that can be a factor of gynecomastia. Atrophy of seminal tissue has also been examined.
Medications may include: Epilim and Tegretol.

### Anti-inflammatory drugs (non-steroidal)

Anti-inflammatory drugs can potentially hide signs of impotency, infection, gynecomastia, prostrate disorders. They can also cause internal bleeding and adversely affect sperm development. The medication Sulphasalazine, used widely for conditions such as inflammatory bowel diseases (Crohn's disease and ulcerative colitis), has been shown to particularly affect current sperm development.

Other anti-inflammatory medications may include: Celebrix, Orudis, and Vioxx. Prednisone- based drugs should be used with care as they also have many known side-effects.

### Anti-hypertensives

High blood pressure medications may cause problems with sperm malformation, lower libido, and contribute to impotence and gynecomastia. Potassium-sparing diuretics that contain spironolactone (Aldactone) have been shown to disrupt the woman's menstrual cycle.

Other types of antihypertensives such as beta-blockers have been identified to lower the energy-producing enzyme Co Q 10 (which is ironically needed for the proper cardio-vascular function), and may hinder sperm motility.

Calcium-channel blockers may also cause the sperm to be sluggish, diminishing their capacity to penetrate and fertilise the egg. Sperm are reliant upon calcium for their motility. Calcium-blockers control the flow of calcium between cells; this can render a man's sperm immobile.

Alpha blockers can lead to problems of retrograde ejaculation. Some also can excessively elevate prolactin production.

Medications may include: Avapro, Capoten, Captopril, Catapres, Cardura, Isoptin, Minipress, Monopril, Norvasc, Renitec, and Zestril.

### Anti-Asthmatic Drugs

Medications such as bronchospasm relaxants may contribute to retrograde ejaculation by relaxing sphincter valves, and if they are steroid based, can cause atrophy (shrinkage) of the testes. Sperm development may also be retarded as some of these medications also affect the balance of the hypothalamic-pituitary-adrenal axis (which is involved with such actions as natural cortisone production, a fair percentage of sex hormones and stress response hormone). This can also cause irregular menstrual cycles dependent on the drug type used.

### Anti-cholesterol Drugs

Drugs that lower body lipid levels may contribute to diminished libido, impotence, and gynecomastia. The body needed cholesterol the manufacture hormones, enzymes and is necessary to cell membrane integrity.
Medications may include: Lipex and Zocor.

### Anti-Gout Medications
Some of the drugs used to control gout contain colchicine, which has been reported to disrupt the genes and sperm. It can damage the DNA and chromosomes therefore affecting the fertilisation of the egg.

Medications may include: Colgout and allopurinol-based drugs such as Zyloprim, which may cause gynecomastia, impotence and infertility.

### Muscle relaxants
Muscle relaxants may contribute to erectile problems, cause impotence and affect the function of ejaculation and urination.

Medications may include: Dantrium and Lioresal.

### Pain-relieving Medications
Some forms of pain-killer drugs that contain Ibuprofen have been known to disrupt ovulation, if used on a regular basis. Others may also cause blood thinning that can potentially lead to haemorrhage problems and can affect sperm count levels and contribute to impotence. Consult with your doctor. Some may recommend that acetaminophen-based medications such as Paracetamol may be safer to use if they are required to be taken.

Medication containing Ibuprofen may include: Advil and Nurofen.

### Roacccutane
Is used to treat severe acne conditions and contains a synthetic form of retinol A. This medication has been linked to many undesirable side-effects such as birth defects including mental retardation. If you are considering trying to have children in the future, please consult with your skin specialist to find a safer alternative; there are many useful natural remedies that can also help.

### Weight Loss Medication
May effect sperm development and ovulation due to avitaminosis nutrient deficiency and lead to other problems such as diminished libido and impotence. If your body weight is outside the current body mass index range, it can cause hormone and fertility problems.

### Ulcer Medications
Some of these drugs work by suppressing digestive enzyme output, which can lead to malabsorption of vital nutrients if used over long periods of time. Cimetidine which is the active compound in drugs such as Tagamet and H2 blockers can impede erections and slow sperm production down.

# Chapter 6

# *Clinical Nutrition*

**'Let thy food be thy medicine and thy medicine be thy food'**
*Hippocrates (460-377B.C)*

The use of diet as a therapy service is the foundation of Natural Medicine. There is an ever-increasing body of knowledge and scientific validation that supports the use of whole foods and nutritional supplementation in the maintenance of health and treatment of disease.

The body is a complex organism that has the ability to heal itself, if only you listen to it and respond with proper nourishment and care. In spite of all the abuse our bodies endure – whether through exposure to environmental toxins, poor nutrition, cigarette smoking, alcohol consumption, or inactivity – they still usually serve us well for many years before signs of illness may start to appear. Even then, with a little help, they respond and continue to function.

The human body is the greatest machine on earth. Nerve signals travel through muscles at speeds as fast as 200 miles per hour. The brain puts out enough electric power to light a 20-watt light bulb. If your leg muscles moved as fast as your eye muscles, you could walk over fifty miles in one day. According to scientists, bone is among the strongest building materials known to mankind; it can withstand nearly as much stretching and bending stress as, and more compression stress than, steel-reinforced concrete can tolerate.

Think of your body as being composed of millions of tiny little engines. Some of these engines work in unison; some work independently. All are on call twenty-four hours a day. In order for the engines to work properly, they require specific fuels. If the type of fuel given is the wrong blend, the engine will not perform its maximum capacity. If the fuel is of a poor grade, the engine may sputter, hesitate, and lose power. If the engine is given no fuel at all, it will stop.

The fuel we give our bodies' engines comes directly from the things we consume. The foods we eat contain nutrients. These nutrients come in the form of vitamins, minerals, enzymes, water, amino acids, carbohydrates, and lipids. It is these nutrients that sustain life by providing us with the basic materials our bodies need to carry on their daily functions.

Individual nutrients differ in form and function, and in the amount needed by the body; however, they are all vital to our health. The actions that involve nutrients take place on microscopic levels, and the specific processes differ greatly. Nutrients have different specific functions; their common function is to keep us going.

Research has shown that each part of the body contains high concentrations of certain nutrients. A deficiency of those nutrients will cause the body part to malfunction and eventually break down – and, like dominos, other body parts will follow. To keep this from happening, we need a proper diet and appropriate nutritional supplements. Brain function, memory, skin elasticity, eyesight, energy, the ratio of lean to fat tissue in the body, and overall health are all indications of how well the body is functioning. With the help of the proper nutrients, exercise, and a balanced diet, we can slow the aging process and greatly improve our chances for a healthier and pain-free – and possibly longer – life.

If we do not give ourselves the proper nutrients, we can impair the body's normal functions causing ourselves great harm. Even if we show no sign of illness, we may not necessarily be healthy. It simply may be that we are not yet exhibiting any overt symptoms of illness. One problem most of us have is that we do not get the nutrients we need from our diets because most of the foods we consume are cooked and/or processed. Cooking at high temperatures and processing destroy vital nutrients and enzymes the body needs to function properly. The organic raw foods that supply these elements are largely missing from today's diet.

'EAT TO LIVE, NOT LIVE TO EAT'! As the ole saying goes, 'you are what you eat', but in actual fact 'you are what you absorb and assimilate'.

The past decade has brought to light much new knowledge about nutrition and its effects on the body, and the role it plays in disease. Phytochemicals, also known as phytonutrients, are one example of the results of this research. These are compounds present in plants that make the plant biologically active. They are not nutrients in the classic sense, but they are what determine a plant's colour, flavour, and ability to resist disease. Researchers have identified literally thousands of phytochemicals and also have developed the technology to extract these chemical compounds and concentrate them into pills, powders, and capsules. These are called nutraceuticals – one of the newer types of modern dietary supplements.

Studies by industries such as the CSIRO have identified that due to inappropriate farming methods since colonising Australia, much of the quality top soils in many areas of the continent have lost massive amounts of vital mineral contents (such as zinc and selenium), approximately 50 – 80 per cent. Therefore, the need for extra quality nutritional supplementation is very essential in these modern times.

Your body's nutritional needs are as unique to you as your appearance is. The first essential step toward wellness, therefore, is to be sure you are getting the correct amounts of the proper nutrients. By understanding the principles of holistic nutrition and knowing what nutrients you need, you can improve the state of your health, ward off disease, and maintain a harmonious balance in the way nature intended. All individuals should take an active part in the maintenance of their health in the treatment of their disorders with the guidance of a health care professional.

The more we take it upon ourselves to learn about nutrition, the better prepared we will be to take that active role. The human body is an amazing machine; approximately 99 per cent of our bodies' cells renew every year. The nutrients that we choose to fuel this machine of ours will have tremendous bearing on the type of body model we will have each year.

An analogy of this may be an example of the type of car you wish to drive. If want an old clunker standard sedan then feed your body poorly, but if you want a top-of-the-line sports model (within reason) then your nutrient requirement needs much more specific attention.

There are various causes and explanations for infertility. One if the most basic is an overall deficiency in nutrients that adversely affects the reproductive system. For instance, the endocrine glands, which secrete and control hormones, depend on a correct supply of nutrients, especially trace minerals. Nutritional deficiencies and harmful chemicals can harm the eggs and sperm even before conception occurs.

Nature teaches us many lessons in the area of nutrition and fertility. For example, in order for a plant seed to grow, the soil needs to be rich in all the nutrients necessary for the plants growth. Mineral deficient soils produce either no crops or below par crops. By adding essential minerals to barren soil, growers can make the soil fertile again. The same analogy is also true for animals.

**Water**

Water is fundamental to all life on earth and it is the universal solvent medium in which all other nutrients are found. Water is the most abundant and important substance on earth and in the human body. It is composed of only three simple molecules, two hydrogen and one oxygen molecule. Our bodies are at least 60 per cent water. It is primarily a component of all the bodily fluids – blood, lymph, digestive juices, urine, tears, and sweat. Water is involved in almost every bodily function. Water is needed to carry the mineral salts (electrolytes) that help to convey electrical currents in the body. Bodily requirements for water vary greatly between individuals; your personal activity level, climate in which you live, your body weight and sex all influence our specific need for water.

## Proteins

Protein is an essential part of nutrition, second only to water in the body's physical composition. Protein makes up about 20 per cent of our body weight and is a primary component of our muscles, hair, nails, skin, eyes, and intestinal organs, especially the heart muscle and brain. Protein molecules are composed of carbon, oxygen, hydrogen, and nitrogen, while fats and carbohydrates are made up of carbon, oxygen, and hydrogen only. All three macronutrients are organic components that are part of living tissue of plants and animals.

Our immune system's defence requires protein, especially for the formation of antibodies that help to fight infection. Haemoglobin, our oxygen carrier, and red blood cells are proteins. Many hormones that regulate our metabolism, such as thyroxine and insulin, also require protein. Biochemical deficiency can occur when there is a lack of enzymes, the protein molecules that catalyse chemical reaction in the body.

Protein is needed for growth and for the maintenance of body tissues. For women, protein intake up to 1-2 years before conception and in the first and last trimester of pregnancy is positively correlated with birth weight, body length, skeletal and organ size of newborns. A low protein diet will also lead to poorer quality and fewer ova (eggs) available for fertilisation. Vegans who eat no animal or dairy products may be low in primary protein intake in their diet. Food combining by adding more nuts and pulses can help to prevent protein deficiency problems.

The body's utilisation of protein is essential to reproductive health. Protein is necessary for the formation of healthy sperm and is involved in the many intricate processes of fertilisation and the development of the embryo. The balance of protein in the body is also important for maintaining the correct acid/alkaline environment; imbalances can lead to a hostile system that can be unfavourable to sperm viability.

After conception has occurred, protein intake should increase by approximately 20 per cent to cater for the increased demands of this major nutrient during the pregnancy. Adequate protein yielding foods may include: fish; free-range eggs; low-fat dairy products; yoghurt; sprouted grains; meat; and nuts. Individuals who choose or prefer a vegetarian or vegan lifestyle can run into some risk factors when trying to conceive, as not all plant-based foods are a complete protein source and certain individual amino acids may be deficient. Correct food combining is needed to create 'primary' proteins.

Proteins are complex molecules comprised of a combination of 22 naturally occurring amino acids (the building-blocks of proteins). Essential amino acids are those our body cannot synthesise on their own and which we must acquire through our diet. The following is a summary of the various types of individual amino acids and their relevant groups.

**Essential**: isoleucine; leucine; lysine; methionine; phenylalanine; threonine; tryptophan; and valine.

**Semi Essential**: arginine; and histidine.

**Nonessential**: alanine; aspartic acid (asparagine); cysteine; glutamic acid (glutamine); glycine; homocysteine; hydroxylysine; hydroxyproline; proline; serine; and tyrosine.

**Others**: These amino acids are not found in body tissues, but contribute to human metabolism: carnitine; citrulline; gamma-aminobutyric acid (gaba); glutathione (a tripeptide); ornithine; and taurine.

**Suggested sources of protein**: White meat chicken (preferably free range, organic feed) with removed skin; white meat turkey with removed skin; turkey leg with removed skin; veal; lean beef; tuna (if pre-packed only in water); boiled/baked fish; small amount of eggs; dry beans; lentils (reduced amount of peas and soybeans); and whey protein supplements.

*Protein: should comprise **12 to 20 per cent** of your recommended daily allowance; 45 – 60 grams or about 200 calories per day.*

## Carbohydrates

Carbohydrates are probably the most important of the three classes of foods since they are our main source of energy and constitute approximately 50-60 per cent of the diet. Carbohydrates are produced by photosynthesis in plants. They can be easily converted to glucose, the energy fuel for the body's cells and each gram of carbohydrate releases four calories, units of heat or energy, for the body.

Carbohydrates are needed to regulate protein and fat metabolism. Many carbohydrate foods are also high in fibre, and fibre is important in the bulking of the stool, which aids in regular elimination of waste materials through the colon.

There are three principal carbohydrates in foods and are classified according to their structure. First are the sugars, both *monosaccharides* (simple sugars), glucose, fructose, and galactose such as those found in honey and fruit, and *oligosaccharides* (multiple sugars), lactose, sucrose, and maltose, such as table sugar and malt sugar, which both happen to be disaccharides (two-sugar molecules).

Then there are the *starches*, or *complex carbohydrates* (polysaccharides – are composed of long chains of glucose molecules), found primarily in vegetables such as carrots, potatoes, and whole grains such as rice and corn. Starches require the enzyme amylase to be broken down into simple sugars for digestion, absorption and utilisation.

Finally, there is fibre, mainly cellulose and hemicellulose, the indigestible roughage found in unprocessed, carbohydrate-containing foods. Some of these forms of fibre may include: psyllium seed husks; pectin; agar; alginate; carrageen; guar gum; slippery elm; and chitosan.

**Suggested sources of complex carbohydrates**: whole-grain pasta; potato (medium sized – baked); rice; oatmeal; cereal (dry); oat, wheat or bran muffins (average one per daily serve); whole-wheat bread (one slice averages one serve per day. If prone to wheat allergies – millet, buckwheat and rye are other alternatives).

*Carbohydrate: should comprise* **45-55 per cent** *of your recommended daily allowance. The average calorie intake from carbohydrates is about 1,200 – 1,400 per day.*

## Fats, Lipids and Oils

Fats, or lipids, are primarily used by the body as a form of energy reserve and for insulation in the body. Fats can be burned from the body stores to make energy, particularly when fats are not sufficient in our diet. Fats are important in transporting other nutrients, such as Vitamins A, D, E, and K (the 'fat-soluble' vitamins). Fats are an essential component of the cell membranes, and internal fatty tissues protect the vital organs from trauma and temperature changes by providing padding and insulation. Fatty tissue, in fact, even helps to regulate body temperature.

Three essential fatty acids are needed biochemically by our bodies: linoleic acid (LA); arachidonic acid; and linolenic acid (LNA). Our dietary requirement for fats varies widely among individuals; the total calorie intake from fats in the diet may be close to the 20-25 per cent range. Persons suffering cardiovascular disease with elevated cholesterol, triglycerides or needing to go on a weight-loss programme may require a dietary range of 10-20 per cent for a time.

Fats are the most concentrated source of food energy, supplying nine calories per gram – more than double the calorie content of proteins and carbohydrates. Fats are commonly divided in to three distinct groups:

**Saturated fats:** are mainly found in animal products; meat; eggs; butter; cheeses; whole milk; and coconut oil.
**Mono-unsaturated fats:** include avocados; eggs; olives; olive oil; peanuts; almonds; hazelnuts; canola; sunflower; and safflower.
**Polyunsaturated fats:** are normally found in liquid form at room temperature and are in margarines; soy bean; fish; walnuts; brazil nuts; corn oils; and sun/safflower.

*Fat: should comprise* **20 – 30 per cent** *of your recommended daily allowance, 40 to 60 grams or 450 – 500 calories per day, primarily from unsaturated fat sources.*

# The Versatile Vitamins

Vitamins are essential to life. They contribute to good health by regulating metabolic processes and assisting biochemical processes that release energy from digested food. Vitamins function as coenzymes helping in a range of metabolic reactions within the body. They are, put simply, helpers in metabolism – essential to growth, vitality and health, and are helpful in digestion, elimination and resistance to disease. Deficiencies can lead to a variety of disorders and general health problems, according to which vitamin is lacking in the diet.

For many decades, orthodox medicine practitioners have played down and even denied the healing benefits contained in vitamins in the treatment and maintenance of good health. It is only in recent years that the use of vitamins in the prevention and treatment of disease is becoming more widely accepted within the medical profession.

Ideally, nutrients should be consumed in wholesome, raw, organically grown foods; due to such a general lack of nutrients in food supplies nowadays, additional supplementation should be a consideration. If we all lived in a pure and untampered-with environment, then modern nutritional supplements would not be necessary, but the sad reality is that our soils are generally poorly managed and the pollution levels are getting worse. There is much debate over the effectiveness of many of these supplements; having said that I still feel there is a place for additional supplementation when other nutrient sources are not ideal.

## Vitamin A (Retinyl palmitate)
Vitamin A is an anti-oxidant nutrient important in detoxification and is one of the fat-soluble vitamin groups. It enhances the metabolic efficiency of essential fatty acids and is required for the maintenance of mucous membranes throughout the body. Vitamin A is necessary for the health of cilia (tiny hair-like projections) inside the fallopian tubes. The cilia work in a wave-like current, which assist the ovum and sperm to travel through the fallopian tube.

Vitamin A is necessary for sperm production, conversion of cholesterol to the male hormone testosterone and the health of the testes. Vitamin A is also important for the proper metabolism of zinc. Vitamin A is essential to good eyesight, especially night vision. It is involved in the rod-and-cone perception of colour and light.

Vitamin A helps to maintain the health of the skin and aids in the repair and growth of new tissue such as epithelial cells of mucous membranes. This assists in protecting the body's immune resistance from unwanted pathogens and enhances proper antibody production. Vitamin A is also involved in the synthesis of steroid hormones (including oestrogen and androgens);

haemoglobin; hydrochloric acid; adrenal hormones; components of the myelin sheath; and the proper growth of bone and teeth require the nutrient.

During pregnancy Vitamin A is needed to help form the baby's teeth enamel, hair and the growth of the thyroid gland.

*Foods high in Vitamin A include:* Cod liver oil; most red, orange and green vegetables; capsicum; carrots; sweet potatoes; parsley; spinach; pumpkin; broccoli; apricots; rockmelon.

*Important note:* Vitamin A is an oil-soluble vitamin and is stored in the body. Dosages of Vitamin A are recommended to be monitored before and during pregnancy, as excessive intake has been linked to birth defects. However, the doses of Vitamin A found to cause foetal abnormalities were in the range of 25,000-500,000 IU (international units) per day. This dosage of Vitamin A is over 100 times higher than the amount provided in most nutritional supplements.

On the other hand Vitamin A deficiency has been linked to infertility, miscarriage and a number of abnormalities such as cleft palate and absence of eyes. Worldwide studies show a lowering of the incidence in birth defects when supplements were given containing levels of Vitamin A (up to 6,000 IU per day). Therefore, supplements containing Vitamin A should *not* be avoided as long as dosage is kept within respected parameters.

## Beta-carotene
Beta-carotene can be used as an alternative to Vitamin A as it can be converted in the body as it is required. It has been found that beta-carotene levels are significantly reduced in immuno-infertile men and that it is an essential nutrient for the normal ovarian function. There are more than 700 different carotenoids that naturally occur in fruit and vegetables, of which at least 50 are estimated to be metabolised by the human body.

Beta-carotene and many of the other carotenoids primarily functions as an anti-oxidant and free radical scavenger, therefore, making them protectors of the body's tissues that may help to prevent various cancers and degenerative ailments.

*Foods rich in carotenes are:* sweet potato; carrots; broccoli; spinach; apricots; pumpkins; rockmelons; pink grapefruits; tomatoes (lycopene); and red capsicum. Supplemental forms of Beta-carotene are commonly derived from *Dunaliella Salina* algae.

## B-Complex Vitamins
B-complex vitamins are the catalytic 'spark plugs' of our body. They function as co-enzymes to catalyse many biochemical reactions and work as a 'team' to restore natural body functions. B vitamins help provide energy by acting with

enzymes to convert carbohydrates to glucose and are also important in fat and protein metabolism.

B vitamins are all water soluble and are not stored very well in the body. Thus, they need to be replenished daily to support the many functions they carry out. Deficiencies of one or more B vitamins can occur fairly easily, especially during times of fasting, weight-loss, stress, or with diets that include substantial amounts of refined and processed food, white flour products, caffeine, oral contraceptive use, tobacco, sugar and alcohol.

### Vitamin B1 (Thiamine or thiamine pyrophosphate)
Thiamine helps a great many body functions, acting as a coenzyme thiamine pyrophosphate (TPP). Though not as directly linked to fertility or reproductive disorders as other nutrients its importance to the holistic function of the body warrants its inclusion. It has a key metabolic role in the cellular production of energy, mainly in glucose metabolism. Thiamine is also needed to metabolise ethanol, converting it to carbon dioxide and water. Vitamin B1 helps in the initial steps of fatty acid and sterol production, helping to convert carbohydrates to fat for storage.

The health of the nerves and nervous system relies on thiamine, possibly because of its role in the synthesis of RNA, DNA, ribose and acetylcholine (via the production of acetyl CoA, an important neurotransmitter). Thiamine is linked to learning capacity (mental functions) and to growth in children. It is needed for the muscle tone of the stomach, intestines, and heart. Vitamin B1 may have a preventative effect on the progression of atherosclerosis due to reducing the accumulation of fatty deposits in the arteries. Thiamine acts as a stabiliser of the appetite by improving the digestion and assimilation of ingested food.

Beriberi is the name of the disease caused by thiamine deficiency.

**Foods high in thiamine include**: whole grains; wheat embryo/germ/bran; brewer's yeast; brown rice; blackstrap molasses; legumes; nuts; egg yolk; fruits; and vegetables.

**Vitamin B1 recommended daily allowances (RDA)**: 1 to 5 milligrams (mg) adult. Therapeutic dosages = (SR): 5 to 150 mg. (adult).

**Note:** using single B vitamins (including folic acids and their group co-factors) individually at therapeutic dosages should always be accompanied with a multi-B-complex to prevent other deficiencies and/or imbalance of metabolic activity. Nowhere in nature does a single B vitamin exist independent from other vitamins of the B group. Therefore, common sense would suggest that if additional supplementation is required they should also be together.

### Vitamin B2 (Riboflavin)
Vitamin B2 deficiencies may contribute to irregular or stoppage of menstruation by altering oestrogen and progesterone levels. Vitamin B2 helps

to maintain normal skin, hair, and nail health. It is essential to cellular respiration and functions as a group of enzymes which helps in the breakdown and utilisation of carbohydrates, fats and proteins. Riboflavin also aids in the manufacture of glycogen (stored sugar) in the liver.

Vitamin B2 functions as a precursor or building block for two enzymes that are important in energy production. It is necessary for red blood cell formation, antibody production and healthy cell growth. Riboflavin also helps with the absorption of iron and Vitamin B6. Together with Vitamin A, it maintains and improves the mucous membranes in the digestive system.

**Foods high in Vitamin B2 are:** avocados; beans; peas; lima beans; almonds; currants; leafy greens; eggs; milk and dairy products; brewer's yeast; organ meats; sprouts; wholegrain cereals; oily fish; legumes; wheat germ; broccoli and almonds.

**Vitamin B2 RDA:** 1.5 to 2 mg. SR: 10 to 200 mg.

### Vitamin B3 (Niacin, Nicotinamide, & Nicotinic Acid)
Vitamin B3 is essential in all living things as Coenzyme 1 (nicotinamide adenine dinucleotide - NAD) and Coenzyme II (nicotinamide adenine dinucleotide phosphate - NADP), are involved in over 200 oxidation-reactions in the body. Vitamin B3 aids in the synthesis of steroidal hormones, lipids and hydrochloric acid (HCA).

The health and function of the nervous system requires adequate levels of Vitamin B3, as does proper cellular and tissue respiration and metabolism. The action of Vitamin B3 is enhanced by other B Vitamins and minerals. Therapeutically, it may also assist in energy production; blood sugar regulation; improving circulation; cholesterol reduction; blood vessel dilation; and membrane formation. All require the need for Vitamin B3.

Niacin supports the health of the skin, tongue, and digestive tract, and is important in the synthesis of sex hormones, oestrogen, progesterone and testosterone, as well as other corticosteroids.

**The best sources of Vitamin B3 are found in**: organ meats like liver; poultry; fish; yeast; dried beans; peas; wheat germ; avocado; dates; figs; and prunes. All contain good amounts of niacin.

**Vitamin B3 RDA:** 15 to 20 mg. SR: 100 – 3000 mg. NAD: 5 – 10 mg.

### Vitamin B5 (Pantothenic Acid)
The name pantothenic acid comes from the Greek word *pantos*, meaning 'everywhere', referring to its wide availability in foods. The main function of Vitamin B5 is in regards to its close inter-relationship with the adrenal gland that is necessary for the production of cortisone, steroids, and other hormones important for health maintenance.

Pantothenic acid as coenzyme A is closely involved in adrenal cortex function and has come to be known as the 'anti-stress' vitamin. Due to its role in adrenal health, Vitamin B5 is also important in the regulation of the stress and central nervous system response in the body. Pantothenic acid may also help to prevent signs of aging such as wrinkles as it is important to the health of the skin and neuromuscular reactions.

Energy production requires adequate Vitamin B5, as does the health of the intestinal tract and cellular structure growth. Cholesterol, ketones, antibodies, acetylcholine, porphyrins, myelin sheaths and fatty acids all require B5 for their synthesis. The health of the testicles also needs good concentrations of Vitamin B5.

Cellular metabolism of carbohydrates and fats to be released as energy require pantothenic acid. B5 is important in maintaining the health of the intestinal tract and it has protective capabilities against potential toxic effects of antibiotics and radiation.

***Foods high in Vitamin B5 include****:* Royal jelly (one of the highest sources); organ meats; chicken; cheese; brewer's and torula yeast; egg yolk; whole grains; beans; mushrooms; wheat germ; peanuts; and various vegetables – sweet potato; green peas; cauliflower; and avocados.

***Vitamin B5 RDA:*** 5 – 10 mg. SR: 20 – 500 mg

### Vitamin B6 (Pyridoxine)
In various research studies, women with pre-menstrual syndrome (PMS) as well as infertility were treated with Vitamin B6 for PMS (100mg-800mg per day) and had their fertility corrected as well.

Vitamin B6 has also shown to be as effective as medical drugs such as Bromocriptine, in lowering elevated prolactin without the potential side effects. Vitamin B6 has also proven to be an effective oestrogen and progesterone balancer.

The liver needs Vitamin B6 to convert excess fat, soluble oestrogen, into water-soluble form. If the body is deficient in adequate supplies of Vitamin B6, this will lead to a build-up of oestrogen in the system. The ovary responds by cutting down its production of progesterone, which can lead to chronic abortion and luteal phase defects.

Therefore Vitamin B6 supplementation would be useful in conditions of low progesterone production. Fluid retention and nausea (hyperemesis gravidarum) may be alleviated with adequate Vitamin B6 during pregnancy. A deficiency may be associated with a higher incidence of gestational diabetes. Vitamin B6 assists the proper absorption of nutrients such as zinc.

Vitamin B6 is needed for the synthesis, breakdown, and absorption of amino acids in the intestine. The balance of potassium and sodium require Vitamin B6, as does the normal functioning of the nervous system particularly the central nervous system (CNS), the muscular system, the integrity of the blood, the pituitary gland and energy creation.

**Vitamin B6 is high in foods such as**: chicken; cereal; brewer's yeast; blackstrap molasses; sunflower seeds; egg yolk; legumes; mackerel; tuna; salmon; lentils; buckwheat; peanuts; wheat germ; and walnuts.

**Vitamin B6 RDA:** 1.6mg -2.6mg. Therapeutic range (SR): 10mg-150mg. Do not exceed prolonged daily doses over 500mg.

### Folic Acid (Vitamin B9, Folate, Folacin, pteroylglutamic acid)

Folic acid is another of the key water-soluble B vitamin group. Its name comes from the Latin word *folium* meaning 'foliage', because folic acid is found in nature's leafy greens. The vitamin PABA, and glutamic acid are part of the structure of folic acid, it is actually a 'vitamin within a vitamin'.

Folic acid is one of the most important pre-conceptual nutrients; folic acid (folate) deficiency can contribute to infertility in many ways. Folic acid is involved in cell division and essential for DNA and RNA formation (compounds of genetic material required for all cellular growth, development, and reproduction). It prevents the breakage and mutation of chromosomes. Folate is the most commonly depleted nutrient during pregnancy.

It is considered to take 2 years to replenish folate stocks after pregnancy and because of this some researchers suggest a 2-year interval between birth spacing, unless a folate supplementation is given. Folic acid is important to take 3 months pre and post conception. Supplementation throughout the pregnancy may also help improve birth-weight and APGAR score at birth.

Folate deficiency is associated with neural tubal defects (NTDs) such as cleft palate/lip, spina bifida, limb deformities, omphalocele, atrial/ventricular septal defects and anencephaly in the newborn. Spina bifida is a condition where there is a split or divided spine and is usually associated with hydrocephalus (fluid on the brain). It is estimated that one in every 700 to 800 births in Australia alone has spina bifida. Anencephaly is a condition that means there is a complete absence or severe underdevelopment of the brain/skull that is fatal. It is estimated that anencephalus accounts for about 30 per cent of NTDs. Studies have shown that supplementation of periconceptional folic acid led to a 50-70 per cent reduction of NTDs.

When taking reasonable amounts of folic acid it is important to balance it with the appropriate amount of Vitamin B12, as this could potentially mask a neural tubal defect. Folic acid improves the health of the ovum and uterine environment. Any singular B group vitamin should really be accompanied with a B complex supplement to avoid any imbalance in nutritional status.

Folic acid is equally as important as Vitamin B12, in the synthesis of haemoglobin and the production of bone marrow and red blood cells. Folate is essential for both mental and emotional health and is involved in the bio-synthesis of neurotransmitters norepinephrine and serotonin. Folate has a stimulating effect on hydrochloric acid production, thus playing a role in increasing appetite and digestion. This nutrient also works with other nutrients (particularly Vitamin B12 and Vitamin C), in the synthesis of amino acids, serine, histamine, choline and in the breakdown and utilisation of proteins.

When folic acid is consumed, it is actively transported into the blood from the gastrointestinal tract, where it acts as a coenzyme for a multitude of functions and is converted to its active form, tetrahydrofolic acid (THFA), in the presence of niacin coenzyme (NADHP) and vitamin C. In the body, folic acid is found mainly as methyl folate, and Vitamin B12 is needed to convert it back to its active form THFA (same and trimethylglycine also work to help convert folic acid).

Extra folic acid is stored in the liver, enough for six to nine months of the vitamin for body use before deficiency symptoms might develop. Folic acid deficiency, however, may still be one of the most common vitamin deficiencies. With increased oestrogen, as in pregnancy or when taking birth control pills, folic acid supplementation helps to prevent deficiency symptoms. More is also required during lactation, which it also aids. Folic acid is often used when there are any menstrual problems.

The 'restless leg syndrome,' which is characterised by creeping, irritating sensations in the legs and occurs most commonly in late pregnancy, is often helped by increasing folic acid, as it may specifically be a deficiency problem. Absorption of natural food sources of folic acid is believed to be approximately 50 to 60 per cent, supplemental sources almost 100 per cent. Heating and processing of foods can destroy up 50 per cent of folic acid content.

Consumption of alcohol also interferes with folic acid absorption. Additional intake of folic acid is advisable at least one to two months prior to conception and during the first trimester of the pregnancy for maximum benefit as it is stored in the body for 6 to 9 months thereafter.

**Folic Acid is high in foods such as:** beans; eggs; green leafy vegetables; spinach; kale; beet greens; beets; chard; asparagus; broccoli; liver; kidney; brewer's yeast; corn; lima beans; green peas; sweet potato; artichokes; okra; parsnips; bean sprouts; lentils; mung beans; soy; whole wheat; milk; oranges; cantaloupes; pineapples; bananas; berries; and fresh wheat germ.

**Folic acid (RDA):** 400ug-500ug (0.4mg-0.5mg) by Australian standards. Therapeutic dosage (SR) may range between 1,000ug-5,000ug, Pregnant and nursing mothers - 800ug.

*Note:* Alcohol, smoking, antacids, aspirin, and contraceptive pill use can inhibit the bodies use of folate.

### Vitamin B12 (Cyanocobalamin)
Vitamin B12 deficiency or pernicious anaemia can lead to infertility in women and men and is reversible with Vitamin B12 supplementation (injections of Vitamin B12 may be required). Vitamin B12 is essential for ALL cells and is the only vitamin that contains essential mineral components.

Vitamins B6, B12 and folic acid combine to reduce elevated homocystine levels, which can cause miscarriage, among other conditions (hypertension, arteriosclerosis, and may prevent pre-eclampsia, toxaemia, and infarction of the placenta). Vitamin B12 is involved in cellular replication (vital for the synthesis of RNA and DNA). A deficiency of Vitamin B12 can lead to reduced sperm count and reduced sperm motility.

In one study, 27 per cent of men, who had sperm counts under 20 million/ml, were given 1,000mcg of Vitamin B12 per day. As a result, they were able to achieve a total count of in excess of 100 million/ml (25). Similar results have also been reported in other studies demonstrating sperm count and motility improvements.

Vitamin B12 is involved in methylation (a form of detoxification) reactions and is required for the synthesis of lipotropic agents (methionine, choline and serine) that protect and repair fatty livers. Vitamin B12 is essential for the development of healthy bone marrow and normal red blood cells. Cyanocobalamin is needed by the central and peripheral nervous systems for the formation and maintenance of the myelin sheath necessary for proper nerve message conduction. Vitamin B12 assists in the metabolism of fats, carbohydrates and proteins.

Vegetarian diets may be compromised by poor Vitamin B12 levels; therefore supplementation may be required to reverse this deficiency. The correct bacteria collected in the gut are also important for Vitamin B production. 'Experimental congenital malformation has been induced with 99 per cent accuracy in animals simply by withholding B Vitamins from their pre-conceptual diet'. (Encyclopaedia of Natural Medicine Vol.2 p.26)

**Vitamin B12 is high in foods such as:** brains; clams; egg yolk; herring; kidney; liver meat; milk; oysters; salmon; sardines; spirulina; and chicken.

**Vitamin B12 (RDA):** 12mg-50mg. Therapeutic ranges (SR) are 300ug-800ug pregnancy, and lactation 2.6ug. Sublingual liquid intake of Vitamin B12 is an effective way of up taking this nutrient if injections or other oral preparations are not available. Folic acid and Vitamin B12 work synergistically together and are usually found in supplementations together.

## Biotin (Vitamin H)

Biotin is a water-soluble sulphur containing Vitamin H, part of the B vitamin family of nutrients. The biotin enzyme participates in many reactions in the body, particularly in the metabolism of fats, proteins and carbohydrates. It also assists in the synthesis of fatty acids and amino acids and in their subsequent breakdown and usage.

It is essential for the introduction of carbon dioxide in the formation of purines, which are constituents of RNA and DNA. Biotin is important in the maintenance and manufacturing of glycogen, therefore required in the creation of energy and storage of energy from food.

The action and activity of insulin is enhanced by biotin. It aids in the synthesis of haemoglobin, antibodies, pancreatic amylase, and Vitamin B3. Capillary walls, cholesterol, skin, hair and the endocrine system all require biotin with other nutrients for their proper function.

Magnesium and phosphorus are essential to convert biotin to its active form. Although biotin is present in the diet, the main source of biotin used by the body comes from the bacteria flora of the digestive system where it is synthesised if the flora is in a healthy state.

*Food sources of Biotin include:* egg yolk; cauliflower; yeast; soy beans; unpolished rice; mushrooms; legumes; and nuts.

*Biotin RDA:* 300 ug. SR: 0.5 to 15 mg.


## Choline

Choline is one of the 'lipotropic' B vitamins that help in the utilisation of fats in the body. Choline as phosphatidylcholine is a base of soy lecithin and thereby helps in the emulsification of fats, triglycerides and cholesterol by helping form smaller fat globules in the blood and aiding the transport of fat through the small vasculature and in and out of the cells. Choline is combined with fatty acids glycerol and phosphate to make lecithin.

Choline is an integral part of the neurotransmitter acetylcholine. Its availability preserves the integrity of the electrical transmission across the gaps between nerves, and this helps the flow of electrical energy within the nervous system. It is also important to the health of the myelin sheaths covering the nerve fibres. Choline helps the liver and gallbladder function and is vital to brain chemistry, as it seems to aid thinking capacity and memory. Choline also helps in the absorption of the fat soluble vitamins.

*Choline RDA:* (male) 550mg. (female) 425 mg. Pregnancy: 450 mg. Lactation: 550 mg. SR: 1 to 3.5 Grams (gm).

## Inositol

Inositol is a part of the B vitamin complex and is manufactured from glucose; it is also closely associated with choline.

Like choline, inositol (as phosphatidylinositol) is also found in lecithin. It primarily functions in cell membrane structures as part of the phospholipids. Inositol is especially important for the cells of the brain, bone marrow, eye tissue, myelin sheath, intestines, and prostate health and may assist with hair growth. Inositol may help to reduce blood cholesterol and aid in the metabolism of fats.

Large quantities are found in the cerebral spinal fluid, and lymph. It also stimulates the intestinal production (flora) of biotin.

***Food containing inositol include:*** whole grains; citrus fruits; brewer's yeast; organ meat; seeds; beans; nuts; lecithin; molasses; milk; soy; oatmeal; and bacterial synthesis in gut.

***Inositol RDA:*** 500 – 1000 mg. SR: 750 – 13,000 mg.


## Para-Aminobenzoic Acid (PABA)

PABA is one of the basic constituents of folate and helps in the assimilation of pantothenic acid (Vitamin B5 and Vitamin B12). PABA can be converted into folate by intestinal bacteria. Para-aminobenzoic-acid stimulates the pituitary gland and can restore fertility to some women who have trouble conceiving. It is also said to be beneficial in the prevention of potential premature births.

PABA also acts as a coenzyme for the breakdown and utilisation of proteins. It plays a role in the formation of red blood cells and is important for health and pigmentation of the skin and hair, (along with Vitamin A, B5, B9, biotin, lecithin and zinc), while also acting as a sunscreen. PABA is involved in the stimulation of the pituitary gland and therefore can assist with oestrogen production.

PABA may also have a protective effect against second-hand smoke, ozone, air pollutants and it can reduce inflammation and enhance flexibility in arthritis. PABA plays its part in helping to fight fatigue and is useful in treating other conditions such as scleroderma, Peyronie's diseases, skin discolouration (vitiligo), thyroiditis and menopausal symptoms. High levels of stress and antibiotics can hinder PABA absorption.

***PABA RDA:*** none. SR: 10 to 100 mg

## Vitamin C (Ascorbic acid, Calcium ascorbate, Sodium ascorbate)

Vitamin C is regarded with high esteem in the human body because it is involved in a number of cellular processes within the body. Vitamin C certainly does have a genuine contribution to reproductive health. Sperm health is

critically dependent upon anti-oxidants, although most free radicals are produced during normal metabolic processes; the environment contributes greatly to the free radical load. Men exposed to increased levels of sources of free radicals are much more likely to have abnormal sperm and sperm counts.
Vitamin C improves all semen parameters; Vitamin C may protect against oxidative DNA damage to sperm (200-1000mg/day) as well as help prevent sperm agglutination (1 gram/day). Positive effects have been shown with Vitamin C and sperm motility and viability.

In the female, Vitamin C is necessary for maturation of the pre-ovulatory follicle. Studies have shown that when dietary Vitamin C was reduced from 250mg to 5mg per day in healthy human subjects, the seminal fluid ascorbic acid level decreased by 50 per cent and the number of sperm with damage to their DNA increased by 91 per cent (Encyclopaedia of Natural Medicine Vol.2 14).

The US Food and Nutrition Board acknowledges that smokers require at least twice as much Vitamin C as non smokers (15). In one study, men who smoked one packet of cigarettes per day received either 200mg, or 1000mg of Vitamin C. After one month, sperm quality improved proportional to the level of Vitamin C supplemented. Another study also showed the non-smokers benefited very well from additional Vitamin C supplementation over several weeks of comparative results.

One of the key improvements that have been observed in these Vitamin C studies, are in relation to sperm and the vast improvements in agglutinated (clumped together) sperm. A major cause of agglutination is due to antibodies produced by the body's immune system binding to the sperm. This could be associated with chronic genitor-urinary tract or prostatic infection. When more than 25 per cent of the sperm are agglutinated, fertility is unlikely.

A study conducted with 3 groups of males with over 25 per cent agglutinated sperm tests were treated with supplemented Vitamin C. After 3 weeks, the agglutinated sperm in the Vitamin group dropped by 11 per cent.

Although this result is significant, the most impressive result of the study was that at the end of 60 days, the entire Vitamin C group had impregnated their wives, compared to none for the placebo group. These findings would suggest that Vitamin C supplementation for infertile males, particularly with antibody problems, may greatly benefit from additional intake of this nutrient.

Vitamin C aids the uptake of iron and studies have shown that Vitamin C is helpful for females to promote ovulation (ovaries are rich in Vitamin C indicating that its presence is strongly needed). Vitamin C is also vital for proper immune system function, hormone, collagen production and connective tissue repair.

Ascorbic acid also aids the metabolism of tyrosine, folic acid, and tryptophan. Tryptophan is converted in the presence of Vitamin C to 5-hydroxytryptophan (5HT), which forms serotonin, an important brain chemical. Vitamin C also helps folic acid to convert it to its active form, tetrahydrofolic acid, and tyrosine needs ascorbic acid to form the neurotransmitters dopamine and epinephrine.

Vitamin C stimulates the adrenal gland function and the release of norepinephrine and epinephrine (adrenaline), our stress hormones; however, prolonged stress depletes Vitamin C in the adrenals and decreases the blood levels. Ascorbic acid also helps the thyroid hormone production, and it aids in cholesterol metabolism. Vitamin C also indirectly assists in protecting the Fat-soluble vitamins.

Vitamin C has been shown to stimulate the immune system to fight infections. Ascorbic acid may activate neutiphils, the most prevalent white blood cells, lymphocytes, for antibody production to defend against various bacteria, viral, and fungal diseases. With high doses of Vitamin C, interferon production can be increased that coordinates cellular immunity to combat may serious diseases. Ascorbic acid can also decrease histamine production, thereby exerting an anti-allergy effect. During pregnancy, Vitamin C is essential of the maintenance of the chorioamniotic membrane. Premature rupturing of this membrane affects 10-20 per cent of all pregnancies and is a major cause of preterm delivery and reproductive system infection. Vitamin C plasma levels decrease generally throughout pregnancies, increased supplementation of Vitamin C would be recommended to enhance protection from premature membrane rupturing.

**Vitamin C is rich in foods such as:** peppers; guavas; parsley; blackcurrant; broccoli; citrus fruit; raw cabbage; strawberries; potatoes; and cauliflower. Iron is high in foods such as prune juice; liver; beef; soybeans; apricots; clams; oysters; parsley; and meats.

**Vitamin C RDA:** 30 to 75 mg. SR: 250 to 10,000 mg.

Vitamin C works hand-in-hand with other nutrients such as bioflavonoids:

### Citrus Bioflavonoids – Vitamin P (e.g. Citrin, Chrysin, Quercetin, Hesperidin, Resveratol, and Rutin)
Bioflavonoids are responsible for the colour of many fruits and vegetables, and are found in grains, nuts, leaves and flowers. Bioflavonoids exert powerful antioxidant and anti-inflammatory actions and have a protective effect over Vitamin C from being oxidised.

They enhance the absorption of Vitamin C into cells and help to improve capillary permeability and integrity, assist to stabilise blood sugar levels and prevent the onset of infection and various allergies. Miscarriage presentation and the stoppage of breakthrough bleeding may be benefited by using bioflavonoids.

**Good sources of bioflavonids** are the white pulp from citrus fruits; blackcurrants; berries; cherries; grapes; buckwheat; apricots; plums; herbs such as echinacea, hawthorn, milk thistle, and bilberry.

*Bioflavonoids RDA:* none stated. SR: 600 to 3,000 mg.

## Procyanthocyanidins (OPCs)

OPCs are potent free radical scavenger nutriceuticals found in pine bark, red wine, grape seed extract and bilberry. Studies conducted using the anti-oxidant called Pycnogenol on sub-fertile males has shown to have marked effect on increasing the health and number of sperm. After a 90-day period of its use, the sperm levels were reported to have climbed by 99 per cent.

*OPC's RDA:* 200 milligrams.

## Vitamin D (Cholecalciferol – D3)

Vitamin D is a group of fat-soluble prohormones, meaning that it has no hormone activity itself, but is converted to the active hormone 1,25-D through a highly regulated synthesis mechanism. Vitamin D is recognised as the sunshine vitamin, since the presence of Vitamin D in nature always appears to require the presence of some UV light.

Vitamin D is essential for calcium regulation and the maintenance of bone health. In adults, Vitamin D deficiency induces secondary hyperparathyroidism, which causes a loss of matrix and minerals of the bones, increasing the risk of osteoporosis and fracture. Deficiency of Vitamin D causes poor mineralisation of the collagen matrix in young children's bones leading to rickets. It is therefore critical for normal skeletal growth during infancy. A woman's Vitamin D requirements increase during pregnancy.

Low birth weight is one consequence of Vitamin D insufficiency during pregnancy. Foetal calcium is supplied by the mother and is dependent upon maternal vitamin D status in addition to calcium intake. Maternal Vitamin D deficiency also increases the risk of Vitamin D deficiency in breast fed infants.

Vitamin D deficiency is becoming increasingly diagnosed during pregnancy, and poses a major health risk. It is especially prevalent in dark-skinned people and those who have reduced sunlight exposure, excessive sunscreen use, alcoholics, avoid dairy product consumption, as well as in infants. Vitamin D is important for overall health and wellbeing, type 1 diabetes, auto-immune disease, multiple sclerosis, rheumatoid arthritis, hypertension, cardiovascular heart disease, and many forms of cancer can be associated with deficiencies of vitamin D.

121

## Vitamin E (Tocopherols)

Vitamin E is an important fat-soluble anti-oxidant vitamin, and is one of the body's great protectors against (free-radical) tissue damage. It is often referred to as the *fertility vitamin* as it is needed by both men and women to maintain healthy reproductive organs. Vitamin E is necessary to ensure conception, healthy pregnancy and delivery. Vitamin E assists in oestrogen level regulation and is helpful for treating PMS. The Greek word *tokos* means 'birth' and *pherein* means 'to carry'.

Vitamin E has had a long history associated with fertility, pregnancy and prevention of habitual (recurrent) miscarriage. It is involved with healthy uterine wall development and increases the health of the placenta. Tocopherol reduces the body's requirements for oxygen and improves circulation.

Vitamin E supplements have shown improvements in sperm motility, sperm count and decreased abnormalities. Vitamin E, together with Vitamin C may help to prevent pre-eclampsia or elevated blood pressure during pregnancy. Vitamin E may help to protect sperm membranes from free radical damage. Studies involved with Vitamin E have shown to enhance the ability of sperm to fertilise an egg in test tubes.

In addition, other studies have also reported high impregnation percentages among trials with infertile couples in comparison to placebo groups. Vitamin E acts as an anti-thrombotic agent, which means it can break up pre-existing clots and protect against excessive platelet build-up without altering the body's normal clotting mechanisms. It assists red blood cells to carry a great quantity of oxygen and greatly enhances immune response factors. Vitamin E exerts a strengthening and stabilising effect on capillaries, membranes, cartilage and other connective tissue.

Vitamin E also helps to protect the body from various types of cancers. With other nutrients, it also offers a protective action to the adrenal and pituitary hormones. Used topically is reduces scar tissue formation and accelerates the healing of wounds and burns. If applied in a suppository form in can help to improve the lubrication of vaginal secretions.

***Vitamin E is high in foods such as:*** whole grains; oatmeal; brown rice; wheat germ and oil; sunflower/safflower; almonds; brazil nuts; walnuts; pecans; cucumber; corn; soy oil; beef; and egg yolk.

***Vitamin E recommended daily allowance (RDA):*** 30mg. Therapeutic dosages: 100mg-1,000mg.

**Note:** Vitamin E should be used at low dosages and raised slowly, particularly if prone to high blood pressure. Vitamin E is required for the metabolism of EFAs and selenium. The best supplemental forms of Vitamin E are natural water-soluble varieties rather than synthetic Vitamin E commonly referred to as DL-Tocopherol. Look for 'd-alpha tocopherol', 'mixed tocopherols and 'mixed tocotrienols'.

## Essential Fatty Acids (EFA)

Essential Fatty Acids are necessary for the formation of the prostaglandins. Prostaglandins have a wide variety of biological functions; they have hormone-like activity and assist in regulating sex gland function. EFAs increase good prostaglandins in the body, which decrease pain, inflammation, cramping, PMS, hypertension and benign breast disease.

These fatty acids are essential for the correct formation of cell walls, the nervous system and foetal brain development. EFAs benefit uterine blood flow and may be protective against cot death (SIDS). EFA derivatives from linoleic acid are found in the Graafian follicles. Graafian follicle is the fluid filled sac that houses the maturing egg in the ovary. Experts speculate that prostaglandin malfunction may cause the fallopian tubes to spasm, throwing off the progression of the egg (ovum).

Another function of the prostaglandins is to induce ovulation. The high level of progesterone characteristic of ovulation triggers prostaglandins and is a sign ovulation has taken place. An imbalance could prevent ovulation.

EFA deficiencies may lead to chromosomal defects, subtle brain dysfunctions, such as dyslexia and attention deficit disorder. Spontaneous miscarriages and delayed labour have also been linked to EFA deficiencies; large amounts are deposited in the last trimester of pregnancy and during early life. Omega-3 fatty acids are especially important for normal cell signalling response, visual and cortical function. Foetal DHA correlates positively with birth weight. Healthy sperm are highly dependent on an adequate supply of Essential Fatty Acids.

Considering the effects of fats and oils on agglutination and cell membrane function, certain fats are definitely good for you and are essential for maintaining optimal general and reproductive health, but there are many others that would be best avoided in your diet. These types of fats include: saturated fats; hydrogenated oils; trans-fatty acids; and cottonseed, coconut and palm oils. Coconut and palm oils are primarily saturated fat, while cottonseed may contain toxic residues due to the heavy spraying of cotton and its high levels of *gossypol*, a substance known to inhibit sperm function. Gossypol is in fact being investigated as a 'male birth-control pill'.

Excessive consumption of saturated fats combined with inadequate intake of essential fatty acids changes the fatty acid composition of the sperm membranes, thus decreasing fluidity and interfering with sperm motility.

Three main factors have been identified that contribute to susceptibility of sperm to free-radical or oxidative damage. Studies have revealed that high levels of free radicals are found in the semen of approximately 40 per cent of infertile men.

- A high membrane concentration of polyunsaturated fatty acids.

123

- Active generation of free radicals.
- A lack of defensive enzymes.

Sperm are extremely sensitive to free radicals because they are so dependent upon the integrity and fluidity of their cell membrane for proper function. Without proper membrane fluidity, enzymes are activated which can lead to impaired motility, abnormal structure, loss of viability and ultimately death to the sperm.

The major determinant of membrane fluidity is the concentration of poly-unsaturated fatty acids, particularly omega-3 fatty acids, such as docosahexaenoic acid, which are very susceptible to free radical damage. The sperm have a relative lack of the superoxide dismutase (SOD) and catalase needed to prevent or repair oxidative damage. Adding to this more susceptible state is the fact that sperm generate high quantities of free radicals to help break down barriers to fertilisation.

*Food sources high in EFAs include:* evening primrose oil (which contains gamma-linolenic acid or GLA); cold water or deep-dwelling fish such as tuna, salmon and cod. Other good sources are: sunflower oil; olive oil; corn oil; butternuts; tofu; walnut oil; linseed (flax oil); and mustard oil. If you consume reasonably large quantities of fish, try to source fish that are lower in the food chain. *(Refer to mercury toxicity, Ch.5).

*Linoleic acid (w6 – EFA):* GLA = 1 to 3 grams.

*Linolenic acid (w3 – EFA):* DHA/EPA = 1 to 3 grams.

*Conjugated linoeic acid (w6 –EFA):* CLA = 1 to 4 grams. CLA is primarily used therapeutically to support in various cancer treatments (breast, colon, liver, lung, leukaemia, melanoma and prostate); inflammatory bowel disorders; type 2 diabetes; glioblastoma; and to assist with weight loss.


**Vitamin K1 (phytomedadione, phytonadione, or phylloquione)**
Vitamin K1 is the form that occurs in green plants, and seems to be the best form of Vitamin k for protecting against osteoporosis. All three forms (K1, K2, and K3) are about equally helpful for blood clotting.

*The RDA for Vitamin K1* is 1 mcg per kilogram of body weight. For an average sized adult approximately 70 to 150 mcg is considered adequate.

# The Magic Minerals

Minerals are basic constituents of all matter and are the spark that keeps our enzymes' engines running. They are part of living tissue as well as existing in their inorganic form in the earth. Approximately 4-5 per cent of the body weight is mineral matter. Minerals are also present in tissue protein, enzymes, blood, and some vitamins.

If the human body were left to decompose completely, most of the organic tissue which we are made up of (proteins, carbohydrates, fats, carbon, oxygen, hydrogen, nitrogen, water, carbon dioxide, and nitrogen) is either evaporated into the atmosphere or enters the soil.

What is left is approximately 5 pounds of elemental mineral ash, of which 75 per cent would be calcium and phosphorus, about a teaspoon of iron, a couple of teaspoons of salt from sodium and chloride, a little more of potassium, and the rest of the ash would contain numerous other elements. There are approximately 103 currently known inorganic minerals on the list of the chemical periodic table.

The average human body is made up of 65 per cent oxygen, 18 per cent carbon, 10 per cent hydrogen, 3 per cent nitrogen, which is contained in protein. Ninety per cent of the oxygen and 70 per cent of the hydrogen combine to make the body's water, which constitutes two-thirds of our body weight. The remaining elements form the organic constituents – proteins, fats, and carbohydrates.

There are approximately 17 essential minerals. (The primary elements carbon, hydrogen, oxygen, and nitrogen, part of all living tissue and food, are not included here). The eight macro minerals are calcium (Ca), phosphorus (P), sodium (Na), potassium (K), chloride (Cl), sulphur (S), magnesium (Mg), and Silicon. The tract elements make up the remaining known minerals, with the majority of them having essential functions in the body also.

Minerals are made up of two main components, an anion and cation for example. Let's look at magnesium, which is the anion component of the mineral; the cation is the other compound that joins with it to give it varied absorption and utilisation capacity such as magnesium oxide, magnesium orotate, magnesium aspartate, magnesium phosphate, magnesium amino acid chelate and so on. These various combinations will also yield differing elemental content of that certain mineral.

***Colloidal Minerals*** are usually derived from pre-historic, vegetated matter. Colloidal mineral supplements are negatively changed, which basically means that the body's absorption and utilisation is very high.

Metallic minerals that you may get in multi-vitamin/mineral supplements, yield much higher mineral element content but are not as well absorbed and utilised.

Colloidal mineral supplements yield a wide spectrum of trace element nutrients (usually over 77) that may no longer be found in our usual food sources.

**Tissue Salts or Colloids** are inorganic salts mineral substances. They are found in human blood, tissue and cells as well as in the ashes of humans after death and in the earth and soil. These salts are present in extremely minute particles in our bodies and are in a simpler form than the minerals found in foods. There are 12 tissue salts, which can be used in various combinations to assist the bodies healing processes in different therapeutic situations.

## Tissue Mineral salts (or Celloids) useful for fertility

- **Women's infertility**

  **PC, IP, MP, S, CF, SP**.
  For psychogenic causes, or where no organic can be found,
  **PP, MP, SP, CP, and IP**

- **Male infertility**
  Where no organic cause can be found,
  **PP, MP, and SP**

## Key Functions

| | | |
|---|---|---|
| • | PC – potassium chloride | Congestion remover & Ph regulator |
| • | IP – iron phosphate | Inflammation remover & Energy transfer |
| • | MP – magnesium phosphate | Neuromuscular Co-ordinator & Energy |
| • | S – silica | Reorganiser & Structure stabiliser |
| • | CF – calcium fluoride | Tissue Strengtheners |
| • | CP – calcium phosphate | Cell builder & Nerve transference |
| • | SP – sodium phosphate | Metabolic acid remover & Ph regulator |
| • | PP – potassium phosphate | Nerve power activator & Energy |
| • | SS – sodium sulphate | Problem fluid remover & detoxifier |
| • | PS – potassium sulphate | Cell oxygenator |
| • | CS – calcium sulphate | Suppuration remover |

## Calcium (Ca)

Calcium is the most abundant mineral in the body. Calcium's optional absorption occurs when adequate amounts of Vitamins A, E, C, D, E, F, magnesium, phosphorus, manganese, iron, lysine, fats and proteins are also present. Calcium is essential for the building and maintenance of all bones and teeth, therefore preventing conditions such as Osteoporosis.

The correct transmission of nerve impulses requires the balance of calcium, magnesium and potassium. The total calcium content of the adult body is entirely renewed over a six-year period.

The body's electrolyte balance and blood Ph (acid base) are regulated by calcium, as are the kidneys. Calcium has also the ability to protect against heavy metal toxicity (esp. arsenic, lead, cadmium, and mercury), particularly through inhibition of absorption by osseous tissue. Calcium and copper are important nutrients in regulating the thyroid gland and a low intake of Vitamin D and Calcium may increase the incidence of breast and cervical cancer. Colorectal cancers have also responded favourable to additional calcium supplementation.

Muscle growth and health is facilitated by calcium, whilst a deficiency may result in pain and muscle cramps. Maintenance of cell permeability and regulation of blood coagulation (blood clotting) are also dependent on this mineral. The activation of several enzyme systems and RNA and DNA structuring are facilitated by calcium. Calcium is necessary for the formation of 'fertile' or stretchy mucus and can also improve the ability of the sperm to swim through it.

A calcium deficiency can lead to nervous tension and fluid retention, and has also been linked to the toxaemia of pregnancy. Calcium supplements must be balanced in a 2:1 ratio with magnesium. Excess intake of chocolate, sugar, alcohol, and salt all cause a severe loss of calcium from the body.

***Calcium is found in food such as:*** unpasteurised dairy products; milk; Swiss cheese; asparagus; figs; buttermilk; sesame seeds; carob; tofu; yogurt; fish (especially sardines); nuts; tahini (ground sesame paste); beans; kale; molasses; rhubarb; cauliflower; and green leafy vegetables.

***Calcium Recommended Daily Allowances (RDA):*** 800 to 1,400 mg. Therapeutic Dosages (SR): 1,000 mg to 2,000 mg.


## Chlorine (Cl)

Chlorine travels primarily with sodium and water and helps generate the osmotic pressure of body fluids. It is an important constituent of stomach hydrochloric acid (HCL), the key digestive acid. Chloride is also needed to maintain the acid-alkaline balance of the body. The kidneys excrete or retain chloride mainly as sodium chloride depending on the body's requirements. Chloride may also help in allowing waste products to be cleared form the liver. The largest amount of chloride in the body is found in the red blood cell.

***Chlorine RDA:*** 750 mg (adult).


## Magnesium (Mg)

Magnesium is a vital catalyst in enzyme activity (it is a cofactor in over 100 enzyme reactions), especially the activity of those enzymes involved in energy production. It is important for the health of every organ in the body and assists in uptake of calcium and potassium. A deficiency of magnesium interferes with the transmission of nerve and muscle impulses, causing irritability and nervousness. Supplementing the diet with magnesium can help prevent depression, dizziness, muscle weakness and twitching, premenstrual syndrome (PMS), and also aids in maintaining the body's proper pH balance and normal body temperature.

Magnesium is especially important to good heart health and for the proper functioning of the neuro-muscular systems of the body.

Magnesium is necessary for the production of oestrogen and progesterone and is involved in the metabolism of carbohydrates. Magnesium may help to prevent toxaemia in pregnancy, muscular contractions/spasms of the uterus and fallopian tubes, which is essential to the proper transport of the sperm and ovum. In the foetus a magnesium deficiency can lead to possible miscarriage, retarded development, low birth weight, and premature labour. Even mild magnesium deficiency can cause free radial damage to the sperm and testes. Magnesium deficiency inhibits the use and excretion of vitamin.

Magnesium and vitamin B1 are needed for cell metabolism and energy production. It is necessary to prevent the calcification of soft tissue. This essential mineral protects the arterial linings from stress caused by sudden blood pressure changes, and plays a role in the formation of bone and in carbohydrate and mineral metabolism. With Vitamin B6 (pyridoxine), magnesium helps to reduce and dissolve calcium phosphate kidney stones, and may prevent calcium-oxalate kidney stones.

Research has shown that magnesium may help prevent cardiovascular disease, osteoporosis, and certain forms of cancer, and it may reduce cholesterol levels. It is effective in preventing premature labour and convulsions in pregnant women. Studies have shown that taking magnesium supplements during pregnancy has a dramatic effect in reducing birth defects.

A study published by the Journal of the American Medical Association reported a 70-percent lower incidence of mental retardation in the children of mothers who had taken magnesium supplements during pregnancy. The incidence of cerebral palsy was 90 percent lower.

Possible manifestations of magnesium deficiency include: confusion; insomnia; irritability; poor digestion; rapid heartbeat; seizures; and tantrums. Often, a magnesium deficiency can be synonymous with diabetes, and are at the root of many cardiovascular problems. Magnesium deficiency may be a major cause of: fatal cardiac arrhythmia; hypertension and sudden cardiac arrest; as well as asthma; attention deficient disorders; chronic fatigue; chronic pain syndromes; anxiety; depression; muscle cramping; hyperinsulinism; osteoporosis; insomnia; irritable bowel syndrome; and pulmonary disorders.

Research has also shown that magnesium deficiency may contribute to the formation of kidney stones. To test for magnesium deficiency, a procedure called an intracellular (mononuclear cell) magnesium screen should be

performed. This is a more sensitive test than the typical serum magnesium screen, and can detect a deficiency with more accuracy. Magnesium screening should be a routine test, as a low magnesium level makes nearly every disease worse. It is particularly important for individuals who have, or who are considered at risk for developing, cardiovascular disease.
This essential mineral assists with the digestion of protein and carbohydrates, protects from heart attack and lymph gland abnormalities.

Research data from the beginning of the 20th century reveals that semen plasm magnesium was then about 30 per cent higher than in the middle of the century, at which time it was lower than normal in 44 per cent of men. The semen magnesium, zinc levels and the acid phosphatase activity are related mathematically. All three correlated with the motility of the sperm.

In the event of a depressed magnesium level, the volume of the testis and the extent of spermatogenesis decreased. High doses of magnesium are necessary to correct chronic magnesium deficiency, which is related to reduced sperm counts and motility. Magnesium deficiency promotes oxidative damage due to iron accumulation in the testes.

It is known that magnesium deficiency is associated with increased smooth muscle reactivity, which may influence patency of the fallopian tube, thereby affecting ability to conceive; it is known that oestrogen receptor binding is a magnesium dependent process, and that magnesium modulates follicle stimulating hormone (FSH) binding to granulosa cell receptors. It is known that magnesium is important in governing key rate-limiting steps in the cell cycle, particularly the onset of DNA synthesis and mitosis (cell division).

***Food sources high in magnesium include:*** unprocessed whole grains (rye, buckwheat, millet); dark green leafy vegies; kelp; nuts; fish; seafood; dried fruits; poultry; beef; pork; lamb; black bean; pulses; brown rice; bananas; soy beans; corn; apples; tofu; molasses; dolomite; wheat germ; and almonds. Magnesium along with potassium can be lost via the renal pathways in urine if you are on certain diuretics or caffeine type beverages.

***Magnesium RDA:*** 350 mg. SR: 300 – 1,000 mg.


## Phosphorus (P)
Phosphorus is the second most abundant element in the body after calcium. Phosphorus is involved in many functions besides forming bones and teeth. Like calcium, it is found in all cells and is involved in some biochemical reactions. Phosphorus is vital to energy production. It provides the phosphate in adenosine triphosphate (ATP), which is the high-energy carrier molecule in the body's primary metabolic cycles. Phosphorus is important in the utilisation of carbohydrates and fats form energy, proteins for growth, and maintenance of all tissue, cells, & nucleic acid in DNA and RNA. Excessive phosphorus intake can lead to a calcium deficiency or malabsorption problem.

Phosphorus combines with the B vitamins to assist in their functions in the body, and is a component of the phospholipids, fat molecules essential to cell membranes. Phosphorus aids muscle contractions, regulated heart beats, involved in the conversion of niacin, and riboflavin to the active forms, and also supports proper nerve conduction. The parathyroid gland regulates the blood levels of phosphorus so it can carry out its essential functions.

*Phosphorus RDA:* 800 mg. SR: 400 to 1,400 mg. (adult).


## Potassium (K)

This mineral is important for a healthy nervous system and a regular heart rhythm. It helps prevent stroke, aids in proper muscle contraction, and works with sodium to control the body's water balance, intracellular fluids and electrolytes. Potassium is important for chemical reactions within the cells and aids in maintaining stable blood pressure and in transmitting electrochemical impulses. Hyper-acidity in the body is counteracted by potassium (particularly citrate). Hormone secretion is dependent on potassium, and can be hyper-secreted during stress states.

A 1997 review of earlier studies showed that low potassium intake may be a significant factor in the development of high blood pressure. Potassium also regulates the transfer of nutrients through cell membranes. This function of potassium has been shown to decrease with age, which may account for some of the circulatory damage, lethargy, and weakness experienced by older people. Together with magnesium, potassium can help prevent calcium-oxalate kidney stones.

Signs of potassium deficiency include abnormally dry skin; acne; chills; cognitive impairment; constipation; depression; diarrhoea; diminished reflex function; oedema; nervousness; insatiable thirst; fluctuations in heartbeat; glucose intolerance; growth impairment; high cholesterol levels; insomnia; low blood pressure; muscular fatigue and weakness; nausea and vomiting; periodic headaches; proteinuria (protein in the urine); respiratory distress; and salt retention. Depletion of potassium can be caused by excess salt; sugar; coffee; alcohol; certain diuretic medications; and sweating.

*Foods high in potassium include:* sea vegetables; fruit; beans; whole grains; dried fruits (particularly bananas); and sunflowers.

*Potassium RDA:* 2 to 5 grams (50 to 125 m Eq/day). SR: 3 to 8 grams.


## Silicon (Si)

Silicon promotes firmness and strength in the tissues. It is part of the arteries, tendons, skin, connective tissue, and eyes. Collagen contains silicon, helping hold the body tissues together. This mineral is also present in chondroitin sulphate of cartilage, and works with calcium to help restore bone. Silicon is also thought to radiate or transmit energy in its crystalline structure, as in quartz crystal. It is said by some to clear stored toxins by being able to penetrate deep into tissues. The 'Silicea' tissue salt is a homeopathic remedy that is described as acting like a 'microscopic surgeon'.

**Silicon RDA:** 9 to 14 mg. SR: 20 to 30 mg


## Sodium (Na)

Sodium is the primary ion found in the blood and fluids. It is also found in every cell in the body, although it is mainly extracellular. It works closely with potassium, the main intracellular mineral. About 60 per cent of sodium in the body is in the fluid around cells, 10 per cent in the cells and around 30 per cent in the bones.

Sodium is an electrolyte, along with potassium and chloride, and is closely tied in with the movement of water. *'Where sodium goes, water goes with it.'*

The body retains approximately 90-100 grams of sodium in the body, in the form of sodium chloride. The salt is a combination of a positive and negative ion combination in crystalline form. Blood pressure can be greatly affected due to the balance of salt status in the body. The shift of sodium and potassium across cell membranes helps to create an electric potential (charge) that enables muscles to contract and nerve impulses to be conducted.

These two minerals also work together to balance the acid-alkaline status in the body via the kidneys. Sodium is also important to the production of hydrochloric acid in the stomach. Sodium is needed to maintain blood fluid volume and is used during the transport of amino acids from the gut to the blood. Aldosterone, a made and secreted by the adrenal cortex, acts on the kidneys to regulate sodium metabolism.

Sodium is present in almost all foods, some of the higher containing ones include: seafood; beef; poultry; celery; beets; carrots; artichokes; kelp; and sea vegetables.

**Sodium RDA:** 1.1 to 3.5 grams. SR: 3 to 9 grams.


## Sulphur (S)

Sulphur is contained in all tissues in the body and is a component of blood haemoglobin, where it acts as an oxidising agent. Sulphur is able to purify and cleanse the digestive tract and prevent the accumulation of waste toxins in the body. Sulphur is needed for healthy blood plasma formation and provides oxygen to the blood. Many of the lipotropic amino acids such as cysteine, taurine and methionine used for liver detoxification contain high amounts of sulphur.

**Foods high is sulphur include:** brazil nuts; green vegetables; onions; garlic; kelp; watercress; Brussels sprouts; cabbage; kale; snap beans; turnips; cauliflower; and kelp. Excessive ingestion of sulphur can potential cause gastro/intestinal upset, including wind and bloating problems.

## Chromium (Cr)

Chromium is vital to blood sugar control. It facilitates the uptake of glucose into cells, and without adequate chromium, the insulin action is blocked. This leads to increased glucose levels and blood sugar fluctuations. This nutrient is critical in cases of debilitated blood sugar metabolism, as it has been shown to lower insulin levels, improve glucose tolerance and decreased fasting glucose levels.

GTF (Glucose Tolerance Factor) is made from a number of nutrients, mainly chromium, also niacin, glycine, cysteine, and glutamic acid. Chromium plays a role in the synthesis of fatty acids and cholesterol. It also has the ability to lower total serum cholesterol and triglyceride levels, while increasing the levels of plasma HDL cholesterol (the good one). It has been suggested that due to its interaction and binding with RNA molecules, chromium may also play a role in protein synthesis.

It competes with iron in the blood in the transport of proteins and also has an amino acid transport capability. The levels of chromium steadily decrease with age. Due to chromium's influence over glucose metabolism, this trace mineral is essential to assist with providing adequate glucose to the brain as a 'fuel' source, and for movement to the nerves and muscles.

A lack of chromium may also predispose the individual to arteriosclerosis, hypertension, and diabetes in later life. Glucose is a vital energy provider to the body, the seminal fluid is bathed in glucose to fuel the sperm's motility and it is essential to the foetal development to have stable supplies of glucose.

**Good food sources of chromium include:** brewer's yeast; corn; clams; nuts; prunes; whole wheat; rye bread; wheat germ; apples; potatoes; eggs; chicken; oysters; wheat bran; beef; fresh chilli; green capsicum; mushrooms; and beer.

**Chromium RDA:** 50 to 200 ug. SR: 100 to 300 ug.

## Copper (Cu)

Both a deficiency and an excess of copper can lead to fertility problems. Nowadays it is rarer to see copper deficiencies due to much of the water supplies being fed through copper piping. However, an excess of copper uptake can contribute to a zinc and Vitamin C deficiency problem.

Copper is a trace mineral, which is mostly stored in the muscles, liver, and bones. It is a catalyst for the formation of haemoglobin (by facilitating the uptake of iron with manganese); elastin (by oxidising Vitamin C and working with it); collagen; melanin (by conversion of tyrosine); phospholipids for the myelin sheaths; and is involved in energy release. The function of the digestive system also requires copper. Copper is necessary for the cellular respiration and the uptake and utilisation of glucose and plays a role in hormone production and breakdown. Protein metabolism, good healing, proper bone formation, all require copper. It also has strong anti-fungal properties.

*Food sources containing copper include:* raw nuts; purple and red onions; almonds; brazil nuts; cashews; legumes; whole grains; and prunes.

*Copper RDA:* 2 to 3 mg. SR: 2 to 5 mg.


## Iodine (I)

Iodine is essential for the correct functioning of the thyroid gland, which controls hormone balance, and to enhance the metabolism. An underactive thyroid may lead to anovulatory cycle (in which no ovulation takes place). Iodine deficiency during pregnancy can lead to damage to the thyroid and cause impairment of brain development in the baby.

Iodine is toxic in excess, but it can be useful in cases of excessive bleeding and polycystic breast syndrome, arthritis, and where increases in mental and physical vigour are needed. Iodine combines with other nutrients such as tyrosine in the manufacturing of the thyroid hormones thyroxine (T4) and triiodothyronine (T3).

Iodine is involved in energy production by encouraging the growth, development and stimulation of cellular mitochondria by increasing the number and size. This trace element also supports the adrenal gland function and is required to maintain both male and female fertility.

Iodine has the ability to excrete arsenic from the body and alleviate certain symptoms of radiation sickness. It is able to also kill several forms of bacteria and fungi. During pregnancy, iodine requirements are increased since in addition to maintaining maternal metabolism, there is increased demand for T4 by the foetus. In the early stages of pregnancy, the foetus is totally reliant on the mother's T4 supply. T4 is needed for foetal central nervous system (CNS) and brain maturation.
Insufficient iodine during early pregnancy and neonatal (e.g. breast feeding) stages can impact on CNS development.

*Food sources may include:* kelp (form of seaweed); dulse; turnips; greens; watermelons; cucumbers; spinach; asparagus; kale; blueberry; peanuts; and strawberries.

*Iodine RDA:* 150 ug. SR: 100 to 1,000 ug.

## Iron (Fe)

Iron store depletion may also be a reason for poor conception. Iron is necessary for the normal formation of haemoglobin (combined with copper and protein) and red blood cells. Excessive tiredness can be a potential symptom of inadequate haemoglobin in the blood. Improper balance of other nutrients such as Vitamin E, calcium, phosphorus, copper and other nutrients are also necessary for effective assimilation and function of iron in the body.

Iron is essential to life and found in every lining cell of the body, particularly the blood. Iron is involved in the strengthening and enhancement of respiration, the immune response, and cellular energy. In order for iron to be properly absorbed, adequate gastric hydrochloric acid and Vitamin C must be present (absorption can increase by 400 per cent). Calcium, copper, and phosphorous are important to be maintained in balance for correct iron absorption. Vitamin E is needed for the proper assimilation of iron also.

Non-heme and heme are the two types of dietary iron that the body can utilise. Non-Heme is found in broccoli; beetroot; peas; raisins; fruits; grains; leafy green vegetables; wheat germ; millet; pumpkin seeds; sunflower seeds; cashews; and brazil nuts.

Excessive amounts of bran fibre, poor gastric acids, anti-acid medications, tea, coffee, unrefined cereals, soy, calcium, and zinc can inhibit non-heme iron absorption. Vegetarians are also at particular risk of low levels of iron if food combining is not balanced.

Heme iron is found in fish, poultry (eggs) and meats. The absorption of iron also relies on the storage capacity within the body. The last trimester of pregnancy is particularly important to have adequate levels of iron as the blood volume in the mother has almost doubled and increased demand for haemoglobin and red blood cells are required.

*Iron is high in foods such as*: prune juice; liver; beef; soybeans; apricots; molasses; almond nuts; lima beans; avocados; rice; kidney; clams; oysters; and parsley.

*Iron RDA:* 10mg-50mg. SR: 15–50 mg. Pregnancy (3rd trimester): 22-27 mg.


## Manganese (Mn)

This trace element is necessary for the utilisation of Vitamins C and E, biotin, thiamine and choline, and as an activator of enzyme systems, including those involved with glucose metabolism, ATP production, free radical scavengers, Manganese is required for normal bone growth and development, lipid fat metabolism, blood formation, pituitary gland formation and the formation of breast milk.

Manganese and zinc may biochemically replace copper levels, thus reducing them. Manganese assists in the synthesis of fatty acids, cholesterol and the thyroid gland hormone thyroxine. It nourishes nerve, brain and connective tissue, maintains sexual hormone production and works well with other B group vitamins.

Manganese is needed for the building and breakdown of protein and nucleic acids (the carriers of genetic information), though protein is important for the proper absorption of manganese. People suffering from diabetes and pancreatic insufficiency may be found to have lower levels of manganese.

This trace element is also involved with effective functioning of the adrenal glands and kidneys. A deficiency of manganese can cause fertility problems such as a total lack of sperm, ovulation and testicular degeneration, spontaneous abortion, infant mortality due to defects in bone heart, and nervous system growth.

Manganese is also said to contribute to the mother's instinctive desire to love and protect her child. Manganese helps to detoxify lead in the body, but excessive intake can interfere with iron storage and absorption.

*Food sources for manganese include:* whole grains; cereals; legumes; nuts; dried fruit; root vegetables; barley; rye; buckwheat; oats; almonds; spinach; beet greens; brussels sprouts; poultry; fish; dairy products; herbs such as raspberry leaf, buchu, bilberry, hibiscus flower, and uva-ursi may also have good manganese content.

*Maganese RDA:* 2.5 to 7 mg. SR: 2 to 50 mg.


## Molybdenum (Mo)

Molybdenum functions as an enzyme cofactor and is an essential trace mineral. It possesses strong antioxidant properties and is involved in regulating the detoxifying chemicals that eliminate purines and pyrimidines from the body.

Studies have shown that animals fed a diet deficient in molybdenum suffer from stunted growth and impaired reproductive characteristics. Molybdenum enhances kidney function and exerts a protective effect against several types of cancers.

*Foods containing molybdenum include:* cauliflower; spinach; fish; liver; peas; beans, legumes; cereal grains; wheat germ; green peas; brown rice; cottage cheese; lentils; split peas; brewer's yeast; potato; molasses; and chicken. These are all good sources of this trace mineral.

*Molybdenum RDA:* 75 – 250 ug. SR: 100 to 500 ug.

## Selenium (Se)

This essential trace element and important anti-oxidant is a potent inducer of detoxification, eliminating many toxic chemicals and heavy metals from the system. The function of selenium is closely related to that of Vitamin E. When deficient it can be associated with decreased sperm motility and increased numbers of sperm abnormalities. The organic form of selenium, such as *Selenomethionine*, is better for incorporation into the sperm. A liquid form of selenium, *sodium selenite* is the best absorbed and utilised version. Selenium helps to protect cell membranes and maintain magnesium levels.

One quarter of infant mortality has been linked to selenium deficiency; it may also be involved in SIDS (Sudden Infant Death Syndrome). Proper selenium status has been associated with lowering multiple types of cancer rates, enhancing immunity, improving thyroid function, preventing oxidative damage to the eyes, and improving cardiac function. Women who have miscarried have shown to have lower levels of selenium comparatively to women who have carried to term.

Selenium is frequently lost through the ejaculate, so replenishment is very important. Selenium's health benefits are far reaching, as it assists in many of the body's systems such as the cardiovascular, digestive, immune, metabolic, muscular skeletal, nervous and not to mention the reproductive. Selenium is an important factor in the health of our thymus gland white blood cells. The health of the hair, skin, and nails also require adequate selenium amounts. Use selenium supplementation wisely as excessive overload can be potentially toxic.

***Food sources that are high in selenium include:*** wheat germ; whole wheat; brown rice; oats; bran; barley; brazil nuts; sesame seeds; tuna; herring; brewer's yeast; wheat germ; scallops; lobster; prawns; crab; oysters; apple cider vinegar; and garlic.

***Selenium RDA:*** 50 to 200 ug. SR: 200 to 600 ug.


## Zinc (Zn)

Zinc is the mineral that has undoubtedly been proven as a mineral of paramount importance with male and female health. Zinc deficiency may be associated with oligospermia, decreased sperm motility and decreased serum testosterone.

High levels of zinc may be lost in male ejaculatory fluids and could exacerbate or bring about a zinc deficiency. Zinc deficiency can cause behavioural and perceptual problems, such as fatigue, depression, and loss of libido (sex drive). zinc is required for the production of sperm and development of the primary and secondary characteristics in the male and in all phases of reproduction processes in the female.

Zinc is commonly deficient, with 67 per cent of Australian men and 85 per cent of women having marginal dietary levels. Zinc is considered to be the single most important nutrient for pregnant women. Deficiencies of zinc can also cause chromosomal aberrations, and lowered testosterone levels.

Zinc status is disrupted by the use of the oral contraceptive pill and copper IUDs, and by the inorganic iron supplements frequently prescribed in pregnancy. Zinc is utilised in the excretion of toxic metals such as cadmium and lead. Zinc is necessary for the formation of elastin chains in connective tissue, collagen. During pregnancy, inadequate zinc leads to common problems such as stretch marks, cracked nipples, and prolonged labour.

More serious problems such as foetal growth retardation and congenital malformations may also result from zinc deficiency. Postnatal depression has been linked with zinc deficiency by several researchers. Zinc-deficient babies cry excessively and are difficult to calm.

The effectiveness of zinc is best illustrated by a study of thirty-seven (37) men who had been infertile for more than five years, and whose sperm counts were less than 25 million/ml. Blood testosterone levels were also measured. The men received a supplement of zinc sulphate (60mg of elemental zinc daily) for 45–50 days. In the 22 with initially low testosterone levels, mean (rate of average) sperm count increased significantly, from 8 to 20 million/ml. Testosterone levels also increased, and nine out of the twenty-two female partners become pregnant during the study time of 50 days. This result is quite impressive given the long-term nature of the infertility and the rapidity of the results.

***Foods containing zinc include:*** whole grains; legumes; unroasted pumpkin seeds; sunflower seeds; wheatgrass juice; oysters; liver; meats; poultry; raw egg yolk; and other nuts and seeds.

Due to the fact the many people don't even consume the recommended daily allowance (RDA) of zinc (15mg), additional supplementation of 45-60mg of zinc per day may appear to be warranted. Combining magnesium and Vitamin B6 with zinc is vital for hundreds of hormones and enzymatic reactions to occur in the body; these 3 nutrients I feel are essential in the correct regulation of the body's hormone and endocrine systems.

***Note***: Zinc Tally or Liquid Zinc Sulphate tests are an effective way of verifying supplemental zinc requirements.

***Zinc RDA: 15 mg or 0.2 mg/kilograms. SR: 10 to 100 mg.***

### Boron (B)

Diets high in boron can potentially double the levels of blood oestrogen. Boron is utilised in the body only in trace quantities for the metabolism of calcium, magnesium, phosphorus and Vitamin D via the parathyroid gland.

It is essential for joints, bone maintenance and metabolism, and raises testosterone, which encourage lean tissue and fat reduction. Boron is often deficient in the western diet.

***Foods that contain boron include:*** apples; pears; rose hip tea; and tomatoes.

### Lithium (Li)

Lithium is a trace element nutrient that has been linked to reproductive and fertility complications in animal studies. It is prescribed in higher doses in the management of conditions such as alcoholism, manic depression/bipolar disease, and attention deficit hyperactivity disorder (ADHD). Lithium is able to enhance the body's immune system and helps to prevent heart attack. Lithium can be toxic in large amounts but in trace quantities it has an effect of assisting other nutrients' absorption into cells and interacts with other trace elements in the body.

***Good sources of Lithium include:*** sea vegetables; sugar cane; drinking water; and some mineral waters.

### Vanadium (V)

Vanadium is a trace element nutrient that has been linked to impaired reproductive capacity. Deficiency states are not very well known in humans, but it is known to play a role in enhancing muscular growth, normalises blood sugar, reduces glycol-sylated haemoglobin in non-insulin dependent diabetics, and adds iodine metabolism and thyroid function. Vanadium should only be consumed in trace element amounts as it can have toxic side-effects if taken in excess.

***Food sources may include:*** fats; black pepper; chicken; dill; corn; linseed; mushroom; parsley; rye; seafood; soy bean; and in supplements as Vanadyl sulphate.

## Amino Acids

### L-Arginine

Arginine is an amino acid that retards the growth of tumours and cancer by enhancing immune function. It increases the size and activity of the thymus gland, which manufactures T lymphocytes (T cells), crucial components of the immune system. Arginine may therefore benefit those suffering from AIDS and malignant diseases that suppress the immune system. It is also good for liver disorders such as cirrhosis of the liver and fatty liver; it aids in liver detoxification by neutralising ammonia. It may reduce the effects of chronic alcohol toxicity.

Seminal fluid contains arginine. Studies suggest that sexual maturity may be delayed by arginine deficiency; conversely, arginine is useful in treating sterility in men. **Doses of up to *4 grams* of l-arginine have been used to greatly enhance sperm count and motility**. It is found in high concentrations in the skin and connective tissues, making it helpful for healing and repair of damages tissue.

*Nitric oxide* (NO) is synthesised from the amino acid arginine by NO synthase (NOS). Increasing the production of nitric oxide in the penis (in particularly the corpus cavernosum, the long cylinders of tissue in the penis that fill up with blood to create an erection), as well as the behaviour circuits in the brain has been shown to improve erectile dysfunction.

Nitric oxide is required for the relaxation of cavernous smooth muscle of the penis is a parasympathetic, nor adrenergic, and non-cholinergic mediated process. Therefore, L-Arginine helps reduce erectile dysfunction stemming from both psychological and sexual asthenia (a medical term for weakness or debility).

Arginine is import for muscle metabolism. It helps to maintain a proper nitrogen balance by acting as a vehicle for transportation and storage, and aiding the excretion, of excess nitrogen. Studies have shown that it also reduces nitrogen losses in people who have undergone surgery, and improves the function of cells in lymphatic tissue.

This amino acid aids in weight loss because it facilitates an increase in muscle mass and a reduction of body fat. It is also involved in a variety of enzymes and hormones.

It aids in stimulating the pancreas to release insulin, is a component of the pituitary hormone vasopressin, and assists in the release of growth hormones. Because arginine is a component of collagen and aids in building new bone and tendon cells, it can be good for arthritis and connective tissue disorders. Scar tissue that forms during wound healing is made up of collagen, which is rich in arginine. A variety of functions, including insulin production, glucose tolerance, and liver lipid metabolism, are impaired if the body is deficient in arginine.

This amino acid can be produced in the body; however, in newborn infants, production may not occur quickly enough to keep up with requirements. It is therefore deemed essential early in life. Studies have also revealed that L-Arginine improves blood flow to the pelvic organs; it increased ovarian response, endometrial receptivity and pregnancy rates in IVF patients.

***Foods high in arginine include:*** carob; chocolate; coconut; dairy products; gelatine; meat; oats; peanuts; soybeans; walnuts; white flour; wheat; wheat germ; and herbs like Astragalus.

**Note***:* People with viral infections such as herpes should not take supplemental arginine, and should avoid foods rich in arginine and low in the amino acid lysine (see below), as this appears to promote the growth of certain viruses. Pregnant and lactating women should avoid l-Arginine supplements. Persons with schizophrenia should avoid amounts over 30 milligrams daily. Long-term use, especially of high doses, is not recommended. One study found that several weeks of large doses might result in thickening and coarsening of the skin.


## L-Carnitine & Acetyl-L-Carnitine (ALC)

Carnitine is not an amino acid in the strictest sense (it is a substance more related to the B complex vitamins). Carnitine is not used for protein synthesis like other typical amino acids.

Acetyl-l-carnitine increases energy via an increase in beta-oxidation. It encourages fatty acids to be catabolised (broken down) in the mitochondria to produce adenosine triphosphate (ATP, the major energy molecule in the body). Carnitine can be manufactured by the liver from two amino acids, lysine and methionine. It is also plays a role in the effect of the thymus gland hormone on the metabolism of cells and white blood cell immune responses.

ALC also serves to protect mitochondrial structure and function. The Electron Transport System that energy is manufactured from is enhanced by ALC. ALC has a regulatory effect on both the cholinergic and dopaminergic systems, while acting as a powerful anti-oxidant. It is considered anti-aging as it reduces lipofuscin and can stimulate the growth of certain brain neurons. Carnitine can improve both sperm count and motility. ALC is also considered anti-hypoxic (improves oxygen uptake), therefore would be useful in cardio-vascular conditions and intermittent claudication. ALC exerts various protective effects over many of the brains and nervous system structures. Multiple cognitive functions could greatly benefit from its use.

The various types of carnitine have numerous therapeutic applications, some of these may include: Alzheimer's disease; depression; memory impairment; aging; Parkinson's disease; chronic fatigue syndrome; ocular protection; enhancing athletic performance; improving verbal fluency; attentiveness; mood; sleep quality; stress response; and co-ordination.

Carnitine concentrations are extremely high in the epididymis and sperm, suggesting an important role in male reproductive function. Epididymis derives the majority of its energy requirements from fatty acids during transport through the epididymis as do sperm. After ejaculation, the motility of the sperm correlated directly with carnitine content. The higher the carnitine content the more motile the sperm. Conversely, when carnitine levels are low, sperm development, function, and motility are drastically reduced.

One clinical study found that carnitine supplementation 1000mg x three (3) times daily led to an increase in sperm count and motility in 37 of 47 who had abnormal sperm motility. Therefore, supplementation of carnitine may help restore male fertility in some cases. Good sources of carnitine are found in beef, liver, and milk.

## Histidine

Histidine is an essential amino acid that is significant in the growth and repair of tissues. It is important for the maintenance of the myelin sheaths, which protect nerve cells, and is needed for the production of both red and white blood cells. Histidine also protects the body from radiation damage, helps lower blood pressure, aids in removing heavy metals from the system, and may help in the prevention of AIDS.

Histidine levels that are too high may lead to stress and even psychological disorders such as anxiety and schizophrenia; people with schizophrenia have been found to have high levels of histidine in their bodies. Inadequate levels of histidine may contribute to rheumatoid arthritis and may be associated with nerve deafness. Methionine has the ability to lower histidine levels.

Histamine, an important immune system chemical, is derived from histidine. Histamine aids in sexual arousal. Because the availability of histidine influences histamine production, taking supplemental histidine – together with vitamins B3 (niacin) and B6 (pyridoxine), which are required for the transformation from histidine to histamine – may help improve sexual functioning and pleasure. Because histamine also stimulates the secretion of gastric juices, histidine may be helpful for people with indigestion resulting from a lack of stomach acid.

Histamine is essential for penile throbbing and vasodilation associated with ejaculation. Though, excessively high levels of histamine levels are associated with premature ejaculation. Histidine is also a useful heavy detoxifier, some it may serve in a duel capacity, as toxic heavy metal overload is a major cause of infertility. Premature ejaculation can be associated with sympathetic nervous system dominance and/or parasympathica insufficiency.

The vitamin cofactors Vitamins B1, B5, and choline are essential acetylcholine precursors and are useful in balancing autonomic activity. Histidine supplementation may also benefit some conditions involving mood changes and free floating anxiety. Persons with manic (bipolar) depression should not take supplemental histidine unless a deficiency has been identified.

***Natural food sources high in histidine include:*** rice; wheat; and rye.

## Lysine

Lysine is an essential amino acid that is a necessary building block for all protein. It is needed for proper growth and bone development in children; it helps calcium absorption and maintains a proper nitrogen balance in adults.

This amino acid aids in the production of antibodies, hormones, and enzymes, and helps in collagen formation and tissue repair. Because it helps to build muscle protein, it is good for those recovering from surgery and sports injuries. It also lowers high serum triglyceride levels. Lysine is also very important for fertility, in particularly to improve sperm motility.

Another very useful ability of this amino acid is its capacity for fighting cold sores and herpes viruses. Individuals who are prone to herpes breakouts may need to avoid or cut down on high arginine foods/supplementation and balance the intake with L-lysine.

Taking supplemental L-lysine, together with Vitamin C with bioflavonoid, can effectively fight and/or prevent herpes outbreaks, especially if foods containing the amino acid arginine are avoided. Supplemental L-lysine also may decrease acute alcohol intoxication.

Lysine is an essential amino acid, and so cannot be manufactured in the body. It is therefore vital that adequate amounts be included in the diet. Deficiencies can result in anaemia; bloodshot eyes; enzyme disorders; hair loss; an inability to concentrate, irritability, lack of energy, poor appetite, reproductive disorders; retarded growth; and weight loss.

***Food sources of lysine include:*** cheese; eggs; fish; lima beans; milk; potatoes; red meat; soy products; and yeast.


## Taurine

High concentrations of taurine are found in the heart muscle, white blood cells, skeletal muscle, and central nervous system. It is a building block of all the other amino acids as well s a key component of bile, which is needed for the digestion of fats, the absorption of fat-soluble vitamins, and the control of serum cholesterol levels.

Taurine can be useful for people with atherosclerosis; oedema; heart disorders; hypertension; hypoglycaemia; fatty/scarred liver infiltration; muscular tics or twitches (with glycine); skin/tissue repair; and to stabilise over-excitable nerve tissue. It is vital for the proper utilisation of sodium, potassium, calcium and magnesium, and it has been shown to play a particular role in sparing the loss of potassium from the heart muscle. This helps to prevent the development of potentially dangerous cardiac arrhythmias. Taurine is also very useful for improving sperm motility.

Taurine has a protective effect on the brain, particularly if the brain is dehydrated. It is used to treat anxiety, epilepsy, hyperactivity, poor brain function and seizures. Taurine is found in concentrations up to four times greater in the brains of children than in those of adults.

It may be that a deficiency of taurine in the developing brain is involved in seizures. Zinc deficiency also is commonly found in people with epilepsy, and this may play a part in the deficiency of taurine. Taurine is also associated with zinc in maintaining eye function; a deficiency of both may impair vision. Taurine supplementation may benefit children with Down syndrome and muscular dystrophy. This amino acid is also used in some clinics for breast cancer treatment.

Excessive losses of taurine through the urine can be caused by many metabolic disorders. Cardiac arrhythmias, disorders of platelet formation, intestinal problems, an overgrowth of candida, physical or emotional stress, a zinc deficiency, and excessive consumption of alcohol are all associated with high urinary losses of taurine. Excessive alcohol consumption also causes the body to lose its ability to utilise taurine properly. Taurine supplementation may reduce symptoms of alcohol withdrawal. Diabetes increases the body's requirements for taurine conversely supplementation with taurine and cystine may decrease the need for insulin.

Taurine is found in eggs, fish, meat, and milk but not in vegetable proteins. It can be synthesised from cysteine in the liver and from methionine elsewhere in the body, as long as sufficient quantities of vitamin B6 are present.

For vegetarians, synthesis by the body is crucial. For individuals with genetic or metabolic disorders that prevent the synthesis of taurine, taurine supplementation is required.


## Antioxidants and other related substances

### Alpha-lipoic acid (ALA)

Lipoic acid is a powerful antioxidant (contains sulphur compound) – both on its own and as a 'recycler' of Vitamin E and Vitamin C. It can restore the antioxidant properties of these vitamins after they have neutralised free radicals. Lipoic acid is classed along with the B vitamin group of nutrients. It stimulates the body's production of glutathione and aids in the absorption of coenzyme Q10, both important antioxidants. Because ALA is soluble in both water and fat, it can move into all parts of cells to deactivate free radicals. Lipoic acid is used by the cells mitochondria to help produce energy and it also stimulates the body's immune system.

Supplemental ALA has been used for almost three decades in Europe to treat peripheral nerve degeneration and to help control blood sugar levels in people with diabetes. It also helps to detoxify the liver of metal pollutants, block cataract formation, protect nerve tissues against oxidative stress, and reduce blood cholesterol levels.

According to Lester Packer, Ph.D, Professor of Molecular and Cell Biology at the University of California, Berkeley, and a leading antioxidant researcher, ALA could play an important role in the prevention and treatment of chronic degenerative diseases such as diabetes and cardiovascular disease. ALA is known also as a metabolic antioxidant, because without it, cells cannot use sugar to produce energy. The body does not produce large amounts of ALA, and since it is found primarily in only a few foods e.g. spinach, broccoli, and organ meats (especially liver), supplementation may be necessary to replenish lost supplies.

**Coenzyme Q10**
Coenzyme Q10 is a fat-soluble antioxidant substance that is structurally similar to vitamin E. It plays a crucial role in the generation of cellular energy/oxygenation, is a significant immunologic stimulant, increases circulation, has anti-aging effects, and is beneficial for the cardiovascular system.

Also known as ubiquinone (from quinone, a type of coenzyme, and ubiquitous, because it exists everywhere in the body), coenzyme Q10 is found in highest concentrations in the heart, followed by the liver, kidney, spleen, lungs, and pancreas and adrenal glands.

Within the mitochondria, the cells' 'energy production centres' where 95 per cent of the cells' energy is created, coenzyme Q10 helps to metabolise fats and carbohydrates. It also helps to maintain the flexibility of cell membranes. The average total body content of CoQ10 is only about 500 – 1500 mg and decreases with age.

Coenzyme Q10 is necessary for the formation of adenosine triphosphate (ATP), a compound which acts as an energy donor in chemical reactions. Apart from producing energy for the body, Co Q10 also protects the body from the damage caused by free radicals. The production of Co Q10 in the body depends on adequate availability of folic acid, vitamin B12 and betaine.

In Japan, coenzyme Q10 has been approved for use in treating congestive heart failure. Various research reports suggest that coenzyme Q10 may also be beneficial in the supportive treatment of various cancers; AIDS; muscular dystrophy; allergies; gastric ulcers; myopathy; periodontal disease; diabetes; and deafness.
Research has shown that low levels of Co Q10 have been identified in women who have recently miscarried. Co Q10 improves blood flow; having good blood flow is a very important function to enhance fertility. Women that are undergoing ICSI procedures would be recommended to take additional Co Q10 supplementation as it may improve fertilisation rates.

*CoQ10 is found in foods such as:* hazelnuts; walnuts; chestnuts; almonds; pistachio nuts; peanuts; mackerel; salmon; sardines; eel; yellowtail; organ meats; soy beans; rice bran; wheat germ; broccoli; spinach; cauliflower; cabbage; garlic; onions; eggplant; and carrots.

There is no standard recommended daily allowance for Co Q10; 100-200mg per daily is a general guide.

Both lipoic acid and Co Q 10 are helpful for enhancing sperm motility and protection, and are important in assisting the mitochondrial function of the aging ovum as well. Other nutrients like alpha-ketoglutarate; carnosine; creatine; trimethy glycine; dimethyl glycine (dmg); and octacosanol may also be worth considering, improving mitochondrial function, sperm motility and slowing various aspects of the aging processes.

## Mucopolysaccarides
These are found in all body tissues, and fluids such as blood group substances, blood vessels, cell walls, connective tissue, tendons, joints, intracellular ground substance and mucous membranes and its function to provide structure.

Chondroitin sulphate is one of the compounds that contain these substances.

Among their many functions these substances are also useful for fertility problems as they are part of the composition of semen fluids and may increase its production. It has also been said that they may also have mild aphrodisiac effects.

*Many sources that contain mucopolysaccharides include:* mussels; raw oysters; aloe vera; ginseng; shellfish; oatmeal; comfrey; wheat germ; cactus; calf tracheal cartilage; and shark cartilage.

## Enzymes
There are over 20,000 different enzymes, which are essential for digesting food, stimulating brain function, supplying cellular energy and repairing tissues, organs and cells. Enzymes are known as the 'sparks of life' and are involved in thousands of biochemical reactions in the body. Enzymes assist may organs to function properly and are involved in elimination of toxic wastes from the body.


# Summary of nutrients for specific sexual organs

**Brain:** B vitamins; choline; calcium; magnesium; potassium; L-amino acids group, and tryptophan.

**Pituitary gland:** B vitamins: pantothenic acid (Vitamin B5): niacin (Vitamin B3): Vitamin E: and zinc.

**Adrenal Gland:** Vitamin A; B vitamins; pantothenic acid; niacin; thiamine (Vitamin B1); Vitamin C; Vitamin E; and essential fatty acids.

**Thyroid gland:** Iodine; B vitamins; thiamine; Vitamin E; and tyrosine.

**Ovaries:** B vitamins; niacin; folic acid; Vitamin E; and zinc.

**Testes:** Vitamin E; zinc; Vitamin A; Vitamin C; and folic acid.

**Sperm:** contains calcium; magnesium; zinc; sulphur; Vitamin B12; Vitamin C. ATP (energy) is an absolute requirement for sperm motility, so nucleic acid and especially inosine, are important for fertility.

# Chapter 7

# *Preparing for Conception*

*'Getting ready for the greatest adventure of your life'*

Ideally, conception should be planned for, with both partners aiming for optimal health by the time of the planned conception. Women should stop using the contraceptive pill at least 3 to 6 months prior to attempting to fall pregnant, to allow hormone level to return to normal.

I recommend that both partners, but especially the female, go on a moderate liver (body) detoxification diet for at least 4 weeks, and eliminate any known allergens from the food intake, to reduce possibility of transferring them to baby via placenta or breast milk.

Both partners need a consistently healthy diet, high in vegetables, protein and fish (low in excessive red meats), high in essential fatty acids (EFAs) e.g. omega 3 and 6; fish oil; evening primrose; linseed (flax); vitamins such as Vitamin A (moderate quantities); B complex especially Vitamin B6 and folate (to reduce neural tubal defects); wholemeal organic oats; Vitamin B12; Vitamin C; Vitamin E; and the minerals like zinc, magnesium, and iron.

### *Fertility-Boosting Smoothie*
1 teaspoon honey (1 teaspoon = approximately 5 grams)
1 teaspoon lecithin powder
1 teaspoon LSA powder (blend of linseed (flaxseed), sunflower seed, & almond nuts in a finely ground powder)
1 teaspoon wheat germ (powder or oil)
1 teaspoon yogurt (acidophilus cultured)
1 raw egg (medium size - organic) (note: only a maximum of 3 per week)
½ medium-sized banana (1/2 a cup of strawberries or mango pieces can also be used together or alternately to vary flavour)
250ml low-fat milk, soy milk, nut milk or rice milk (preferred)
Options: 1 tablespoon x low-fat ice cream, sorbet or gelato (preferred); carob powder is also highly nutritious and can add additional flavour and texture to the mixture.
Blend & Serve – approximately every second day
This drink is highly nutritious, packed with protein and makes a delicious refreshing liquid snack.

### Baby-Making Juice

2 carrot sticks (average size)
2 celery sticks (average size)
¼ raw beetroot (average size)
¼ apple (preferably peeled Red Delicious variety)
Options: small amounts of broccoli; brussels sprout; silver beet; kale; cabbage; wheat grass; barley grass; ginger; cranberries; or a pinch of parsley.
Blend all with a vegetable juicing machine & dilute the remaining juice with 50% water (half and half) to makes approximately 250 ml of juice that can be served daily. Do not store for long periods of time as the vital enzymes can be lost via oxidation, best to make and drink as you go!

Freshly made juices are nourishing, living foods in liquid form, providing the body with a rich assortment of vitamins, minerals and abundant enzymes. Raw juices require minimal digestion and can be assimilated by the body very easily.

Juice therapy is a method of detoxifying and cleansing the body of unwanted chemicals, wastes and toxins and supplying beneficial nutrients needed to fight disease. Fresh juices provide a superior vehicle by which unusually high quantities and concentrations of the food's life force can be consumed.

Veggie juices to assist with menstrual problems include: beet; beet greens; swiss chard; and water cress.
Impotence problems: alfalfa sprouts; kale, lamb's quarters, and wheatgrass.
Prostate problems: asparagus; parsley; cherry; pear; strawberry; and watermelon.
Pregnancy: alfalfa sprouts; bean sprouts; beet; beet greens; carrot; kale; lamb's quarters; parsnip; swiss chard; grapefruit; peach; and watermelon.

## Foods to reduce for improving your fertility

*Artificial sweeteners* – there are still few conclusive studies that have been conducted to prove if artificial sweeteners have negative effects on reducing fertility. Products that contain *saccharin* and *aspartame* such as NutraSweet or Equal may best be avoided to be on the safe side. Aspartame is converted to formaldehyde (a poison) once it reaches temperatures in excess of 30°C (86°F); this occurs once it has been ingested. It is then converted to formic acid, which is a very highly toxic substance; aspartame is potentially one of the deadliest neurotoxins in the world. *Sucralose* has a chlorinated base similar to DDT and is linked to auto-immune disease. *Asculfame K* is also quite nasty as it is linked to causing cancers and leukaemia.

*Caffeinated foods and drinks* – if you really can't do without your morning cuppa, I would recommend trying to switch coffee products for tea as a starter. Tea as a rule normally contains a quarter to half the amount of caffeine than most coffee-based products.

Tea also contains several chemical compounds such as aromatic polyphenol and hypoxanthine that may have some benefits for fertility. Having stated this, it is still warranted to keep caffeine intake to very moderate amounts. De-caffeinated products may also be considered as an alternative. Caffeine can also be in various medications, stimulants like No-Doz, weight loss pills, and herbs such as guarana and kola nut. Check product packaging details to verify caffeine content. Also back-off milk /dairy products as much as possible!

**Lunch meat products** – many of these foods contain nitrates and nitrites which are linked to increasing certain cancer growth.

**Food additives and preservatives** – Monosodium glutamine (MSG) and BHA are well known for causing sensitivity reactions and affect body hormone activity and receptability. Hormones such as oestrogen can be particularly imbalanced, which can reduce fertility and/or foetal development. MSG is found as an additive in a lot of foods such as: Chinese take-aways; flavoured chips (crisps); meat seasoning; and packaged soups.

**Peas and soybean products** – can potentially have an effect on fertility as these foods contain phyto-oestrogens. Phyto-oestrogen-containing foods have been extensively studied and are proven to exert numerous health benefits particularly for menopause symptoms and on hormone-dependant cancers, but in excessive amounts these phyto-oestrogen foods exert oestrogen-mimicking-like effects that can be undesirable when trying to fall pregnant.

These foods can possibly unbalance other reproductive hormone levels. Peas contain a natural chemical called *m-xylohydroquinone,* which has been shown in studies to exert a contraceptive effect and can reduce sperm production. Also check on product packaging as these foods can be hidden or are major components of other food preparation.

**Peanuts and spinach** – excessive intake of these foods can possibly reduce body calcium levels, which in turn can affect other nutrient balances and your baby's growth.

**Sweets (lollies), Soda (soft drink) and refined-sugar products** –
excessive intake of these items can contribute to blood sugar fluctuation problems such as *hypoglycaemia* (low blood sugar), which in turn can affect other reproductive hormone levels. Sugar leaches the body of precious vitamins and minerals due to its effect on the body's acidity (ph balance) and increased demand on the detoxification and elimination systems. Every organ in the body can be affected by sugar.

**Saturated fats** – excessive saturated fat consumption needs no great explanation about its negative effects on health and wellbeing. We have all heard how it can contribute to conditions such as: obesity, heart disease, cancer and oestrogen overload. Particularly try to avoid fried food and coconut oil.

*Rare red meats* – uncooked meats can carry contaminates and viruses such as *toxoplasmosis* that can potentially affect the health of baby during gestation.

## Mother Nature giving Cupid a helping hand -'*Feeling Frisky'*

*From Aphrodite to Venus - foods used through-out history to get you in the right mood for love:* alfalfa sprouts; almonds; aloe vera; apples; apricots; artichokes; asparagus; avocados; baby spinach; bananas (if there was ever a 'phallic symbol' of the male appendage – men may not choice the lady finger variety – size matters); beans (though can be a passion-killer if you are prone to gas/flatulence); beetroot; betel nut; berries; broccoli; cabbage; carrots, celery; cauliflower; chives; chocolate; coconut; cucumber; fennel; figs; grapes; garlic (best not to breathe on any one); honey; onions; oysters; peach; pecans; pine nuts; pomegranate; pumpkin seeds; spinach (makes you strong like pop eye); sunflower seeds; pure seafood. Shellfish (eg mussels, scallops and anchovies); quince; snow peas; truffles; raw organic eggs; vanilla; walnuts; wheat germ; and yams.

*Almond Milk* - Nuts, seeds and pulses contain plant chemicals called phytosterols, which are known to promote testosterone production. Nuts also contain magnesium, which balances levels of hormone prolactin, which can compete with testosterone. Almonds are regarded as the most nutrient-containing nut high in important reproductive system nutrients including zinc and L-arginine. Sunflowers also regarded as the most nutrient-containing seed.

*Asparagus* – You're not alone if long, firm, tender stalks evoke erotic images. Nineteenth-century bridegrooms were served three courses of asparagus due to its supposed lover-giving powers.

*Caviar* - Is reputed to have been the virility booster for both Casanova and Rasputin. You too can be a 'Sexual Adonis'.

*Champagne* – known for centuries as the drink of love, moderate quantities of champagne can lower inhibitions and cause a warm, glowing feeling. Just check out the famous lover Casanova – he used champagne to conquer his many lovers.

*Chocolate* – 'Aztec viagra' a renowned aphrodisiac, it may be because of the feel-good chemicals it releases. Chocolate / pure cacao is high in the mood-enhancing amino acid DL-phenylalanine, Phenylethylamine (PEA) which improves opiate (eg Dopamine) responses in the brain. Its benefits may be a combination of aroma, taste, texture and appearance that excites the senses. Chocolate is both a sedative that relaxes, and a stimulant that increases desire.

*Celery seeds* - soaked in water (an infusion) and washed over the male reproductive organ prior to intercourse is said to help in maintaining full erection. The ancient Romans had the right idea when they dedicated celery to

Priapus, their god of fertility and virility. This veggie contains androsterone, a male hormone which, according to researchers, attracts women.

**Fresh Figs** – ancient Greeks celebrated seasonal crops in a frenzied copulation ritual. Many believe the shape of the figs represent womanhood. The legendary Cleopatra's favourite fruit was said to be the fig.

**Garlic (Allium sativum)** - in studies garlic was given in drinking water at doses of 100mg per kilogram of body weight per day over a 3-month period. Results showed that there was significant increase in the weight of seminal vesicles, epididymides and the sperm counts were also significantly elevated.

**Herbs and Spices** – throughout history, various herbs and spices have been used to stimulate the libido, so why not add asafoetida, basil, cloves, garlic, ginger, ginseng, pepper, and cardamom to your menu?

**Honey** – Sweet, spreadable and smoothing, honey is the ultimate love food. While Egyptians offered it to the god of fertility, other cultures encouraged newlyweds to lick honey off each other's palms, ensuring a sweet life together.

**Onion juice** – combined with honey is said to support sperm production.

**Oranges** – age-old customs say lovers who bathe in orange-scented water after the first time they make love will have a long and lust-filled union. Oranges soaked in Grand Marnier liqueur and dipped in chocolate are said to set the loins on fire.

**Oysters** – were another favourite of Casanova who reputedly ate 50 raw ones every day in the bath, with his lady of the moment. They're high in zinc and mucopolysaccharides – essential for the production of sex hormones – and the repeated changing of the oyster's sex from male to female gives it sexual mystique.

**Walnuts** – are a good source of copper, and were used by the Romans to increase libido and sexual desire. They were thrown at newlyweds to increase fertility. If you suffer from an under-active thyroid condition excessive ingestion of walnuts may potentially worsen the condition by increasing the clearance of the thyroid hormone, thyroxine, from the body, though they may benefit those with an overactive thyroid condition.

A dry Martini, shaken not stirred. *Bond....James Bond* (need I say more)!

## Getting your body into good condition

I recommend a moderate exercise program, especially for the ladies, though, if hubby is a self-made man but has been using the wrong materials for the last few years and is now more stomach than man, then this is an activity you can both participate in.

*Regular exercise* makes you feel great, keeps your body flexible and supple, and promotes longevity and healing. Exercise also has a powerful effect on the mind by enhancing the release of pain-relieving and mood-elevating substances in the brain called endorphins and also described as some of our bodies 'happy hormones'. Moderate exercise helps to improve sleep, reduces stress, increases self-esteem, promotes good circulation, enhances cardio-vascular fitness and tones and strengthens the muscular/skeletal systems. It must be remembered that too much exercise can be just as dangerous to our health as too little exercise, so find a happy balance.
*'Those who think they have no time for bodily exercise will sooner or later need to find time for illness'.*

*A spinal check* from your chiropractor or osteopath might also be worth looking into. Over the years, I've observed that pelvic stagnation problems and a tilted uterus can indeed lead to reproductive dysfunctions. *Pelvic congestion* can also occur when the breathing cycle is interrupted. When we breathe, our lungs not only expand and contract, but every part of our body moves subtly, in a rocking fashion, including the pelvis. The subtle rocking of the pelvis causes an expansion and contraction of the muscles within the pelvic walls and the muscles, in turn pump the lymphatic fluid. If the lymphatic pump is slowed down, the pelvis will become fixed and unable to move properly, leading to congestion of the lymph fluids within the pelvis. Injuries to the lower vertebrae of the back and sacro-iliac joints may need to be investigated and treated to restore correct function.

*Regular body-work* such as massage is also good to promote deep relaxation, blood and lymph flow throughout the body.

*Non-essential medications* and drugs such as tobacco, alcohol and coffee would be best avoided or kept to a very minimum. You don't want me rousing on you for that. Check with your doctor first to rule out what can go and what should stay. Diet should be wholesome and as fresh as possible. Periodic mini-fasting on vegetable juices for 3–5 days can be useful, with periods of 2–4 weeks on an adequate protein (mostly vegetarian) diet. Moderate amounts of soy foods are a good choice of protein for females, as they contain phytoeostrogens.

The diet should include plenty of raw and conservatively cooked vegetables; various fresh fruits; plenty of clean (filtered) water (approximately 2 litres daily); seaweed; seeds; nuts; beans; fresh wheat germ; lecithin; LSA (linseed, sunflower seed and almond nut powder); and whole grains. These are all necessary to build a healthy foundation to your diet regime. Try to source organic foods when possible as the nutrient content is very high (in many cases thousands of times higher than other foods) and are void of the harmful pesticides and herbicides.

Also don't forget the basics:

### Getting moderate full-spectrum sun light exposure

*'Let the sunshine in';* the light we are exposed to on a day-to-day basis has an influence on ovulation and reproductive hormones. Lack of adequate sunlight can result in depression, which in turn can suppress fertility. Avoid excessive artificial light sources.

Inadequate full spectrum sunlight exposure effects eye (retinal) – pineal gland and hypothalamus-pituitary hormone production. Gonadotrophic hormones, growth hormones (the youth and regenerating hormone), melatonin and sex hormones can all be disrupted affecting the correct function of the endocrine system. Melatonin is produced by the pineal gland that regulates our circadian rhythm; if you have ever experienced jet-lag or are a shift-worker you will know what it feels like when it's out of balance. Sunlight is needed to recharge the bodies' cellular batteries. Try to get at least 20 minutes of quality sunlight every day and leave your sunglasses at home.

### Getting quality sleep

It helps to restore and rejuvenate the brain and organ systems including the reproductive system. Lack of sleep may even lead to menstrual irregularities that may be a factor in delaying conception. It appears that the hormones that trigger ovulation, and even the sperm maturation process, are somehow tied into the body's biological clock.

The release of sleep-wake hormones such as melatonin, serotonin and cortisol is triggered, in part, by information given to the brain by its 'light meter' the pineal gland usually involving light reception on the retina of the eye. The same part of the brain that regulates sleep-wake hormones also stimulates daily pulses of reproductive hormones for men and women via a feedback cycle.

Remember the rule of thumb of having eight hours of sleep, eight hours of work, and eight hours of play. It has been reported that the best quality of sleep is achieved prior to midnight, therefore try to get into a routine of getting to sleep earlier.

Some natural remedies to improve sleep quality include: Nutrients - Calcium, magnesium, niacin (B3), B6, B12; Adenosine (the sleep molecule of the brain) – at 100 to 200mg sucked sublingually under the tongue nightly; supplemental melatonin – starting at 3mg daily dosage; Tryptophan or 5-hydroxytryptophan (5-HT) precursors to the 'happy happy joy joy' chemical – serotonin, taking in the morning.

Herbal remedies may include: Valerian spp, chamomile, corydalis, lavender, pulsatilla, jamaica dogwood, lemon balm, california poppy, passionflower, polygala, skullcap, kava, hops, oat green / seed, withania, and zizyphus.

### Get plenty of pure 'negatively charged' unpolluted air

Good quality air is necessary to balance our oxygen and nitrogen for cells to regenerate. Life doesn't exist without it. Avoid long-term exposure to air conditioning systems.

### Electromagnetic fields (EMF)

Try to avoid as much EMF exposure as possible. Some evidence suggests that humans may actually require a low-level field of EMF exposure in order to reproduce (the earth's core and thunderstorm naturally radiate low-field EMF). The type that is detrimental to our health is the low-field ionising EMFs, which we are exposed to from X-rays and air travel (cosmic radiation).

Non—ionising EMFs are not fully understood in regards to their effects on reductive function. This form of EMF is sourced from radio frequencies, microwaves, lasers, and electric appliances, high voltage lines and power outputs. To be on the safe side it is probably best to minimise your close proximity to power point outlets and switch off as many non-essential appliances as possible, including the bedside clock, electric blankets, video display units and computer monitors.

Studies have revealed that women who worked in an environment high in EMF exposure were three and a half times more likely to have impaired fertility from endometriosis, and two and a half times more likely to have cervical factors (which could impede the sperm ability to penetrate) in comparison to other women not exposed to similar working environments. This also applies equally to men as well.

Reishi mushroom, burdock and grapeseed are good examples of some phytoceuticals that may help to protect the body from the effects of radiation. Epsom salt (magnesium sulphate) can absorb radiation, as do cactus plants. The spider plant, or African violet, is also believed to be a natural detoxifier that can absorb ions and naturally balance humidity. Its hairy leaves can trap dust particles and remove toxins. The geranium scent it emanates is refreshing and is said to harmonise negative emotions as well!

Crystals such as amethysts and quartz combat atmospheric pollution and electro-magnetic fields; they are also said to be beneficial when promoting healing. A good idea to put next to your computer or other high-radiation output area!

Last but definitely not least, **a positive mental attitude**. The essence of life! Attitude is also an important factor in the process of health maintenance and healing. We must have a positive state of mind in order to bring harmony to the body. The realisation that the body (lifestyle), spirit (desire), and mind (belief) must come together is the first step to better health.

# Getting the Body Detoxified

The Detoxification Phase is the first stage in the fertility program and an important step in preparing conception. Males will need some 90 days to make complete new sperm. It may seem like a long time, but the sperm made today only become available in 90 days from today. Females need a minimum of 50 days; 3 months is recommended. You may feel okay, even though your body may be extremely toxic. However, when the body detects too many toxins in the bloodstream, it sounds 'warning bells'; this is medically called the 'Herxheirmer effect' (which is more commonly referred to as a 'Healing Crisis').

This detoxification reaction may not be apparent in some individuals for up to several weeks after commencing a detox program. The type of symptoms that may be experienced can closely mimic those of a common cold, for example: fatigue; bad breath; headaches; some muscle aches and pains; smelly perspiration; stronger-smelling urine; increased bowel movements; increased menstruation with dark blood and clots; and running nose can all be part of this process of eliminating toxins from the body systems.

Even at the time, for some people the 'Healing Crisis' symptoms may feel severe, but it is well worth the effort to see the process through this cleaning phase. The general results in the end are like feelings of renewal with boundless energy to burn like they haven't had in years.

There are a number of various detoxification therapies and techniques that can be used to assist in enhancing your cleansing process.

***Chelation therapy*** is a method used by some doctors, which requires the administering of intravenous solutions (through the veins, in a drip). The most common chelating agent is a type of amino acid called ethylene-diamine-tetra-acetate (EDTA). The molecules of EDTA bond to and chelate (remove) many toxins and heavy metals from the body, via the kidneys. Chelation helps to remove lead, strontium, aluminium, cadmium, mercury, and other toxins. This technique is quite invasive and can also lead to the leeching of vital nutrients as a casualty of the process.

Other less invasive and natural methods of detoxification may include the use of some of the following techniques and or agents:

- Drinking plenty of pure, filtered water; at least eight glasses (2 litres) is required daily. Personal factors may vary this amount.

- Cut out caffeine beverages such as coffee and black tea. Dandelion tea or coffee is an excellent substitute during a detoxification program particularly as a liver cleanser.

- Taking a fibre supplement such as: psyllium seed husks; slippery elm; guar gum; pectin; rice bran; and marshmallow root helps to improve the evacuation of toxins through the bowel.

- Foods that support the body's detoxification processes may include:

    Vegetables: broccoli; cabbage; cauliflower (from the Brassica food family); garlic; onions; asparagus; avocado (source of glutathione); kale (source of B vitamins); globe artichoke (Cynara scolymus) (natural detoxifier particularly for the liver and gallbladder); beetroot; carrots; sweet potatoes; pumpkin; spinach; celery; watercress; parsley; coriander; and zucchini. Wheat grass juice is an excellent detoxifier and rejuvenator.

    Fruits: apples; pears (high in pectin); apricots; peaches; mangos; melons; papayas; pineapples; bananas; kiwi fruit; all berries (high in antioxidants; lemon; pulses; whole grain rice; millet; and olive oil.

- Reduce orange and orange juice consumption.

- Colon irrigations and enemas are also other techniques that can be introduced into a detoxification regime.

- Extra Vitamin C and bioflavonoids may be required during the cleansing process and may assist in minimising rebound healing crisis symptoms.

- Having an Epsom salt bath (magnesium sulphate) on a daily basis helps to relax the muscles and draw the toxins through the skin.

- Dry skin brushing using long strokes all over your body towards the heart helps to move lymph, improve circulation, exfoliate (remove) dead skin and open pores so impurities can escape.

- Make sure you are getting plenty of rest and quality sleep.

- Get into vegetable juicing (similar to the recipe mentioned earlier).

- Drink 2 glasses of lukewarm pure water with a squeeze of lemon and/or lime daily. Then you could also add two teaspoons of genuine maple syrup and a $1/10^{th}$ of a teaspoon of cayenne pepper to increase the detoxification process. (This is also known as one of the Hollywood detox diets). Adding 2 to 4mls daily of liquid zeolite supplement is helpful in eliminating heavy metals and other toxins from the body, as well as protecting the body from radiation.

- Another drink to help clean the colon may include a combination of: 1 tablespoon of bentonite clay powder, 1 teaspoon of psyllium husks, ½ cup of apple juice, ¼ cup of aloe vera juice, and ½ cup of warm water.

- Massage and other body work techniques are very useful to have during your cleansing phase as they assist in manually draining toxins out of the tissues and help to energise the body. Aromatherapy oils assist in relaxation, rejuvenation and detoxification.

- Herbal remedies/teas may include: alfalfa; bupleurum falcatum; dandelion root (taraxacum officinale radix); ginger; green tea (camellia sinensis); red clover; rosehip; chamomile; lemongrass; milk thistle or St Mary's thistle (silybum marianum); schizandra chinensis; turmeric (curcuma longa); and peppermint.

- Herbs to flush the colon may include: aloe vera; cascara sagrada; dandelion root; flaxseed; red raspberry; rhubarb; butter nut; senna and triphala (an ayurvedic combination of three fruits – amla, bihara, and harda). Look after your colon, and your colon will look after you!

- Consume reasonable qualities of super-greens and foods such as: garlic; apple pectin; wheatgrass; barley grass; sea kelp; spirulina; and chlorella.

- Activated charcoal tablets help to remove poisons, miso paste can remove nicotine and other toxins, amino acids L-cysteine (remove mercury), and L-methionine, taurine (liver detoxifier), glycine, L-lysine and glutathione also remove numerous toxins and heavy metals.

- Bentonite clay used internally and externally draws toxins out.

- Nutrients may include: Minerals - calcium and magnesium chelate; potassium; chromium; copper chelate; iron; zinc chelate; and rutin. Vitamins – Vitamins B1, B5, B6, B12, folic acid, Vitamin C, and choline. Anti-oxidants may include: N-Acetyl-Cysteine (a precursor to Glutathione); Glisodin (Cucumis melo juice) contains Superoxide Dismutase enzyme; selenium and co enzyme Q 10.

- Eat small meals regularly throughout the day and avoid high simple sugar-containing foods and foods that may cause potential allergy reaction such as dairy and wheat based products.

- Hydrotherapy and thermal heating and cooling effects of water are responsible for its therapeutic effects in healing. It is great at enhancing circulation and hence removing toxic wastes through the mobilisation of white blood cells.

- Alternating between hot and cool can help to open blood vessels, enhance lymphatic drainage and draw out impurities throughout the body to improve organ function. Once you have triumphed your way through this cleansing process you will gain a much greater feeling of overall health and wellness.

157

# Chapter 8

# *Plan B: Alternative and Complementary Therapies*

**'Back to the Future.' The low-tech, low-invasive approach to boosting your chances of success**

This following chapter will explore the many and varied types of complementary therapies that are available today that can be utilised in the treatment process of reproductive and related conditions. Many of these therapies have been adapted over a rich history of hundreds to thousands of years of therapeutic application. If you are considering taking a more pro-active role in the treatment process to help restore and resurrect your general wellbeing and reproductive functions, then this section of information will help to demystify and familiarise you with the many beneficial uses that alternative and complementary medicine systems have to offer.

## Acupuncture

### *Pinpointing the problem*
Acupuncture originated in China over five thousand years ago. The philosophical foundation of acupuncture is the same as described in *Traditional Chinese Medicine*. There is a growing understanding and respect in Western cultures of the immense therapeutic benefits that acupuncture has given Asian culture for centuries.

Acupuncture treatments involve the insertion of special needles (or more recently laser beams, ultra sound waves, sonar rays, and electro stimulation) into the various *acupoints* (just under the skin) within the *meridian* system. There are over one thousand of these points throughout the body. By stimulating these specific locations the flow of *qi* and body's electric current is enhanced to help correct and restore the balance of health.

In addition to the use of needles, other forms of treatment are applied to acupoints. Heat is used by burning a herb called *Moxa (jiu)* made from mugwort (artemisia vulgaris) above the point to be treated (moxibustion). The mugwort herb is used because of its unique properties that can stimulate acupoints and hasten the healing process. In acupuncture, the practitioner may burn a pinch of moxa on a slice of ginger atop an acupoint, or alternatively, placed directly on the point and removed quickly as soon as the point feels too warm to the patient.

Mugwort is also used in a form which is rolled into a cigar-shape called a moxa stick and waved in a rotating manner about one inch away from the skin over the deserved acupuncture point.

Another traditional technique used in treatments is called *cupping* which involves utilising glass or bamboo cups that create a suction vacuum over the acupoint or painful muscle area and draws blood to that particular site.

Acupuncture can be applied for numerous health ailments and can help to promote a general sense of emotional and physical wellbeing. The acupuncturist may assess for example that a women's uterus may be in a 'cold' state that may manifest as menstrual irregularity, pelvic inflammation, abnormal vaginal discharge, depressed liver function, and so on. Treatment may in this instance be focused on stimulating the various points needed to re-balance the menstrual hormones, strengthen the kidney function and improve blood and energy flow, to nourish the uterus. This can assist in the 'absorption' of the yang energy of the sperm in enhancing conception.

Studies have shown the positive therapeutic effectiveness of acupuncture on both male and female reproductive dysfunctions. Recent clinical trials in Germany and China found acupuncture given for 25 minutes pre and post embryo transfer during IVF procedures improved conception rate almost *2-fold*. 26.3 per cent of control group conceived in comparison to 42.5 per cent of the acupuncture group.

There are twelve major meridians, or channels, that run throughout the body. Each channel is associated with a specific Organ system. The twelve main channels are usually described in pairs, reflecting the link between energy systems and organs in Traditional Chinese Medicine. These pairs (and abbreviations) are as follows.

| Yin Organ | | Paired Yang Organ | |
|---|---|---|---|
| Lung | Lu | Large Intestine | Li |
| Spleen | Sp | Stomach | St |
| Kidney | Ki | Urinary Bladder | UB |
| Liver | Lv | Gallbladder | GB |
| Heart | Ht | Small Intestine | SI |
| Pericardium | Pc | Triple Warmer, or San Jiao | SJ |

**Note**: These points and others (and/or abbreviations) will be referred to throughout various sections in this book.

**In TCM (Traditional Chinese Medicine) terms infertility is basically divided into two main categories:**

1. Hormonal; and
2. Structural (i.e. obstructive).

Of these two major categories TCM further differentiates the cause of infertility into:

1. Deficiency syndromes; or
2. Excess syndromes.

The deficiency category (i.e. hormone imbalance) is subdivided into:

1. Kidney Essence deficiency / Qi-Blood dual deficiency; or
2. Liver Qi stagnation (liver qi stagnation can be either a deficiency or excess syndrome type).

The Excess category comprises the following:   Phelm-Damp retention and/or blood stasis.

In reality, individuals present with a mixed-matched combination of these syndromes. A skilled Acupuncturist/Traditional Chinese Medicine (TCM) practitioner recognises these differing patterns and adapts appropriate treatments to bring about a state of harmony and balance back within the body.

*Kidney Essence Deficiency* – In basic terms, the reproductive aspect of kidney essence includes all of the tissues and fluid secretions that are involved in human reproduction. This portion of kidney essence controls sexual maturation, fertility and the capacity to reproduce. Kidney essence requires constant replenishing, which is provided by the spleen activities. Kidney essences can become depleted when other aspects in excess e.g. overwork, overuse of alcohol, drugs, excessive sexual/physical activities, (work hard, play harder), inadequate rest. Deficiencies of the Zang organs such as the spleen and lung, chronic illness, and day-to-day life processes will also cause insufficiency of kidney essence.

Kidney essence deficiency usually manifests as a predominant deficiency of the Kidney YIN or deficiency of the Kidney YANG.

*Kidney Yang-Essence Deficiency* –
Characterised by *Cold* signs: Late/long menstrual cycle (can be amenorrhea, scanty, or pale flow); general intolerances to cold; cold extremities; cold lower abdomen; sexual hypofunction; low libido; lack of vaginal secretions; copious and clear urination; pale swollen and moist tongue; deep, weak and slow pulse; usually severe fatigue; dizziness; and depressed mood.

160

**Treatment principles**: To warm and tonify the Kidney Yang and enrich the Kidney Essence. TCM herbal formulas may include: BA JI YIN YANG WAN (Morinda formula) or YOU GUI WAN (Right turning formula).

### Kidney Yin-Essence Deficiency –
Characterised by *Heat* signs: Short/early menstruation (can be light-coloured flow, absence of clots); general intolerance to heat; dry mouth; night sweats; thirst at night; red tongue with little to no coat, dry and may have cracks; pulse thready and rapid; increased libido; and frequent sexual dreams.

**Treatment principles**: To nourish the Kidney Yin and enrich the kidney essence. TCM herbal formulas may include: ZUO GUI WAN (Left returning formula) with SI WU WAN (Danggui four combinations).

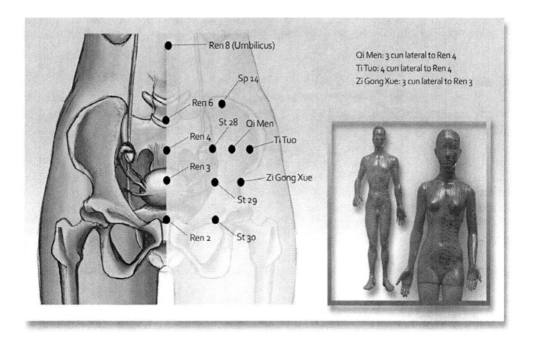

*Figure.14. Acupuncture Meridian Points*

## Points that help to regulate hormonal imbalances

## Women

### Conception Vessel 4
This point is located five-finger widths below the navel on the mid-line of the belly. Tonify this point to invigorate the blood and regulate menstruation.

### Spleen 6

This point is located four finger widths above the interior anklebone, in the shallow hollow just behind the tibia. Disperse this point to regulate chi and the blood in the uterus. *DO NOT use these two points if you are, or may be, pregnant.

### Spleen 10

If the menstrual cycle tends to be short: bend the leg at a right angle of 90 degrees. Get someone to place the finger of their opposite hand, right on left, and vice versa along the front of your kneecap, and stretch the thumb backwards towards your groin. The tip of their thumb will be on Spleen 10, 5 cm above your knee. Disperse to circulate chi and blood.

### Stomach 36

Bend your knee as for Spleen 10. Catch your kneecap between index finger and thumb. The middle finger is in the outside of your shinbone, and Stomach 36 is at the tip of this finger, outside the tibia. Disperse to circulate chi and blood.

### Kidney 1

The kidney meridian governs sexual energy, and the end of the meridian is a powerful point in fertility. This point is at the centre of the ball of the foot. Disperse this point with your thumb for help in conceiving.

## Men

## Conception Vessel 6

On the vertical line, two finger widths below the navel, tonify this point; **CV 4** – as before, four finger widths; **CV 2** – on the same line, at the crest of the pubis.

**Governing Vessel 4** – Between the third and fourth lumbar vertebrae.

## Bladder 31, 32, 33, 34

Along each side of the sacrum to the tip of the coccyx. These four points run down either side of the spine, parallel to the four fused vertebrae of the sacrum. The points are three finger widths on each side of the backbone.

**Spleen 6, Ren 12, Ren 4** – stimulated with moxibustion may also benefit improving sperm activity and quality.

**General reproductive system acupuncture points**:

These points when stimulated regularly may help to improve hormonal responsiveness, increased blood flow and boost efficiency of the reproductive organs.

### Ear Triangular Fossa

This point is located in the upper, inner part of the ear.

### Ear Intertragica Notch
This point is located just above the earlobe in the crevice between the two cartilaginous areas in the lowest point side inside the ear.

### Epang II: (Scalp Reproductive Points)
These points are found above the forehead within the scalp, just inside the upper corner of the hairline above the outside of the eyebrow, or where you feel sensitivity.

### Zigong: (Palace of the Child)
This point is located four inches below the navel and three inches lateral to the midline.

### Ren 3: (Central pole of the conception meridian) – This point is located on the midline, four inches below the navel.

### Ren 4: (Origin of the source of the conception meridian)
This point is located on the midline, two inched below the navel. Ren 4 represents the source of life point and is called the *Dan Tien*.

### Stomach 30: (Rushing Qi)
This point is located on the lower abdomen, five inches beneath the navel and two inches lateral to the midline, just above the superior border of the pubic symphysis.

### Kidney 16: (Vital Shu)
This point is located one inch on either side of or level with the umbilicus.

Studies have shown the acupuncture treatments impacts on B – endorphins, which in turn affects the levels of gonadotrophin-releasing hormone (GnRH), and has been used in an attempt to regulate hormonal imbalance and specifically to adjust FSH and LH levels.

In Traditional Chinese Medicine (TCM) a creative substance called *'Jing'*, is believed to be the creative energy that is passed from the parents to the child at conception, this is said to fortify our constitutional health.

# Ayurvedic Medicine

Ayurvedia is an ancient and comprehensive system of complementary medicine that originated in India over five thousand years ago, though it is believed that the true origins many even date back as far as forty thousand years. Ayurveda (Ayu = life/longevity) (Veda = Science) meaning the *science of life*. Ayurveda places equal emphasis on body, mind and spirit, and strives to restore the innate harmony of the individual.

The keystone of Ayurvedic medicine is the belief of *constitutions* that refer to the concept of metabolic body types or *Doshas,* which consider an individual's overall health profile, including strengths and susceptibilities. The subtle and often intricate identification of a person's constitution is the foundation to this critical process of matching treatment protocols to the individual's correct constitutional type.

The three metabolic body types are known as **Vata, Pitta**, and **Kapha.** They include distinction of physique to the Western view of body types as thin, muscular, and fat. In Ayurvedic medicine these constitutions are recognised as having a far greater influence on a person's overall health and wellbeing than is adopted by Western medicine.

The Ayurvedic body typing could be likened to a blueprint which outlines all the innate tendencies built into a person's system. Most people are a mixture of *dosha* characteristics (such as Vata–Pitta), with one usually more predominant than another. Each of the body types flourishes under a specific diet, exercise plan, and lifestyle. When there is balance of the doshas in accordance with an individual's constitution, the body, mind and spirit will also be in harmony and balanced, therefore, resulting in vibrant health and energy.

When the doshas are imbalanced (*Vikriti*) or are not in equilibrium, then the mind and body becomes susceptible to negative stressors and 'dis-ease' will follow.

In Ayurveda the 'Dosha' is an interpretation of constitutional energy, which can assist in also showing what certain seasons may be best to attempt conception. The sacred ceremony for impregnation is known in Ayurveda as *Garbabhana samskara.*

**The various body types or *prakrita* include:**

| | |
|---|---|
| Monodoshic | Vata = V or Pitta = P or Kapha = K |
| Bidoshic combinations | VP, VK, PK, PV, KP, or KV |
| Tridoshic combination | VPK |

## The *Vata* Body Type

The Vata metabolic type is changeable, unpredictable, and various in action, mood and shape.

- Thin; bony; elongated face; light in weight; tall or short in build; skin is dry and coarse; extremities are cold; low endurance; hyperactive. The Vata is good at initiating things but is poor at finishing them.
- Small deep-set eyes, close together or far apart, dark sclera (white part of the eye); vivacious; eats and sleeps at all hours (erratic); imaginative; impulsive; nervous disorders; teeth are very small or protruding, crooked, and easily cracked.
- Prominent features; joints are loose or rigid and are pronounced; hands/ fingers are very long or very short; hair is thin, coarse, dry and wiry.
- Prone to constipation; cramps; insomnia; premenstrual syndrome; tongue is rough, cracked or 'geographic'; body odour has little to no smell or perspiration; they tend to skip meals; sleep lightly; are restless; learn very easily though has poor long-term memory, but good short-term memory,
- The personality of the Vata is enthusiastic, performs activity very rapidly and has fluctuating energy and moods. They are also intuitive people and anxious by nature.

## The *Pitta* Body Type

The Pitta metabolic type is relatively predictable and is of medium build, height, strength and endurance. Their body weight is stable, moderate and is proportionately maintained.

- Often fair, frequently have red or blond hair, thin, fine, soft and may grey or bald early; the face is oval, angular and medium in shape; skin is sensitive, warm, perspire heavily, slightly oily, moist, delicate, and freckly, prone to acne; haemorrhoids; ulcers; stomach ailments such as heartburn.
- Extremities are usually always warm to hot; the eyes are sharp with an intense, penetrating gaze and are sensitive to light; the sclera is yellowish to red; teeth are moderate size and yellowish.
- Hands/fingers are medium length and oval shaped; nails are slightly oily and a pinky or copper colour; joints are smooth and flexible; chest is medium and ribs are not so visible; body odour is strong; tongue is pink, reddish and soft pigmented.
- The Pitta personality is often orderly; efficient; intense; short tempered; can be critical; doesn't usually miss meals (eats regularly and have a strong digestive capacity); sleeps regularly; lives by the clock; has good short- and long-term memory; intelligent; warm; loving; articulate; passionate; is usually described as being impatient; and is a 'perfectionist'.

## The *Kapha* Body Type

The Kapha metabolic type is solid, heavy set, and strong, with a tendency towards being overweight. Everything about Kapha is slow and relaxed.

- Hair is thick and glossy, wavy; face is round; full, stocky and large framed; skin is cool, thick, pale and oily; body temperature is cool; great endurance; eyes are large, attractive, with long, thick lashes; the eyes are moist and tend to be teary; the sclera is white and glossy.
- Hands/fingers are thick, stubby and fleshy; teeth are white, strong and large; nails are thick, well rooted, soft glossy and white; joints are strong; body odour is usually nil; tongue is thick, pale pink, fleshy and moist.
- Kaphas are slow to anger; eat slowly; appetite is mild; sleep long and heavily; are slow to act; plethoric.
- The Kapha personality is known to procrastinate and be obstinate; they are affectionate; compassionate; very patient; tolerant; forgiving; steady mood, not easily flustered or hurried. The Kapha type is prone to high cholesterol; obesity; allergies; and sinus problems.

## Ayurvedic Medicine and the management of disease

There are 4 basic principles that Ayurvedic medicine applies in the treatment of disease and imbalance.

### *Shodan* or Cleansing and Detoxifying
Correct detoxification in the treatment of disease is placed in very high esteem in the Ayurvedic system of medicine. Purifying techniques collectively called *pancha karma* are commonly adopted to assist in removal of toxins that are considered the root of disease state.

### *Shaman* or Palliation
This stage in the management of disease is used to assist the balance the bodily *doshas. Shaman* is a combination of healing modalities that include using herbs, fasting, chanting, yoga, breathing techniques, meditation, exercise, and limited sun exposure. Palliation also focuses on the spiritual level of healing; *Shaman* emphasises the preventative and curative cycle of the healing process.

One method that is used for Kapha and Vata types is known as 'kindling the fire'; this technique stimulates the gastric function using a combination of honey, and herbs such as long pepper, ginger, cinnamon, and black pepper.

### *Rasayana (ra-sign'-ana)* or Rejuvenation
This phase of the healing process is the tonification stage. Tonification means enhancing the body's inherent ability to function, and could be likened to a physiological tune-up/service. This level of healing focuses on restoring virility and vitality to the reproductive system, counters sterility and infertility, helps

improve sexual performance, and enhances the health of future progeny. Rasayana is also employed to slow the biological processes of aging. The treatments used at this stage of healing may include herbal remedies prepared in pills, powders, and tablets, mineral remedies, exercise, special yoga positions and breathing techniques, which are matched to the specific requirements of the individual's *dosha* type to rejuvenate and restore the body's tissues and organs.

### Satvajaya (Sat-va-j-eye'-a) or Mental Hygiene (Spiritual Healing)

The Satvajaya techniques of healing focus on the higher level being the spiritual and mental functions. This method involves the use of *Mantra* or sound therapy, for the vibration pattern of the mind; *Yantra,* to take the mind out of its ordinary modes of thinking by concentrating of geometric figures. *Tantra* helps to alter the state of one's consciousness; decongests and refreshes the mind to direct energies through the body and rid the body free of negative emotions and thought patterns. This is achieved with meditation, gems, crystals, colour, light therapy and other techniques and natural medicines.

Ayurveda is comparable or very similar to the philosophies and practices of other holistic health care modalities such as Traditional Chinese Medicine (TCM).

Like TCM, Ayurveda also believes in the theory of the **Five Great Elements (Panchamahabhuta)** as follows:

Space (Akash); Air (Vaya); Fire (Agni); Water (Jala); Earth (Prithivi).

### The Four Aspects of Life (AYU)

Atma:     The Soul
Mamas:     The Mind
Indriya :     The 5 Senses
Sharira:     The Body

### The Tridoshic Theory

*Dosha* - the functional intelligences within the body

**Vata** (Space, Ether, and Air): energy of movement; communication; transport. Emotions.

**Pitta** (Fire and Water): energy of digestion; conversion; hormone; metabolism; and enzyme activity. Intellect.

**Kapha** (Water and Earth): energy of structure; cohesion; liquidity; lubrication; Anabolic.

## Greco–Roman 'Humoral' Theory

The ancient 'Humoral' theory evolved over thousands of years from Greco-Roman origin. This system of medicine parallels close similarities to that of the ancient Traditional Chinese Medicine and Ayurvedic system of medicines and philosophies. The Humoral theory was developed with many interlocking governing laws based on four fundamental interacting and opposing elements.

Humours refers to the 'semi-gaseous' fluids or 'body fluids' (however, in modern medicine science does not equate to identified body constituents). Like other holistic systems, the humours are represented as being in a state of balance when the person is healthy. Ill-health is represented when one of these humour elements is relatively to dominate in respect to the other humours.

### The four humours are recognised as:
Blood, Phlegm, Yellow Bile, and Black Bile. (These humours are believed to arise from the liver and represent various degrees of ingestion, digestion, absorption and elimination of food and nutrients.)

### The four governing elements are recognised as:
Air, Earth, Fire and Water

### The four governing qualities are recognised as:
Cold, Dry, Hot and Moist.

These give each individual their unique constitution or temperament personality type.

### The four temperament types are recognised as:
Choleric, Melancholic, Phlegmatic and Sanguine.

The primary generative energy or *vital force* of this Greco-Roman 'Humoral' theory is known as **Pneuma**.

## The Humours

### Blood
The humours theory represents the blood as being made from the best quality, and thoroughly digested food. It is transmuted into fresh, normal body secretions such as breast milk, menstrual blood and sperm. Blood is the humour for *digestion*.

### Phlegm
The phlegm humour is made from second-best quality nutrients and digestion. It makes the digestive juices, mucus, saliva and sweat. This humour assists with *elimination* of wastes from the body.

### Yellow Bile

Yellow bile is thought to be made from the coarser and less-refined nutrients; it makes the bile and enhances ingestion and assimilation of nutrients.

### Black Bile

This humour is composed from the least digestible and least nutritious part of food. Black bile is believed to be stored in the spleen and improves the ability to absorb and retain food until properly digested.

## The Temperaments /Constitutional types

### Choleric

A choleric individual is described as quick to anger; bilious; impatient; irritable; and passionate. Choleric types are governed by the fire element and have hot and dry qualities. This person is inclined to a sallow complexion, and is slender in physical build. The choleric women may be subject to heavy, periods with fiery, hot red blood.

### Melancholic

Melancholics are governed by Black Bile, the element Earth, and the Cold and Dry qualities. This temperament type is creative, intellectually gifted, and inclined to be spiritual. The melancholic is inclined to frequent illness, depression, and physical weakness. Women of the melancholic constitution type are believed to have heavy menstrual periods and have more difficulties with fertility.

### Phlegmatic

The phlegmatic is a serene and even-tempered individual. Physically, phlegmatic are usually of average build. This type is governed by the Water element and the Cold and Moist qualities.

The phlegmatic woman's periods are not excessively troublesome and the flow of the blood is neither too light or too much.

### Sanguine

The sanguine individual is described as amorous, courageous, hopeful and optimistic. This constitution is related to the Blood humour, the Air element that is comprised of the Hot and Moist qualities. Sanguine females are usually well-mannered individuals who are believed to suffer from few gynaecological problems and the menstrual periods are usually normal.

# Herbal Medicine

### Botanicals used for reproductive health
### 'The Gift from Mother Nature – spicing things up'

There is currently a renaissance occurring in the appreciation of plants as medicinal agents. Public demand for access to natural remedies and alternatives in treatment for health concerns is increasing at a massive rate. This is an area within the broad spectrum of medicine where natural medicines are at the forefront of the health revolution.

Herbs and botanical plants have provided mankind with medicines from the beginning of civilisation. Throughout history, various cultures have handed down accumulated knowledge of medicinal plant use to successive generations. This vast body of information serves as the basis for much of traditional medicine today.

Phytomedicine is a more recently used term to describe whole-plant preparations of herbal medicines, rather than just using the single isolated (usually synthetically created) chemical compound that is characteristic of orthodox medical drug preparations. By utilising the whole extract of the plant rather than an isolated part of it, herbalists believe there is a more synergistic and counterbalancing effect with the other active ingredients contained within the plant that nature has provided.

Approximately 25 to 50 per cent of all prescription drugs contain ingredients isolated from herbs and plants. There are estimated between 250,000 to 500,000 plants remaining on the earth today (the number varies depending on whether subspecies are included). This illustrates the need for modern science to turn a wider attention to the plant world to investigate and seek the answers to our growing health care questions. Considering 121 prescription drugs come from only 90 species of plants, 74 per cent of these were discovered following up folklore claims. Approximately 25 per cent of all fertility prescription drugs are still derived from trees, shrubs and herbs. Due to the massive daily loss of forestation due to industry, it is vital that more research and investigation be focused on locating and regenerating threatened varieties of plants. Logic would suggest that there might still be more invaluable therapeutic treasures out there?

The World Health Organisation (WHO) has estimated that two thirds of the world population still uses traditional complementary therapies as their primary treatment protocol for health complaints in comparison with orthodox medicine (allopathy). The use of herbal/phyto medicines makes up a very large proportion of this number. Herbs are the world's original pharmaceuticals; modern medicine today would not have evolved without botanical medicine first showing us the way.

All animal life on earth has evolved from a food chain based on plants. Humans, like other animals, eat plants and other animals in order to nourish and replace body cells and create life force. This evolution within the living surrounding of other plants and animals means that human beings are biologically compatible with plants because they derive from the same source. All the nutrient ingredients necessary to create and maintain life in its healthiest form are contained within living matter. Life is derived from and maintained by chemical reactions and life is designed to be health.

*'He causeth the grass to grow for the cattle and herbs for the service of man.'*
**Psalms 104:14**

## The Therapeutic Action of Herbal Medicine

Orthodox medicine uses a lot of big, technical and complicated words to describe various disease names, drugs and procedures. Herbal medicine also has its own in-house lingo that explains the pharmacology and actions that medicinal plants can have on directly affecting the physiology of the body.

These therapeutic actions may be due to a specific chemical present in the plant or it may be due to a complex interaction between various constituents of the plant. These various actions have been categorised into groups that depict their potential therapeutic applications, the many and various types of herbal medicines may have numerous crossover actions and be used and interchangeable in a number of differing health conditions.

Here is a basic crash course of some of these major categories and terminology used to describe herbal actions:

- **Adaptogenic**: a substance that increases the body's resistance to physical, environmental, emotional or biological stressors and promotes normal physiological function.
- **Alterative** (also referred to as depurative, blood purifiers): a substance that improves detoxification and aids elimination to reduce the accumulation of metabolic waste products within the body. Alterative also help to gradually restore proper function of the body and slowly change the course of a disease. These substances are largely used to treat chronic skin and musculoskeletal disorders.
- **Anti-inflammatory**: a substance that reduces inflammation.
- **Analgesic** (also referred to as Anodyne)**:** a substance that relieves pain.
- **Antiandrogenic**: a substance that inhibits or modifies the action of androgens (male sex hormones).
- **Alkaloids**: a plant originating nitrogenous compound that has numerous physiological effects.
- **Antiemetic**: a substance that reduces nausea and vomiting.
- **Antacid**: a substance that counteracts or neutralises acidity in the gastrointestinal tract.

171

- **Antimicrobial**: (also referred to as Antiseptic) a substance that inhibits the growth or destroys micro-organisms. Others that fall into this category are anthelmintic (worms); antibacterial (bacteria); antifungal (fungi); antiparasitic (parasites); and antiviral (viruses).
- **Antioxidant**: a substance that protects against oxidation and free radical damage.
- **Aphrodisiac**: a substance that stimulates sexual desire.
- **Anxiolytic**: a substance that alleviates anxiety.
- **Astringent**: a substance that causes constriction of the mucous membranes and exposed tissue, usually by precipitating proteins (this action has the effect of producing a barrier on the mucus or exposed skin).
- **Anabolic**: a substance that assist the body the build up tissue.
- **Bitter tonic**: a substance that is bitter tasting that stimulates the upper gastrointestinal tract via stimulating the bitter-taste buds in the mouth.
- **Carminative**: a substance that relieves flatulence and soothes intestinal spasm and pain, usually by relaxing intestinal muscle and sphincters.
- **Cathartic** (also referred to as a Purgative)**:** a substance that assists or induces evacuation of the bowel (having a strong laxative action).
- **Cholagogue**: a substance that increases the release of stored bile from the gallbladder.
- **Choleretic**: a substance that increases the production of bile by the liver.
- **Circulatory stimulant**: a substance that improves blood flow through body tissues.
- **Counter-irritant**: a substance that produces a superficial inflammation of the skin so as to relieve a deeper inflammation such as muscles, joints and ligaments.
- **Demulcent**: a substance that has a soothing effect on mucous membranes.
- **Diaphoretic**: a substance that promotes sweating and thereby controls a fever.
- **Diuretic**: a substance that increases urinary output.
- **Emmenagogue**: a substance that initiates and promotes menstrual flow.
- **Expectorant**: a substance that improves the clearing of excessive mucus from the lungs by either altering the viscosity of the mucus or improving the cough reflex.
- **Galactagogue**: a substance that increases breast milk production.
- **Hepatic:** a substance that improves the tone, vigour, and function of the liver.
- **Immune enhancing/stimulant**: a substance that enhances immune function.
- **Immune modulating**: a substance that modulates and balances the activity of the immune system.
- **Lymphatic**: a substance that assists detoxification by its effect on lymphatic tissue.
- **Mucolytic:** a substance that helps to break up and disperse sticky mucus, usually in the respiratory system.

- **Ovarian tonic**: a substance that improves the tone, vigour, and function of the ovaries.
- **Oxytocic**: a substance that causes contraction of the uterine muscle in association with giving birth.
- **Parturifacient**: a substance that induces and assists in the efficient delivery of the foetus and placenta.
- **Partus preparatory**: a substance then in preparation for labour and childbirth. Usually treatment begins after the end of the first trimester.
- **Progesterogenic**: a substance that promotes the effects or production of progesterone.
- **Sedative**: a substance that reduces activity, particularly in the nervous system and decreases nervous tension.
- **Nervine tonic (Nervine)**: a substance that improves tone, vigour, and function of the nervous system, both relaxes and energises the nervous system.
- **Spasmolytic**: a substance that reduces or relieves smooth muscle spasm (involuntary contraction).
- **Stimulant**: a substance that heightens the function of an organ or system.
- **Styptic**: a substance that stops bleeding when applied locally.
- **Thymoleptic**: a substance that elevates mood.
- **Tonic (general)**: a substance that improves the tone, vigour, and function of the whole body.
- **Trophorestorative**: a substance that has a healing and restorative action on a specific organ or tissue.
- **Uterine tonic**: a substance that increases the tone of the uterus muscles.
- **Vulnerary**: a substance that promotes the healing of wounds.

Botanical medicines are dispensed in various standardisations of strengths and potencies. The different forms that herbal preparations are available in may include: powder; tablet; capsule; infusion (such as herbal teas); decoction; and fluid tincture extracts.

Because herbal medicines usually exert multiple therapeutic actions many are able to be utilised in a variety of different ailments simultaneously. Herbal medicines work best when combined with other compatible herbs to provoke a synergistic reaction in the biochemical and physiological processes.

This following section will delve into the world of botanical and herbal medicines that can be used for reproductive related disorders. For those who are considering trying herbal medicines treatments or are currently undergoing treatment from your naturopath or herbalist and are wanting to know more about how these herbal medicines work, then the information will give you a very comprehensive overview of these individual botanicals and the research behind why they are recommended for reproductive health care.

# Herbal Medicines used for Male Infertility

## *Tribulus Terrestris/Pratense (Caltrops) (Bai Ji Li)*

Tribulus is considered a reproductive tonic in Ayurvedic medicine and is used to treat impotence, libido and infertility of both genders. Tribulus contains the steroidal furostonal sappanin protodioscin. Research shows the herb stimulates sperm production and increases the quality, motility and survival time of sperm in male infertility. Preliminary research suggests Tribulus increases the endogenous production of luteinising hormone. It is speculated that increased luteinising hormone will in turn stimulate endogenous testosterone conversion to dihydrotestosterone (DHT) and therefore increases in sexual performance and desire (libido) in both males and females may be seen. Dihydrotestosterone (DHT) also increases the production of red blood cells and muscle development.

Luteinising hormone is a hormone produced by the hypophysis that stimulates development of the interstitial cells (sertoli and germinal cells) of the testes and secretion of testosterone by those cells thereby improving spermatogenesis. In the female this hormone, working in conjunction with follicle stimulating hormone (FSH), is responsible for maturation of the follicle of the ovary, and its rupture and transformation into the corpus luteum.

Tribulus may help to increase FSH and Oestradiol in women, with a minor effect on testosterone. For this reason, Tribulus may be considered for irregular menses, an invigorating tonic for post-partum women and menstrual difficulties such as menopausal symptoms and poly cystic ovarian syndrome (PCOS).

The active constituents in Tribulus have shown to assist in dilating coronary arteries, improving coronary circulation and reducing angina symptoms.

Tribulus also has actions on the liver where it may help to improve cholesterol and protein metabolism, therefore enhancing energy production. The kidneys may also benefit from the diuretic actions of Tribulus by preventing and reducing kidney stones. Dysovulatory disorders and infertility may be normalised with Tribulus when administered daily from day 5 to 14 (only) of the menstrual cycle. Males who suffer from Kleinfelter's syndrome (a chromosomal abnormality leading to hypogonadism) have experienced improved libido and potency when using Tribulus.

In Traditional Chinese Medicine (TCM), Tribulus is used in cases of ascendant liver yang, characterised by headaches, vertigo, and painful red eyes; it is said to calm the liver and anchor the yang. The herb dispels wind and stops itching of skin lesions. In PMS (Premenstrual Syndrome) it constrains liver Qi, which can cause symptoms such as tender breasts, pain in the flank, cramps, and mental distress. It may also help for conditions such as elevated blood pressure, insufficient lactation, and where there is pain and distension in the chest.

Tribulus should be taken in a standardised extract form called *Tribestan* which contains no less than 45 per cent of the saponin protodioscin.

### *Epimedium Sagittatum / grandiflorum – (Horny goat weed)*

With a name like horny goat weed it doesn't take much imagination to guess what it is used for. Horny goat weed was traditionally employed to treat impotence, spermatorrhea, frequent urination, forgetfulness, weakness and painful cold lower back and knees. Horny goat weed had been used as an agent to increase sexual desire (aphrodisiac), performance capability and assist in the correction of sexual dysfunction (loss of libido, impotence, frigidity, and premature ejaculation).

In TCM Epimedium or Yin Yang Huo (Xian Ling Pi) is used as a tonifier of the kidneys and fortifies the Yang, strengthens and warms the reproductive system. Epimedium can be used also be used for female conditions such as irregular menstruation. Some of the isolates from Epimedium have shown anti-platelet and bone-sparing activity.

Horny goat weed may help to increase sperm production and stimulate the sensory nerves, with a moderate androgen-like effect on the levator ani, testes and prostate. Epimedium may help in the prevention of osteoporosis after ovariectomy and has shown to improve quality of life in patients suffering chronic disease. It is also has some mild antibiotic, expectorant, immune-modulating, and anti-tussive (anti-cough) properties.

### *Liriosma Ovata – (Muira Puama)*

Muira Puama has a long history in traditional indigenous Amazon culture for treating sexual debility; impotency; grippe; rheumatism; neuromuscular problems (neuralgias, locomotor ataxis); gastro-intestinal problems; paralysis; and beriberi. Researchers have validated the traditional claims of Muira through investigations and support its historical uses.

Muira Puama seems to have two particular effects on reproductive problems:

1. Increases libido. Muira Puama is rich in naturally occurring sterols, which are possible building blocks for hormones such as testosterone. Muira Puama contains beta sitosterols, campesterol, and lupeol. Another chemical helps to create hormones. Beta sitosterol may assist in activating the body's receptors for hormones such as testosterone, revving our hormonal engines and leading to both heightened libido and enhanced performance. Also contained in Muira are other chemicals and volatile oils like camphor, which help restore the sex drive. These active chemical compounds enhance mental ability to become sexually aroused and stimulate nerves to carry messages to pleasure centres in the brain.

2. The second of Muira Puama's main effects is that it helps to increase penile hardness; this may stem from its apparent effect on circulation. Although the full mechanism of how this process works is not totally understood,

those who have used this herb have laid claim to many testaments of its benefits.

In one study, 262 males who were experiencing an inability to attain/ maintain an erection and had a lack of sexual desire were given Muira Puama. 62 per cent (who had loss of libido) felt the herb 'had a dynamic effect' and 51 per cent (with erectile dysfunction) thought the extract was beneficial. Another study indicated that Muira Puama had a positive psychological impact when trialled on 100 men with sexual asthenia.

### *Serenoa Serrulata – (Saw Palmetto)*
This herb has been extensively researched and is more effective than most conventional drugs in the management of prostatic enlargement. Accumulation of testosterone in the prostate quickly transforms the testosterone into the hormone Dihydrotestosterone (DHT).

This hormone is responsible for accelerated multiplication of the prostate cells, nuclei and resulting hyperplasia. The fatty acids in saw palmetto combat this powerful form of male hormone, first by limiting the conversion of normal testosterone to DHT, then by preventing DHT from binding to prostate cells and triggering excess growth.

Advanced Benign Prostate hyperplasia (BPH) is one of the leading factors in less-than-firm erections as men age. Although BPH is more prevalent in men over 45, younger men may also notice subtle changes in their ability to perform. If your bladder feels full because an enlarged prostate is pushing against it, it is difficult to keep your mind on the situation at hand. The pressure that arises from BPH detracts from the inner tension that many men say they feel arousal and ejaculation. In this way, BPH can detract not only from sexual performance, but from the pleasure as well.

Saw palmetto is highly regarded as a general tonic with applications of debility, functional impotency, male senility, and the feeling of being run-down both physically and mentally. It is also used in atrophy conditions of the testes and ovaries. The berries of saw palmetto are also believed to increase sperm production. Recently, studies have shown saw palmetto also possesses anti-oestrogenic effects. Oestrogen apparently inhibits hydroxylation and elimination of dihydrotestosterone. This herb is also used as a tonic, diuretic, sedative, and endocrine agent. It is said to slightly enlarge breasts in women and is considered an aphrodisiac.

Historically, saw palmetto has been time honoured for its usefulness as a fertility enhancing agent. Many of the most respected eclectic herbalists swear by its benefit for both male and female fertility. In TCM this herb nourishes the reproductive Qi, fortifies the Kidney Yang and Spleen Qi. It may influence the pituitary function via its hormonal influence on the endocrine glands, including the ovaries, testicles, thyroid and breasts. Traditionally, saw palmetto is used for impotence, amenorrhea, long menstrual cycles, and lack of sexual desire.

### Morinda Officinalis – (Ba Ji Tian)

Morinda officinalis is an important Chinese herb; it is a kidney tonic, and therefore strengthens the yang. It is also used as a sexual tonic, treating impotence and premature ejaculation in men, infertility in both men and women, and a range of other often hormonally related conditions, such as irregular menstrual cycles. Ba Ji Tian is also affective in regulating urinary dysfunction, and pains in the lower back and pelvic regions.

### Panax Ginseng (Korean ginseng) (Rhen Shen)

It's hard to find any single food or herb with enough nutrients to meet all the body's endurance needs and bring the body into harmony. Based on its reputation and much scientific research behind panax ginseng perhaps it comes close. Over the centuries, the reputation of ginseng as a 'sexual rejuvenator' or 'aphrodisiac' has been well claimed. Ginseng's botanical name 'panax' comes from the same word as the Greek goddess Panacea, healer of all.

Recent studies have shown that ginseng enhances libido and copulation performance. These effects of ginseng may not be due to changes to hormone secretion, but its ginsenoside components' effect on the central nervous system and gonadal tissue. Clinical trials and studies have also confirmed that ginseng does have a significant role to play in the treatment of male sexual and infertility problems; panax has significant stimulating and arousing actions.

In one example of an open study, 66 male patients were treated with ginseng extract, of whom 20 were control, 30 had idiopathic low sperm count and 16 had a low sperm count associated with varicoceles. All received 4 grams of ginseng extract per day for three months. Sperm count, total testosterone, sperm motility, free testosterone and dihydrotestosterone (DHT) rose in all groups after 3 months' treatment.

Panax is an adaptogen, which means that it has a non-specific action on improving the body's general resistance to stress and fatigue. It improves energy metabolism – particularly during prolonged exercise and under the challenge of stress. It spares glycogen in muscles during exercise, preventing fatigue and lactic acid build-up and encourages the use of fatty acids as energy.

Ginseng has the potential to heal virtually all tissue types and inhibit the aging process. It enhances antibody responses, cell-mediated immunity, natural killer cell activity, production of interferon and phagocytic function.

Ginseng acts as a general tonic with protective effects on the cardiovascular and hepatic systems. Panax influences the hypothalamic-pituitary-adrenal axis, thus having a modulating effect on various aspects of the endocrine system.

Panax's other therapeutic applications may include: alcoholism; arrhythmia; asthma; epilepsy; pregnancy; cancer; depression; drug abuse; myocardial infarction; regulates blood pressure; blood sugar control; chronic immune disorders; helps to protect from arterial disease; reduces menopausal symptoms (it exerts a mild oestrogenic effect); and acts as a general tonic.

Panax should be avoided if the individual if very hypersensitive to stimulation and allergies. Younger people should use panax on a sporadic basis due to its effect of potentially depleting Qi energy flow with over-use.

### *Panax Quinquefolium (American Ginseng)*

American ginseng is another variety of ginseng, closely related to the Korean ginseng variety, but is less stimulating on the nervous system, (therefore, more useful than panax if you suffer nervousness, and insomnia problems) and is said to have greater application in immune and learning disorders. In TCM, Panax (Ren Shen) is considered more a 'Yang' herb or warming and energising. American ginseng is considered more 'Yin' cooling and rejuvenating. Not only does American ginseng have its place in male fertility, it also helps female fertility by stimulating the growth of the uterine lining.

### *Withania Somnifera* – Ashwaganda, Winter Cherry (referred to as 'Indian Ginseng')

Withania has adaptogenic potential regarded as equal to panax ginseng in terms of this tonic, stamina-improving properties. Withania retards various aspects of the aging process; stimulates the endogenous production of melanin, improves sexual performance and increases general resistance to stress (including physical, chemical, and biological). Its Hindi name means 'horse smell', and refers not just to its odour but to it giving one the strength of a horse.

Withania is the herb of choice in cases where 'burn out' from stress and the exhaustion stage has been reached. It also has its place in treating connective tissue disorders, hypotension, and has anticancer/tumour actions.

Ashwanganda is highly praised in Ayurveda Medicine and has broad application for multiple ailments such as Alzheimer's disease; anaemia (iron); HIV; immune deficiency; inflammation; tumours; arthritis; fatigue; and as a tonic from chronic illness and aging to name a few.

Considering that the Ayurvedic (Indian) culture was the one that gave to the world the first sex manual, the *Karma Sutra*, all those years ago and the country has such a massive population, it might be wise to consider the advice from this ancient traditional system of healing.

The use of withania for reproductive system conditions such as low sperm counts would be greatly benefited by this herbal medicine. Withania also exerts anti-inflammatory, hypotensive, hepatic-protective (liver), and anti-bacterial actions. It is high in nutrients such as iron, arginine and ornithine.

One of the main active chemicals in withania is the substance called withanolides. These compounds exert a weak steroidal-hormone-like effect and can help to mimic the body's naturally occurring hormones, such as testosterone and progesterone. Withania also appears to have a circulation stimulatory action by relaxing the blood vessels. By improving the body's circulation chemical messages are able to get to the necessary locations throughout the body so it can do its job more efficiently.

Research into withania's anti-anxiety action is believed to be primarily through the herb's active compounds mimicking a naturally occurring chemical in the brain called gamma-amino-butyric acid (GABA) (not the cricket ground!). GABA has a role of decreasing the effect of stimuli that reach the brain, therefore, if you are experiencing a lot of stress particularly you would describe it as feeling like you're 'burning-out'.

By balancing this transmitter in the body, the feelings of being overwhelmed and physical manifestations of stress and anxiety can be prevented such as heart palpitations, hyperventilations and those butterfly feelings in the stomach and when your heart feels like it's in your throat. Withania's aphrodisiac reputation may be mainly due to its ability to restore and stimulate an overall sense of wellbeing.

### Schizandra Chinensis - Schisandra (Wu Wei Zi)
Schisandra is primarily used as a blood purifier where the liver is under-functioning and it is applied in cases of both acute and chronic liver disease, particularly when the liver requires protection and detoxification. Schisandra may be employed in stress conditions, to improve memory and brain functioning, co-ordination, improves sensory functions, and by apparently acting on the central nervous system it is also reputed to exert an adrenal gland tonic action.

Other conditions that may benefit from using schisandra include: wheezing; spontaneous sweating; nocturnal emission; chronic diarrhoea; insomnia; and forgetfulness. Considered a harmonising tonic in Chinese medicine, with a long history of uses including: adaptogen; hepatic and renal aid.

In TCM, the kidneys are the primary system that regulated the flow of Qi through the body and treatment is focused towards the kidney and spleen with reference to improving reproductive health.

Schisandra is one of the top herbal medicines for enhancing sperm production; studies have shown to increase RNA, glycogen and enzymes to the kidneys and gonads when taken over a 3-month period.

### Gingko biloba leaf (also referred to as Maidenhair tree)
Gingko has been historically praised as an overall balancing tonic herb, particularly for the elderly. Gingko has been used in traditional Chinese medicine since 2,800 BC and is a species of the world's oldest living tree. With thousands of year of empirical observation and more than 400 studies to validate its reputation, gingko biloba has become one of the most prescribed

herbal medicines throughout the world, particularly in Europe. Gingko leaf extract has received much attention as a result of research that documents its ability to improve memory function.

The hallmark of gingko's effects is that it improves circulation, and it does this by dilating/relaxing cerebral blood vessels and arteries making them work more efficiently, which increases blood flow to the brain. The active ingredients of gingko are flavone glycosides; ginkolides; bioflavonoid (especially quercetin); heterosides; sitosterol; lactones; and anthocyanins. Ginkgo contains more of a chemical called terpene lactone than other plants; this substance is known to also enhance circulation. Scientific research also has shown how gingko can improve the circulation to peripheral tissues to supply blood to men's and women's sex organs.

Studies using gingko extract have shown its usefulness where men suffered erectile problems due to insufficient circulation. Other research has stated that gingko can enhance sperm production, as a result of its potent antioxidant action and nutrients that are provided by the herb.

Ginkgo may help to control nocturnal emissions by modulating tissue sensitivity and improving muscle tone. There has also been marked improvement in cases of involuntary or premature ejaculation. This could be a result of improved focus and mental clarity. Gingko can significantly increase the production of brain neurotransmitters, such as dopamine, and adrenaline which are associated with increased alertness and pleasure arousal.

Gingko has shown that it can normalise the acetylcholine receptors in the hippocampus (a part of the brain), and it enhances the utilisation of oxygen, glucose, and activates the sodium/potassium pump (essential to proper cellular functioning) and nerve cells.

Conditions that gingko could also be used for may include: Alzheimer's; senility; tinnitus (ringing in the ears); vertigo (dizziness); certain types of depression; headaches due to vascular origin; cognitive memory loss; hearing loss; dementia; senile macular (eye) degeneration; diabetic retinopathy; impotence; PMS; asthma; and allergies (due to its ability to inhibit platelet activating factor-anti-PAF).

It takes about 50 pounds of gingko leaves to create one pound of standardised gingko biloba extract (GBE). Before purchasing gingko in tablet or capsule form ensure that they contain at least 24 per cent flavone glycosides, and 6 per cent terpene lactones (mainly ginkgolides).

### Astragalus Membranaceus – (Huang Qi)
Astragalus has a revered reputation as an adaptogen for chronic stress and a specific tonic for strengthening resistance to disease. It has anti-viral activity, enhances the production and secretion of interferon and increases the function of natural killer cells. This herb has shown to increase IgA, IgE, and IgM

antibodies. It has an invigorating effect on cell metabolism and aids adrenal function.

Astragalus is used in states of chronic debility, fatigue, and where restoration to immune function is required. It is also reputed as an anti-aging tonic, assists in relieving menopausal symptoms such as night sweats, and has applications in supporting cancer treatments. Studies using extracts of astragalus on sperm production has shown outstanding results. Some investigations have yielded results using astragalus outperformed all other herbal medicines in the output of sperm number and motility.

Astragalus helps to expel toxins and pus, it is a lung and cardiac tonic, and has application in conditions such as nephritis, hypoglycaemia, and fungal infections. Research has shown sperm motility increased by 150 per cent when the males were treated with the astragalus herb. In TCM, astragalus tonifies the Spleen Qi, raises Yang Qi, and augments protective Qi. It has also been traditionally used to help the body to mend and heal such as after surgery.

### Avena Sativa – (Oat seed)
Oat seed is considered one of the best remedies for 'feeding' the nervous system – especially in cases of depression, exhaustion, and nervous debility. Oat seed has beneficial application in reproductive dysfunction particularly where the nervous system involvement and tonifying of the genito-urinary system is indicated. Oats have a strong reputation for promoting deep relaxation, and have been used throughout the centuries to treat conditions such as anxiety, insomnia, stress and more recently, tobacco and drug withdrawal. Other medical uses include treatment for connective tissue tone; gout; kidney and gallbladder disorders; arthritis; constipation; diarrhoea; fatigue; and coughs.

Oats also are reputed to be a sexual stimulant in both humans and animals. It is said that horses that eat wild oats are more likely to mate, and with more vigour. Old phrases are still used today that depict the historical belief in the use of oats. Terms such as 'feeling his oats' and 'sowing wild oats' should need little explanation. Chemically speaking, oats contain a number of constituents: vitamins; minerals; proteins; and polysaccharides, which are carbohydrate sugar chains that are used by the immune system and as a fuel sources. In addition, oats supply active compounds such as steroidal saponins, which are believed to influence hormonal balance. Beta-sitosterol structurally resembles testosterone, oestrogen, and progesterone and is believed to modulate hormone levels, directly or indirectly.

The seeds are rich in iron, manganese, and zinc (refer to nutrition section for further information on these important nutrients regarding reproductive health). Alkaloids such as gramine, avenine, fatty acids and B-vitamins are also contended in the humble oat. These alkaloids are believed to attribute to the relaxation effect of oats.

In TCM oats provide nourishment to the endocrine, nervous, and immune systems and it tonifies Qi, Blood, and Essence.

### Eleuthrococcus Senticosus – (Siberian Ginseng)

Siberian ginseng has a long reputation as a rejuvenator of general health, memory restorative, and increases longevity. Siberian ginseng reduces the activation of the adrenal cortex in response to stress and prevents thymus and general lymphatic damage. The herb allows subjects to withstand greater levels of stress inducing stimuli from adverse physical conditions; affects increased mental activity, improved tissue oxygenation, endurance and athletic performance.

Siberian ginseng has been shown to increase reproductive capacity and sperm counts, scavenger free radicals, and stimulate cellular repair enzymes.

Compared to panax (Korean) ginseng, Siberian ginseng is less stimulating on the nervous system, but may be more beneficial at reducing fatigue and enhancing chronic immune function. Siberian ginseng like other varieties is classified as an adaptogen. This action may indicate its usefulness on blood pressure and in part its ability to improve kidney function.

Eleuthrococcus demonstrates activity as an immune stimulant – most notably increasing helper T-cells and natural killer cell activity. (Siberian ginseng and astragalus both work well together in chronic immune/disease conditions). Siberian ginseng is also used in conditions such as male impotence (stimulate male sex glands); stress (adaptation); fatigue; debility; drug withdrawal; adrenal gland exhaustion; radiation protection; colds; chest problems; and as an appetite stimulant.

Chinese experiments using Siberian ginseng in humans have shown:
Increased production of luteinising hormone (LH) produced by the pituitary gland in the brain, which stimulates progesterone in women; increased testosterone secretion in men and women; and improved muscle development.

Animal studies using ginseng also shows increased fertility and productivity: Cows produced more milk, bees produced more honey, bulls' production of semen up to 28 per cent higher, and mice even grow heavier testicles.

### Morinda Citrifolia (Noni)

Noni is the juice from the tropical fruit Morinda Citrifolia. Noni is one of the most commonly used herbal medicines among the Pacific Islanders and has been used in traditional healing practices for thousands of years. Noni is emerging as one of the best and most diverse natural remedies currently available today. Increasing scientific research into noni has yielded what traditional healers have known for generations, *it is a remarkable medicinal plant.*

Impressive results have been observed in conditions such as allergies; arthritis; bruises; mild depression; diabetes; poor digestion; high blood pressure; headaches; heart disease; menstrual cramps; burns; mental activity; obesity; migraines; pain; sexual and reproductive disorders; sleep problems; stress; poor energy; parasite infestation; cancer support; and immune dysfunctions.

Noni juice is an excellent source of vitamins, minerals, trace elements and amino acids. Xeronine is an enzyme produced in the intestines, which is believed to be necessary for proper cellular function. Xeronine enhances nutrient transport into, and out of, cells. It is involved in enzyme and hormone regulation, antibody function, protein structures and reducing inflammation. Availability of xeronine is enhanced in noni by the abundant presence of proxeronine, which is converted in the large intestine to xeronine. Noni also contains proxeronase which catalyses the conversion of proxeronine to xeronine.

Some of the other important compounds found in noni include: asperuloside; scopoletin; phytoserols; damnacanthal; and anthraquinones. Over 150 isolated nutraceuticals have been identified in Noni which is unique to the plant species; this supports its impressive and multi-faceted actions for a broad range of conditions and general health maintenance.

### Turnera Diffusa - (Damiana)
Damiana has a long-term reputation as an aphrodisiac and sexual tonic. It is beneficial to the endocrine system – improving hormone function. Helps to enhance mood and is a urinary remedy. The alkaloids in damiana are thought to have a testosterone-like effect and the cyanogenic glycoside provides a relaxing influence.

Damiana is an excellent nerve tonic and strengthener that makes it a choice herb to assist in conditions such as depression; anxiety; hysteria; convalescence after debility; and individuals with 'feeble' libidos.

### Pygeum africanum – (Pygeum)
Pygeum has a broad pharmacological activity. Its most prevalent clinical uses are to treat prostatitis, male infertility, impotence, and benign prostatic hyperplasia (BPH). Pygeum contains three different categories of fat soluble lipophilic compounds. The phytosterols are the plant equivalent to animal cholesterols.

These active constituents have marked anti-inflammatory properties and interfere with inflammatory-producing prostaglandins. The terpenes have an anti-swelling effect and ferulic esters that can reduce prolactin and cholesterol levels. Pygeum has been shown to indirectly reduce testosterone levels, through a fatty acid called *N-docosanol*. This potent cumulative combination of these actions means that pygeum is a very versatile herb.

### The rainforest herb – Iporuru

Iporuru is a unique traditional treatment for males in that the female partner rather than the man takes it. A plausible explanation for this effect is that the herb increases the receptivity of the cervix to sperm cells. The herb is also taken by men to increase their fertility.

French scientists have proposed that men taking iporuru would have more viable sperm (and increased potency) through the action of yohimbine, a compound found in both iporuru and yohimbe (Pausinystalia yohimbe) bark (also a potent male reproductive system herb).

### Cinnamon Twig and Poria Pill

A traditional Chinese herbal formula that treats infertility due to varicocele, it may also be useful for increasing sperm count, sperm motility and improves circulation in the lower abdominal region.

### Hochu-ekki-to

A Japanese herbal formula that helps sperm cells to develop properly, Hochu-ekki-to has shown to raise both testosterone levels and sperm counts. It may also be effective in alleviating infertility caused by the cancer treatment doxorubicin (Adriamycin). A study using this formula has shown an overall improvement in sperm count, motility and reduced abnormalities by approximately 50 per cent.

### Emblica Official – (Indian Gooseberry, Amalaki)

Indian gooseberry has a traditional role in Ayurvedic medicine as a rejuvenating herb, with major uses in conditions such as cancer, heart disease, and lowering of cholesterol. Indian gooseberry is a main ingredient in the famous Ayurvedic formula, Chawan Prash, which was formulated thousands of years ago. It is revered as a major therapeutic herb in India with reputations as an anti-aging tonic. It applications are definitely diverse, and male reproductive health is one of it additional applications.

### Mucuna Pruriens – (Kapi Kachu, Atma Gupta, Velvet Bean, Cowitch, Cowhage) seed

In Ayurvdedic medicine, mucuna is one of the premier rejuvenation herbs for men and women. Its reputation as a powerful aphrodisiac dates back thousands of years, and is still used today as an enhancer of sexual potency and to help treat infertility.

Atma gupta is held in high esteem as a tonic herb to reverse the aging process; its nutrient profile is very impressive with over 25 per cent being made up of protein, with a rich complex carbohydrate, alkaloid, and fibre content. Atma gupta has a natural ability to generate L-Dopa, which is deficient in conditions such as Parkinson's disease, and it is also used to help with diabetes mellitus (reduced blood sugar levels). L-Dopa improves dopamine production, which may also be useful for improving attention deficit hyperactivity disorder (ADHD) and sleeping problems.

Velvet bean exerts a testosterogenic action to improve libido, muscular mass, strength and healing effect on bone fractures. Mucuna pruriens may help the body also increase human growth hormone (HGH), somatotropin production, thus contributing to linear skeletal growth as well as burning fat from fat cells.

Mucuna pruriens is traditionally combined in formulas containing other popular Ayurvedic rejuvenating herbs including ashwaganda (withania), shativari, and/or amalaki.

### Nelumbo Nucifera (Sacred Lotus)
Sacred lotus is another Ayurvedic herb that combines well with Velvet Bean; it is a nutritive tonic, rejuvenating, aphrodisiac, and a nervine. Useful for males and females as a pre-conception tonic, and it is used in spermatorrhoea, impotence, leukorrhea, venereal disease, diarrhoea, bleeding disorders like menorrhagia, heart weakness, fatigue, and is good for decreasing anxiety and improving concentration.

### Alfalfa (Medicago)
Alfalfa grows abundantly in the wild and is cultivated extensively for animal foods. It is best known as an overall nutritive herb. It is rich in trace elements needed by the glandular system and contains high amounts of beta-carotene, the precursor to vitamin A. It also helps to purify the blood, particularly because of its high chlorophyll content.

Using alfalfa is a good way to supply extra nutrients necessary for the health of the glandular system (particularly the pituitary). It is also an excellent source of Vitamin K. Alfalfa means 'best food'. It contains an abundance of alkaline minerals, proteins, Vitamins C, B group vitamins with traces of B12. There are at least eight enzymes that enhance healthy digestion and provide new life to the body cells.

Sprouted seeds are one of the best sources of 'live enzymes'. Enzymes are the catalysts for all living development. There are very few foods in the world which are able to supply the amounts of B vitamins, Vitamin C, Vitamin E, Vitamin G, Vitamin K, Vitamin U, and amino acids.

### Kelp
Kelp-like alfalfa is rich in trace minerals and is also nourishing to the glandular system. Kelp is native to the Pacific coast, although other related species of seaweed are native to the Atlantic coast. Kelp, because of its iodine content, is sometimes used as a blood purifier and contains significant amounts of iodine, calcium and potassium. Kelp as a nutritional supplement is helpful for those with first-degeneration hypothyroidism (under active thyroid), a common cause of miscarriage and elevated prolactin levels. Iodine is also important to foetal development in trace amount.

## Bee Pollen

Bee pollen is produced by the male part of flowering plants. Bees carry the pollen from flower to flower, an action which cross-pollinates and fertilises seeds. The bees carry some of the pollen on their back legs to the hives where they use it for food. The pollen is then made into royal jelly, to be fed to the young developing bee larvae.

The Hunza, who live in the Himalayan mountains and the Caucasus people of Russia, both renowned for their health and longevity, eat above average quantities of bee pollen and honey.

Many athletes and other health-conscious individuals consume bee pollen as an energy-promoting food supplement and is regarded by many as the 'perfect food'.

Bee pollen is composed of 10 to 15 per cent protein and also contains 18 amino acids, 28 minerals, 11 enzymes and 14 fatty acids, as well as B complex vitamins; Vitamin C; carotene; calcium; copper; iron; magnesium; potassium; manganese; sodium; plant sterols; and simple sugars.

Among the many health benefits of pollen are claims that it balances glandular activity; is useful in combating certain cancers; protects the body from pollution and radiation; enhances endurance and stamina; reduces fatigue, depression and colon disorders; improves immune function; reduces prostate enlargement; slows down the process of aging; and in some cases increases fertility.

According to a report regarding infertile men with low sperm counts, those who took supplemental bee pollen proved to solve the problem. After taking bee pollen the men reported improved health in general, an increase in sexual activity and improved sperm production.

Another study in Yugoslavia showed how bee pollen corrected various menstrual problems. Half of the study group of women with menstrual complaints were given bee pollen with Royal Jelly and the other half were given a placebo. Almost all the women on the pollen-jelly regimen showed marked improvement or a disappearance of their menstrual problems, whereas the placebo group showed little change.


## Chlorophyll

Chlorophyll is the green pigment found in plants and is referred to as the 'blood of plants', as chemically it is very similar to that of human blood (haemoglobin). Chlorophyll is an excellent body cleanser. It is available supplementally in a liquid form. It is abundant in phyto-nutrients such as spirulina; beetroot; chlorella; wheat grass; and barley greens for example. It helps to regulate menstruation, cleanses the liver, builds the blood and has many other beneficial effects on the body and overall health.

### Polygonum Multiflorum (He Shou Wu, Fo-ti-teing)

Polygonum is a popular herb in Chinese herbal medicine. It has always been considered a rejuvenating and vitality-enhancing herb, helping to prevent aging and encouraging longevity. Traditionally much folklore is attached to He Shou Wu and the large old roots are thought to have remarkable powers.

He Shou Wu is thought to concentrate Qi (vital energy). Medicinally, Polygonum is used for: toning properties; lowering cholesterol; as a nerve tonic; decreasing dizziness; neuritis; neurasthenia (nerve pain); epilepsy; and tinnitus. It helps connective tissue to repair and is believed to increase both male and female fertility.

He Shou Wu also remedies the liver and kidneys, counteracts infections such as tuberculosis bacillus and malaria, and is used to improve blood sugar levels and is a tonic to the blood. Studies have demonstrated polygonums' beneficial effects on enhancing fertility and other female functions involving ovulation and Corpus Luteum formation in animals.

### Psoralea Corylifolia (Bu Gu Zhi)

Bu Gu Zhi in Chinese tradition has been considered a yang tonic remedy and is valued in Chinese medicine to treat impotency, premature ejaculation and to improve vitality. The seeds are used to counter debility and other problems reflecting 'kidney yang' deficiency such as lower back pain, frequent urination, incontinence and bed-wetting. Bu Gu Zhi is also used in tincture form externally to treat skin conditions e.g. psoriasis; alopecia (loss of hair); vitiligo (loss of skin pigmentation); and rheumatism.

### Cordyceps sinensis (Cordyceps) (Tochukaso, Dong Chong Xia Cao)

Cortises grows 10,000 feet up on the Himalayan slopes, where native Tibetans search for one of the most treasured herbs in Traditional Chinese Medicine. As a tonic herb, cordyceps mushroom is prized for its ability to restore vitality, increase sexual potency, clear the lungs and enhance endurance.

This mushroom is one of the secret weapons of the Chinese Olympic athletes, and has been known for centuries to: increase endurance and stamina; aid recovery; ease stress; invigorate libido; supplement both yin and yang; strengthen the lungs; replenish life essence; and replenish kidney yin and yang.

Cordyceps is the premier kidney tonic and is a potent specific herb for all kidney diseases and related diseases such as diabetes, infertility and leukaemia. Contemporary therapeutic indications include: chronic bronchitis; chronic fatigue syndrome; nephritis; heart arrhythmias; and impotence; and are a valuable support during radiation and chemotherapy.

Cordyceps is commonly combined with other exceptional medicinal mushrooms (particularly for immune disorders and to support cancer treatments); these include: Shiitake (Lentinula edodes); Maitake (Grigolia frondosa); Reishii

(Gandoderma lucidum); Coriolus Versicolor (Karawatake PSK); and Snow fungus (Tremella fuciformis).

### Pausingstalia Yohimbe (Yohimbie bark)

Yohimbe works on nerve activity as an alpha-adrenergic blocker which normally constricts the blood vessels. By blocking this nerve activity, vessels are allowed to dilate, therefore resulting in increased blood flow, while reducing blood pressure and enhancing the ability to get erections. Yohimbe may be effective in treating erectile dysfunction of both physical and psychological origin.

Studies have shown that yohimbine (alone) is successful in 34-43% of cases of both organic or psychogenic erectile dysfunction and impotence. Yohimbe, combined with L-arginine (amino acid), have also yielded positive results for enhancing female sexual arousal. Yohimbe may also aid in weight loss by suppressing the body's ability to store fat. The isolated active alkaloid for Yohimbe has been used pharmaceutically in medicinal drug form for erectile dysfunction conditions.

Yohimbe has been referred to as 'Natures' Viagra'.

*Warning*! Excessive intake is known to be linked to some side effects such as, anxiety; panic attacks; hallucinations; blood pressure elevation; increased heart rate; dizziness; headaches; and skin flushing.

If standard dosage of yohimbe is observed (approximately 15-20mg) potential side effects would be greatly minimised. Yohimbe bark extracts are available in low dose homeopathic preparations.

### Smilax Species (Sarsaparilla)

Sarsaparilla is widely used commercially as a flavouring and foaming agent in food. The herb is therapeutically considered as an excellent general tonic for both males and females. Natives of various cultures claim its benefits as an aphrodisiac agent.

Researchers have claimed that two particular compounds in sarsaparilla (sarsapogenin and smilagenin) possess hormone/steroid-like actions in the body similar to that of testosterone, progesterone and cortin. Sarsaparilla is anti-oxidant, anti-inflammatory, antiseptic, anti-rheumatic and alterative (blood purifying properties).

Therapeutically this herb has been used to increase energy; protect the body from radiation exposure; hormone regulation; heat rash; hives; eczema; psoriasis; premenstrual syndrome; frigidity; impotence; itchy skin; fungal conditions; infertility; arthritis; and tumour growths.

### Garcinia Mangostana (Mangosteen)

Mangosteen is another of the tropical fruits that has emerged as one of the most successful food supplements, which is being supported with credible scientific evidence to match a wealth of anecdotal claims from traditional folk medicine. Prized among many cultures, in Asia it is called 'the Queen of fruits' and in the French Caribbean, 'the food of the gods'.

The phytoceuticals of the mangosteen have been widely studied by medical and pharmacological researchers. Xanthone is a newly discovered class of active compound among many other compounds isolated from mangosteen. The list of potential therapeutic applications and actions is very impressive.

Mangosteen, like noni (morinda citrifolia) and other similar medicinal foods such as Himalayan goji berry juice (lycium barbarum) would be worth consideration to support more specific treatments, particularly due to their general tonic effects.

### Rhodiola Rosea (Rhodiola root, Sedum roseum, Golden root, rose root, Arctic root, Russian Rhodiola)
Rhodiola root has been used in traditional medicines of countries throughout Russia, Scandinavia and Middle Asia. The therapeutic actions of rhodiola mimic many of the actions of the ginseng variety of medicinal plants.

Rhodiola has been used to increase physical endurance; mental performance; male sexual function; liver protection; reduce fatigue; and as a supportive treatment of cancer. Rhodiola combines well with other adaptogen and tonic herbal medicines to support treatments for male infertility.

### Long Jack (Eurycoma Longifolia Jack Radix, Tongkat Ali root)
Eurycoma can help to naturally unbind bound testosterone to increase free testosterone. It also has shown to increase ATP production, which reduces fatigue and enhances energy and stamina. Eurycoma influences pheromones in the body thereby having an effect on increasing sexual desire.

### Red Kwao Krua (Butea superba)
The tubers of Red Kwao Kruda constitute a traditional Thai plant medicine that has a long history of treating male sexual dysfunction. In a three-month randomised, double-blind clinical trial on volunteers with erectile dysfunction, the results revealed that eighty-two per cent improved significantly and, in addition, did not experience side-effects.


### Other important herbal medicines to consider in treating male fertility:
Abuta; aloe vera; Chinese wolfberry (lycium chinense); deer antler; codonopsis (codonopsis pilosula), eurycoma longifolia; willow herb (epilobium spp); chuchuhusai bark (maytenus krukovit), garlic (allium sativum); gota kola (centella asiatica); lesser periwinkle; lepidium satiuvm; muira puama (ptychopetalum olacoides); salix nigra (black willow); seabuckthorn seed; sariba (hemidesmus indicus); suma (Brazilian ginseng); nettle root (urtica dioica); buchu (barosm betulina); pimpillella; and hydrangea.

TCM herbs – lycium seed (Gou Qi Zi), cuscuta (Tu Si Zi) and fleece flower root many benefit improving sperm counts. Cornus (Shan Zhu Yu) may benefit improving sperm motility.

Yi Kang Tang (Yi Kang Decoction) has been studied by the Department of Reproduction, Zhejiang Hospital, Hangzhoa, China, and proven to have many benefits for male immune infertility (e.g. anti-sperm antibody AsAb and mycoplamsa), better than Prednisone. Zengjing Granule (ZJG) TCM composition has shown to improve sperm quality by restoring epididymal gland wall thickness.

Other supplements may include: Royal jelly (super food); wheat germ (high in Vitamin E and octacosanol); pycnogenol (a superantioxidant in pine bark and grape seed); and pumpkin seeds (rich in zinc) also have known benefits for male fertility. Though some people may have potential allergies to these supplements, it is best to avoid them if you are particularly allergy prone.

### Ferulic acid
is a substance found in many plants that has been shown to have anti-oxidant properties. Preliminary studies have shown that it improved sperm motility, but this was measured by external application to the sperm. Future studies may also show it to be promising when used internally for improving fertility.


## Herbs to avoid for Male Fertility

*Jambul, Neem and Vitex* in low doses may have some male therapeutic system applications, in high doses may potentially cause fertility problems.

*Echinacea* in high dose extracts have been reported to potentially affect fertility; echinacea appears to affect the DNA of sperm that can change the enzymes necessary for sperm to penetrate through the egg's shell. Though, in low doses echinacea may have therapeutic benefits if underlying infections require treatment.

*Ginkgo Biloba* has also shown that its use in high doses can affect sperm from penetrating that egg outer surface. Again, gingko biloba can also have other therapeutic uses in lower dosages as it is a potent antioxidant that can have a protective effect on sperm and can assist peripheral circulation to the brain and penis.

*St John's Wort* in lab studies has identified that this herb contains chemicals that reduce the sperm's ability to penetrate the egg, but have not been proven yet in human trials.

*Hibiscus flower* has been shown to reduce pituitary hormones that are necessary for fertility and may also reduce sperm production.

# Herbal Medicines used for Female Infertility

Fertility drugs may not be for everyone. Some women have to stop taking them because their ovaries have become hyper-stimulated (a severe health-threatening condition) or they have developed other problems such as cysts. Other issues that may play a major factor in your choice to use fertility drugs is the high statistical odds that approximately 50 per cent of conceptions may end up miscarrying with Clomid or the elevated chances of multiple births with the use of certain medications like Menotropins. Mother Nature has also provided use with a plethora of alternatives that yield less potential risks and side effects to choice from.

## *Vitex Agnus – Castus – (Chaste tree/berry) fruit*
Vitex exerts a balancing action on the female sex hormones. Research has revealed that vitex affects the diencephalon-hypophyseal system. Here it causes increased luteinising hormone (LH) production and inhibits the release of follicle-stimulating hormone (FSH). This leads to a shift in the ratio of oestrogens to progesterones, in favour of progesterones and hence a corpus luteum hormone effect.

What is obvious is that this herb is more phyto-progesteronal than oestrogenic and that it is more effective in troubles building up to menstruation, rather than starting with or following it, which points to an effect in support of, or mimicking, corpus luteum (thus, is a promoter of prolactin). Symptoms of pre-menstrual syndrome (PMS) that respond well to chaste tree include reduction in headaches; pressure and tenderness in the breasts; bloating; acne; carbohydrate cravings; oedema (fluid retention); irritability; and mood fluctuations.

New research challenges the conventional wisdom that vitex can increase prolactin production. It is now known that vitex has *Dopaminergic activity*, which can explain its success in treating numerous gynaecological conditions, many of which may be related to high prolactin levels. Dopamine and compounds of similar molecular structure inhibit prolactin secretion from the anterior pituitary. Increased prolactin inhibits corpus luteal development, thereby indirectly reducing the secretion of progesterone in the luteal phase of the menstrual cycle. Therefore, vitex may increase progesterone by reducing prolactin rather than by increasing LH as past research suggests.

Vitex, also known as 'monk's pepper' can suppress testosterone levels, thus having an anti-aphrodisiac (decreased libido) effect; so if you are looking for some hanky-panky best not to over do it with Vitex. Prior to ovulation, vitex can assist with ovary maturation, combined with herbs such as blue cohosh (caulophyllum thalictroides), chaste tree works in a similar manner as medical drugs like Clomid (but without the long list of side effects) to enhance conception by stimulating ovulation of the ovum/s, (eggs). Vitex supports the release of gonadotrophins from the pituitary gland and decreases the symptoms of dysmenorrhoea (menstrual period pain).

It is recommended to avoid vitex during pregnancy (except under practitioner supervision) as it interacts with various endogenous hormones. Chaste tree lengthens the duration between periods if irregular, restores regularity in those afflicted with endometriosis and helps to alleviate menorrhagia (heavy menses) and secondary amenorrhea (absence of menses) (especially where due to a luteal phase defect).

Vitex may benefit during menopausal change and assist the body in regaining a natural balance after childbirth and after the use of the birth control pill. Vitex is recognised as a hypothalamic-pituitary-ovarian axis regulator, but caution should be exercised in women under 20 years of age when hypothalamic-pituitary axis is easily disrupted.

Vitex also has a galactagogue action, which means it promotes the production or flow of breast milk. Other conditions vitex has application for include: benign breast disease; cystic hyperplasia; post-natal depression; endometriosis; fibroids; follicular/ovarian cysts; latent hyperprolactinaemia; luteal phase complaints; metrorrhagia; infertility resulting from decreased progesterone levels; corpus luteal insufficiency; threatened miscarriage; and dysfunctional uterine bleeding.

Investigations into vitex have indicated that, if it is taken in high doses early in the menstrual cycle it may potentially suppress ovulation, though other investigations state that the use of vitex can actually assist in the ovulation (egg release) phase of the cycle and increase luteinising hormone levels.

When vitex is taken during the luteal phase (after ovulation) it may help to regulate and lengthen the cycle. This action can benefit an implanting embryo to give it a better chance of taking to the uterine wall. Vitex is relatively slow acting therefore it may take several months of use before optimal effects occur.


### Chamaelirium Luteum – (False Unicorn Root, Helonias)
False unicorn root is one of the most highly reputed female reproductive system herbal medicines (though, the lack of in-depth phyto-chemical research and quality clinical trials is still required to fully appreciate false unicorn root's therapeutic applications). What is known of this herb is that it exerts a menstrual cycle regulation effect, is a uterine tonic, and improves the secretory responses and cyclical functions of the ovaries; it appears to have an adaptogenic effect on this organ.

It contains phyto-oestrogenic precursors and thus is beneficial for conditions that require oestrogen normalisation such as in menopause. Hedonias is also known to be diuretic, a digestive tonic, and anthelmintic (eliminates parasites). False unicorn root is used for infertility caused by dysfunction in follicular formation.

The list of therapeutic applications that helonias could be applied to include: adenomyosis; amenorrhoea; anorexia; cystic hyperplasia; digestive weakness; dysmenorrhoea; endometriosis; fibroids; infertility; chronic pelvic inflammation; leucorrhoea; symptoms of menopause; menorrhagia; menstrual irregularity; threatened miscarriage; erratic ovulation; polycystic ovarian syndrome; nausea in pregnancy; to prepare the uterus for labour during pregnancy; dysfunctional uterine bleeding; post-partum haemorrhage; weight loss, corrects sexual debility; and sensations of downward pressure in womb.

False unicorn root is almost extinct in the wild because of excessive collection. So its use should be restricted until cultivation occurs. (Paeonia Lactiflora may prove a suitable and cheaper substitute).

### Aletris Farinose – (True Unicorn Root)
True unicorn root is a bitter tonic digestive herb and a uterine tonic. This herb combines well with false unicorn root and its used in dysfunctional uterine bleeding conditions. Other applications for this herb may include: 'idiopathic' infertility; anorexia; cystic hyperplasia; digestive weakness; flatulence; and pelvic congestion.

### Angelica Sinensis – (Dong Quai, Dang Gui) root
Dong quai is considered one of the 'Emperor' remedies for its ability to restore blood, regulate menstrual rhythm and strengthen the uterus. In China, it has been used for more than 2,000 years, and is referred to as *female ginseng*.

It builds blood the way astragalus (Huang Qi) builds Qi, bringing warmth and nourishment to the viscera as well as the skin, muscles and flesh. By quickening the blood, it banishes cold, wind, and dampness.

Dong quai benefits the liver, heart, spleen, and drives away the pain of obstructive stagnation (e.g. blood clots). Dong quai strengthens immunity and benefits the circulatory system. Research shows it increases utilisation of oxygen in the liver, calms the central nervous system and relieves pain associated with neuralgia (nerve pain), ischemia (lack of oxygen), and rheumatic or osteoarthritis.

Due to its ability to nourish blood and mobilise circulation, dong quai promotes the healing of wounds, ulcers, and inflammations. The remedy possesses immune-regulating properties and may be used for acute viral infections such as colds and influenza.

Dong quai had been used to assist fertility for many hundreds of years in traditional Chinese medicine, and is said to regulate uterine function by stimulating smooth muscle, compounded by a complementary relaxing influence possibly associated with dysmenorrhea (painful periods – particularly of a dragging-down nature); amenorrhea (no menses flow); scant menstrual flow; abnormal menstrual cycle; moderate uterine bleeding; PMS; infertility; and menopause symptoms.

Clinical studies using a combination of herbs including dong quai, corydalis, white peony, and ligusticum wallichii demonstrated a 93 per cent improvement rate for treating dysmenorrhoea. In another study, infertility resulting from tubal occlusion was treated for up to 9 months with uterine irrigation (douche) of dong quai extract. Nearly 80 per cent of patients regained tubal patency, and 53 per cent became pregnant.

Male infertility has improved with dong quai, sperm motility and viability both increased with its use. Dong quai also helps to alleviate liver disorders, lung problems, and it potentates Vitamin E activity. Dong quai can also be applied in conditions such as digestive weakness and allergies (sensitivities).

Dong quai contains many nutrients, such as: cobalt; copper manganese; calcium; potassium; Vitamin E; Vitamin B12; plant sterols; coumarins; essential oils; and various flavonoids. The plant-sterols in dong quai are in one way as powerful as animal-based estrogens, but they can pack enough punch to give it a dual effect in the body.

The herb can lower excess oestrogen activity in some women, while stimulating oestrogen activity in those who need it, resulting in a balance in both groups. The plant sterols in dong quai weakly mimic oestrogen in the body and trigger competition among oestrogen tissue receptors, resulting in a diluting effect.

In women with low oestrogen, the active constituent combines with women's naturally occurring hormone to activate oestrogen receptors that otherwise might not be stimulated. Correct oestrogen balance is required for enhanced sexual responsiveness.

The essential oils in dong quai have anti-spasmodic properties; studies using dong quai have shown that its pain-killing effects in reducing menses pain were measured at 1.7 times the effect of aspirin medication. These properties would also be applicable in other cases where mild pain relief is requires such as headaches and arthritis.

Dong quai has also been used for allergies; anxiety; water retention; mood swings; fibrocystic breast disease; poor circulation; and high blood pressure. Dong quai has an effect as a mild 'blood thinning' agent and should not be used during very heavy periods and when taking certain IVF or prescription blood thinning medications such as warfarin.

### Paeonia Lactiflora – (Paeony, white Peony, Bai Shao) root
Paeonia is a wonderfully diverse herb primarily used in Chinese medicines for at least the last 1,500 years and is one of the top herbs used in female infertility and reproductive system disorders. Paeonia is an anti-spasmodic /mild skeletal muscle relaxant, soothes smooth muscle spasms, especially useful for dysmenorrhoea, angina, and migraine headaches. In traditional Chinese medicine it is considered as a blood and Yin tonic and is used to help

'blood deficiency'. It is mildly 'phyto-oestrogenic', and exerts anti-convulsant, anti-inflammatory, anti-allergic, immune and cognitive enhancing actions.

Various applications that peony may be used for include: anaemias; menstrual dysfunction; infertility; leukorrhea; uterine bleeding; spermatorrhea; neurasthenia; muscle cramps; epilepsy; polycystic ovary syndrome (in combination with liquorice); fibroids (in combination with pareunia suffruticosa, poria cocos, cinnamomum cassia, and prunus persica); endometriosis; androgen (hormone) excess; benign breast disease; irritable bowel syndrome; poor memory and concentration; ringing in the ears; dizziness; blurred vision; hot flushes; night sweats; menorrhagia; metrorrhagia; threatened miscarriage; myalgia; erratic ovulation; toxaemia; and restless foetus in pregnancy.

Peony is also a regulator of the hypothalamus-pituitary-ovarian axis, and is a good substitute for other herbs like false unicorn root and shatavari. Traditionally, paeonia was also one of the herbs used to make a famous women's tonic remedy called 'Four Thing Soup' together with rehmannia (rehmannia glutinosa), chuan xiong (ligusticum wallachii) and Chinese angelica (angelica sinensis).

### Cimicifuga Racemosa - (Black Cohosh, Sheng Ma) root and rhizome
Black cohosh is a popular herb used to normalise the female reproductive system. It is effective in the treatment of dysmenorrhea, amenorrhea, menopausal symptoms, cramps, ovarian dysfunction and insufficiency. Traditionally it was employed for uterine and rectal prolapse, relief of spasms, sciatica, tinnitus, rheumatism and osteoarthritis. Black cohosh has a tonifying effect on the uterus and allays nervousness and coughing.

More commonly used up help soothe the symptoms and depression of menopause, black cohosh does have its place in treating conditions that may contribute to infertility, some of which may include: hypothalamic-pituitary-ovarian axis dysfunction; fibroids; endometriosis; polycystic ovarian syndrome; and idiopathic infertility. In TCM, black cohosh raises the Yang Qi, having an energetic lifting effect.

Black cohosh has also been shown to have potential applications in male infertility. The viability of sperm cell and motility increased with the use of this herb.
**NOTE**: Due to black cohosh's emmenagogue action (increases the strength of uterine contraction) it is not recommended to be used in the early stages of pregnancy (if required to use only under practitioner supervision).

### Asparagus Racemosus - (Shatavari, wild asparagus root)
Shatavari is another of the prime rejuvenating (rasayana) Ayurvedic herbs. It is considered particularly helpful in conditions affecting both the female and male reproductive systems. Shatavari is reputed as an aphrodisiac and promoter of fertility, which is said to 'give the capacity to have a hundred husbands'.

One of its names means 'having one hundred roots', which also bespeaks its reputation as a fertility-enhancing plant. Shatavari has notable nutritive properties, and is excellent for nursing mothers to encourage to quantity and quality of breast milk (galactagogue). Preparations based on shatavari are often recommended for threatened miscarriage.

Shatavari is also used as a digestive said (particularly as an anti-diarrhoea agent). It exerts a cooling action useful for condition such as heartburn; irritable bowel syndrome; hot flushing; menopausal symptoms; PMS; irritability; cystitis; and recovering after illness.

### Caulophyllum Thalictroides (Blue Cohosh – Squaw root)
Blue cohosh is an anti-spasmodic to the female reproductive system with a tonic effect on the uterus and fallopian tubes. Blue cohosh is well applied in combination with other herbal medicine, for example, vitex agnus castus to assist with the promotion of ovulation and other herbs where uterine weakness; false labour pain; menopause; dysmenorrhoea; fibroids; amenorrhoea; ovarian/pelvic inflammation; and uterus atony are indicated.

Like black cohosh, this herb also has emmenagogue and oxytocic actions, therefore should be best avoided in the early stages of pregnancy.

Traditionally, blue cohosh was used throughout pregnancies to help prevent threatened miscarriages, but I would be conservative and remain cautious in using blue cohosh too early in the pregnancy.

### Lepidium Megenii (Maca root)
Maca is a rainforest herb that is a member of the cruciferous potato family. Maca is an important food in the diet of native Peruvians and is believed to have been used as a medicinal food for more the ten thousand years. It is rich in amino acids, high in proteins, calcium, magnesium, potassium and other nutrients. Maca root has been referred to as *Peruvian ginseng* and like other ginseng herbs, maca is known to increase energy and supports the immune system. Maca root is a super rich source of glucosinolates, which are known to be highly protective of carcinogens or cancer causing agents. Maca is reputed to be very supportive in treating for stomach cancer.

Maca has been used therapeutically for: anaemia; chronic fatigue syndrome; impotence; improving ejaculate volume; osteoporosis; menopausal and menstrual problems. Maca has been shown to influence the hypothalamus-pituitary axis, thus influencing the endocrine system function. Studies have discovered that maca can increase progesterone and testosterone levels in women, making it potentially useful in luteal insufficiency (short-luteal-phase dysfunction). In Ayurvedic medicine, maca root is regarded as a 'rebuilding tonic', strengthening the nervous system and brain via its effect on kidney energy. Harmonising of all endocrine functions and enhances emotional stability.

## Entada phaseoloides (Matchbox Bean)
Australian Aborigines use the seeds to treat female sterility and indigestion, and as a painkiller.

## Royal Jelly
Royal jelly is another panacea for health and longevity seekers. Worker bees make this exotic substance for their queen bee, and all of us want to be queen or king bees of course. The amazing size, fertility, and life-span of the queen bee is attributed to its dietary food source of royal jelly.

Royal jelly is definitely an energiser. It is high in certain unique fatty acids, simple carbohydrates, and pantothenic acid, which is supportive of the adrenals. It also contains the other B vitamins especially Vitamins B1, B3, B5, all of the essential amino acids, and many minerals, such as iron, calcium, silicon, sulphur, and potassium.

Royal jelly has been used to support weight loss, as it is a rich and energising nutrient yet low in calories (20 calories per teaspoon), and to treat problems such as fatigue; allay body aches; boost adrenal gland function; relieve insomnia; digestive disorders; infertility; ulcers; and cardiovascular ailments.

Whether this mysterious substance really is a great rejuvenator and supporter of youth and longevity will need to be studied. But many people, especially women, experience an uplifting feeling when they take either liquid or encapsulated royal jelly.

## Glycyrrhiza glabra (Liquorice root)
Liquorice likely has the most celebrated herbal past, extending thousands of years, beginning in the Orient and progressing around the world. It has many actions and clearly many uses. Also known as sweetwood or sweetroot, the 'great detoxifier', and the 'great peacemaker', this root contains many steroidal-like chemicals related to adrenal and ovarian secretions. Historically it was used for colds and coughs, and it has become popular as a laxative and for use in children, who tolerate its sweet flavour more readily than bitter herbs, with problems such as fever, colds, and constipation.

Liquorice root has many apparent actions. It is an antitussive and expectorant, anti-inflammatory and anti-arthritic, antitoxic (through liver support and protection) and antibiotic, possibly anti-cancer (recent research has shown liquorice's inhibitory effect in some tumour growth), and a laxative. It also acts as a demulcent and emollient, meaning it softens and soothes tissues and mucous membranes.

Liquorice further offers adrenal support with its mineralocorticoid-like substances and contain estrogenic chemicals such as beta-sitosterol and stigmasterol. Its adrenal stimulation allows it to be an anti-stress herb and to be helpful in inflammatory problems, such as arthritis, and in hypoglycaemia, which is a problem related to weak adrenals.

The estrogenic support allows its use in women as a sexual and uterine tonic and for problems of infertility. A study combining liquorice and white peony over 24 weeks using equal amounts of 6 grams of the herbs daily successfully treated women with infertility due to poly-cystic ovarian syndrome (PCOS); many of the women were recorded at the 12-week mark as being positively diagnosed pregnant. Serum levels of testosterone and free testosterone were significantly decreased after 4 weeks in 90 per cent of the women, and 25 per cent had fallen pregnant within 12 weeks of the 24-week trial. However, testosterone levels after 12 weeks were lower only in the pregnant group. At the end of the 24-week trial, the LH/FSH ratio was significantly lower in the treated group.

Liquorice root has been used as a stomach and intestinal remedy for problems such as indigestion; nausea; constipation; for infections of the respiratory tract, including colds and flu; hoarseness, sore throat and wheezing; hepatitis; ulcers; haemorrhoids; skin problems; muscle spasms and fevers associated with sweating; and general weakness. Liquorice has also been suggested for people with high blood pressure, yet there is a concern here since excessive intake can elevate blood pressure.

It appears that the whole root or deglycyrrhizinated liquorice (DGL) is safe and has the positive attributes of liquorice extract without side effects. DGL has been the subject of recent interest and research, and it apparently still helps in healing ulcers. Usually liquorice root is used in herbal combinations and not by itself; it also balances the flavour of these formulas. In Chinese herbology, liquorice is one of the most commonly used herbs, along with ginger.

### Barley grass
Barley grass helps to boost energy levels. The chlorophyll found in barley grass assists the oxygen-carrying capacity of the blood. It is a rich source of vitamins; minerals; amino acids; antioxidants; chlorophyll; beta-carotene; SOD (super oxide desmutase); and live enzymes.

SOD found in barley grass helps the body detoxify chemicals and foreign substances, thereby helping to prevent the onset of disease.

### Spirulina
Spirulina is a form of micro-algae rich in vitamins, minerals, chlorophyll, and protein. It is recognised as a whole food source. The concentration of nutrients in spirulina is like no other grain, herb or plant and is highly digestible and assimilative.

Spirulina contains gamma-linolenic acid (GLA); linoleic acid and arachidonic acid; very high in alkaline protein; essential amino acids; Vitamin B12; iron; the nucleic acids RNA and DNA. Spirulina supplies all the necessary nutrients to cleanse and heal the body; the high protein contents helps to stabilise blood sugars; reduce appetite; boost energy; reduce elevated cholesterol; protect the immune system; and enhance oxygen transport throughout the body. Spirulina is truly a wonder food.

## *Wheat Grass*

Wheat grass is another of the super foods and is an energy-packed food containing an immense array of over 100 vitamins, minerals, chlorophyll, laetrile, and other trace elements. Wheat grass is used to increase the health of the immune system; lower blood pressure; detoxify the liver, colon and kidneys; improves circulation; nourish and carry oxygen to the body cells; protect chromosome damage; rid the body of the toxic effects of pollution; and has potent antioxidant properties.

The juice from wheat grass is a favourite among people who are into fresh raw juices and is a very supportive food source used by people combating cancers. Wheat grass has been linked to enhancing FSH production in the body, therefore improving the quality and protection of the eggs (ova) in the reproductive system; as yet these early investigations have not been validated. Wheat grass is highly regarded in TCM for supporting fertility health.

## Other Phyto-Medicines that may be considered for female infertility problems:

anise (pimpinella anisum); viburnum opulus (cramp bark); diosceria villosa.spp (wild yam); glycyrrhiza glabra (licorice root); aloe vera; zingiber officinale (ginger root); anemone pulsatilla (pasque flower - use low dose, only with care); leonurus cardiaca (mother wort - use with care); capsella bursa-pastoris (shepherd's purse); ligusticum wallichii (cnidium; chuan xiong); nettle leaves; mitchella repens (squaw vine); alchemilla vulgaris (ladies mantle); ashoka (saraca indica); lamium album (white deadnettle); black haw (viburnum prunifolium); beth root (trillium erectum); mugwort (atremesia vulgaris – use with care); red raspberry leaf (rubus idaeus/r.strigosus); red clover (trifolium pratense); chamomile (matricaria recutita, chomomilla); and snow peas.

A TCM recipe called Nuzhen Yunyu Decoction (NYD) was studied by Xiyuan Hospital, Chinese Academy of TCM, Beijing. The conclusions to the study showed NYD significantly improved reproductive system blood circulation. This promoted a holistic regulation of the reproductive system and enhanced ovulation. Bushen Huoxue Decoction has also be used to treat ovulation dysfunction.

Two natural products developed in the USA by Selmedica HealthCare™ are claiming extremely high success rates in enhancing fertility. The male fertility enhancing product is called **AMBEROZ**™ which has shown to increase sperm counts by over 300 per cent in *93.7 per cent* of males using the product. The female fertility enhancing product is called **OVULEX**™ and Selmedica HealthCare claims that using this product has a *92.7 per cent* success rate.

I know of the herbal active ingredients used in these products; some are very well documented for their therapeutic applications enhancing fertility, some of the other herbal ingredients used in these formulas are unusual as to the significance of why they are included in fertility-enhancing products. Having said that, given these natural products claimed success in fertility they may be worth checking out.

## Herbs to avoid during pregnancy

Even though herbal medicines are *'natural'* it does not mean they cannot cause harm. There are a large number of botanical medicines that also contain potential active constituents that are known to possibly cause problems with conception and can increase the risks of miscarriage occurring.

This is a list of some of the main herbs that should be avoided. If you are uncertain about a particular herbal medicine you wish to use please seek further advice from a qualified herbalist for appropriate guidance: adahota; arbor vitae; barberry; broom; blood root; celandine; feverfew (in large doses); golden seal; hibiscus; juniper; mandrake root; mugwort; neem; nutmeg (in large doses); pennyroyal; poke root; senna; southernwood; tansy; wormwood; and zoapatle.

## Natural Treatments for Hormone Imbalances: Ovarian Hormones

*Phyto-oestrogens* e.g. alfalfa; black cohosh; ginseng; anise; dong quai; parsley; soya (beans, sprouts, milk); red clover; sage (salvia officinalis); fennel; flaxseed; cucumber; beans; lentils; grains; cabbage family; tofu; tempeh; sunflower seeds; millet; sesame seeds. Moderate amounts may be helpful to balance excessive/deficient oestrogen, but don't correct the underlying problem. *Be cautious with over-consumption of phyto-oestrogens (coumestans, isoflavones, lignans and sterols) as they can have a potential contraceptive affect on both men and women.*

*Ovarian tonic herbs* e.g. false unicorn root; dong quai; saw palmetto; black cohosh; shativari; paeony; true unicorn root; lady's mantle; liquorice; St John's wort; wild yam for oestrogen production and balance. Possibly ginsengs (esp. panax), though this may act through adrenal gland stimulation. Nutrients: Vitamin E, zinc, Vitamin C and magnesium for oestrogen balance.

*Progesterone supportive herbs* (through ovarian activity – there are no 'true' phyto-progesterones). Herbs of choice may include: vitex agnus castus, lady's mantle (and traditionally, sarsaparilla, wild yam, beth root, yucca, mistletoe, blue cohosh, fenugreek, though there is no conclusive confirming data on the latter). Nutrients for progesterone may include: Vitamin B6/ pyridoxal-5-phosphate, magnesium. Other ovarian tonics are damiana and golden seal.

**Progesterone creams** containing synthetic progesterone derived from extracts of herbs such as *wild yam* may be worth considering as the newer generation of these cream preparations is showing much promise in their relief of menstrual and menopausal symptoms.

Their benefits in enhancing fertility are still to be greatly investigated, but the early observation I have seen and reports from other practitioners appears to be very encouraging. Synthetic hormones can interfere with the body's natural hormone balance and can block possible ovulation when used during certain times in the menstrual cycle, but when used at the appropriate times to enhance ovulation and prevent low progesterone shortfalls it could be very helpful not only to fertility, but in preventing possible threatened miscarriage.

### Pituitary Hormone – Prolactin
Elevated levels of prolactin can be reduced through vitex agnus castus (chaste tree), Vitamin B6 or pyrodoxal-5-phosphate (activated B6) (in reasonable doses, under practitioner supervision). Medically drugs such as Bromocryptine (ergot derivative) may be considered.

### Luteinising Hormone (LH)
 - Elevated levels can be reduced with bugleweed (form of kelp); black cohosh; paeony; and hops. Low levels can be increased with vitex agnus castus.

### Follicle Stimulation Hormone (FSH)
 – Elevated levels reduced with bugleweed; paeony; and vitex. Low levels increased with black cohosh.

### Testosterone (T)
 - For elevated levels (in females) vitex and liquorice may lower testosterone. Other anti-androgenic herbal medicines are saw palmetto and paeony.

### Thyroid
 – Thyroid dysfunction can lead to miscarriage; the blood pathology tests for these hormones and various others have come under criticism as being relatively unreliable as a diagnostic tool. Basal temperature and physical characteristics may be useful indicators. When the thyroid function is in a state of balance this is referred to as *euthyroid*.

Thyroid imbalance is a relatively common problem affecting one out of eight females that are diagnosed at some point in their life. Males are also affected, but in comparison females are five to eight times more likely to have thyroid dysfunction. The thyroid gland can either under function known as hypothyroidism or over function known as hyperthyroidism.

Thyroid problems are normally diagnosed via thyroid function blood pathology: elevated thyroid stimulating hormone (TSH) may indicate hypothyroidism, as doe's decreased thyroxine (T3) and T4 levels. Hypothyroidism may also cause and increase in prolactin hormone production that can also decrease fertility.
A simple home test that you can perform using a basic glass mercury thermometer is a usual indicator of thyroid activity. Firstly, shake down the

mercury in the thermometer and place by the bed to be used first thing in the morning. On waking in the morning before getting out of bed place the thermometer under your armpit for 10 to 15 minutes. Do this every morning for three days.

If your average temperature is **36.5 degrees C (97.8°F)** or lower then you may well have an underactive or sluggish thyroid. This simple test may sometimes help to show underlying problems that may not necessarily have shown up on a blood test. Follow-up temperature readings over the full monthly cycle may give a more accurate indication of how the thyroid is performing.

During pregnancy the mother's thyroid function is very important for correct neural formation and activity of the developing foetus. Imbalances can lead to numerous potential cognitive and behaviour problems of the child.

***Hyperthyroid (high temperature)*** – e.g. *Grave's Disease*, may require prescription medication, radiation, radioactive iodine, and/or a medical thyroidectomy procedure (to cut it out)! Some of the signs and symptoms of suspected hyperthyroidism may include: rapid heartbeat (palpitations); increased sweating; anxiety; irritability; increased sensitivity; and weight loss. An overactive thyroid condition can lead to a greater conversion of androgens (male hormones) to oestrogen that can cause menstrual dysfunction caused ovulatory failure.

Medical drugs may include propylthiouracil which prevents the utilisation of iodine similar to isothiocyanates found in goitrogen foods.

Some of the natural treatments for hyperthyroid conditions may include: Herbal remedies - bugleweed (lycopus spp); vervain; lemon balm (melissa officinalis); lithospermum officinale; rehmannia; vitex (in high dose - but use only under supervision of practitioner). Cabbage, soya and walnut may also lower free thyroxin levels.

***Hypothyroid (low temperature)*** – e.g. *Hashimoto's Disease*, may require medical drug therapy such as thyroxine (Oroxine - from bovine source). T4 preparations such as: Synthroid, or Levothyroid; desiccated thyroid, and synthetic mixtures of T3 and T4: Liotrix or Thyrolar. Hypothyroidism can cause inadequate sex hormone levels and relative oestrogen excess. Some of the signs and symptoms of suspected hypothyroidism may include: low energy-fatigue; weight gain; water retention; low libido; irregular menstrual cycles; hair loss in major cases; dry skin; brittle nails; feeling cold in normal temperatures; depression; high cholesterol; and mental fogginess. An under-active thyroid condition can cause lower levels of sex hormone-binding globulin (SHBG), which leads to an eventual increase in oestrogen; this can also contribute to ovulatory failure. The armpit temperature of someone with hypothyroidism is regularly lower than 96.6 degrees F. Hypothyroidism early in pregnancies is linked to both increased risk of miscarriage and impaired neurological development in the unborn child.

Some of the natural treatments for hypothyroid conditions may include: bladder wrack (form of seaweed); poke root (only ever use under supervision and at low dosage, avoid in pregnancy); blue flag; astragalus; bupleurum; sarsaparilla (smilax spp); coleus forskohlii; morinda officinalis; l-tyrosine; potassium; iodine; natural desiccated thyroid gland extract; kelp; Vitamin B6; Vitamin C; choline; selenium; dehydroepiandrosterone (dhea); and lecithin.

Vitamins such as A and E are also important for the health of the pituitary gland and for correct thyroid-stimulating hormone (TSH) production. Vitamin D is an immune modulator and has a place in treating auto-immune thyroid dysfunction. Tyrosine and iodine are essential for the function of throxine; selenium is needed for the conversion of T3 to its active form. Hashimoto's thyroiditis is a T helper 1 (Th1) immune-dominant condition. The Central American fern polypodium leucotomos is an effective remedy to quench the excessive Th1 cytokine response (Leucostat is a product available through Metagenics).

Exposure to substances such as pesticides and PCBs (polychlorinated biphenyls) can decrease T4 levels and interfere with Vitamin A status in the body. These chemicals can also initiate autoimmune reactions against the thyroid gland.

The low temperature associated with hypothyroidism may inhibit cell division. The application of circulation stimulants may help to raise basal temperature, and thus, help to prevent threatened miscarriages. Some examples include: Cayenne (Capsicum spp), and Ginger (Zingiber officinal).

Other nutrients useful in hormonal imbalances are: Vitamin E; essential fatty acids (EFAs); B complex vitamins especially with Vitamin B6 (or pyridoxial-5-phosphate); Vitamin C; zinc; magnesium; calcium; and chromium.

**Natural Medicines that may benefit conditions contributing to infertility:**

*Uterine Dysfunctions - (poor circulation to the placenta, fibroids, endometriosis, threatened miscarriage):*
Black haw (viburnum prunifolium); cramp bark (viburnum opulus) (good for menstrual cramping); false and true unicorn root; wild yam (dioscerea spp – it is anti-inflammatory, a nervine tonic and uterine anti-spasmodic among other actions).

Wild yam may possibly affect the body's hormone levels (oestrogen, progesterone, and DHEA); paeonia (also affects the hormone levels); lady's mantle, shepherd's purse and beth root (are good anti-hemorrhagics to settle down excess bleeding); and vitex (may also have a place in helping these conditions).

Raspberry leaf and squaw vine: These two herbs have been traditionally used to improve preparation for labour; their applications in the first trimester (3 months) of pregnancy is questionable, therefore may be best avoided until later in the pregnancy.

Nutrients such as Vitamin C, bioflavonoids, Vitamin E and essential fatty acids (EFAs) also have their roles to play in these situations to strengthen capillaries, modulate prostaglandins, and improve circulatory function of the uterus.

### Allergies and Auto-Immune Disease:
Herbs such as hemidesmus (indicus) (benign immune suppressant); albizzia (lebbeck) (anti-allergic); rehmania (benign immune suppressant); bical skullcap (scutellaria baicalensis – * it may possibly have a teratogentic effect); and feverfew (tahacetum parthenium) are contraindicated to use during pregnancy.

Other herbs include: perilla fruteseen seed (control T-Helper 2 lymphocytes); polypodium leucotomos (control T-Helper 1 lymphocytes); chamomile (matricara recutita)- Chen Pi; picorrihiza kurroa; bupleurum falcatum; boswellia; nettle leaf; gingko biloba; and typlohora indica (use only under supervision of practitioner).

Nutrients such as: Vitamin C; Vitamin D; bioflavonoids; quercetin; rutin; hesperidin; bromelains; cetyl myristoleate (CMO); and reishii mushroom (gandoderma lucidum).

### Immune Dysfunction
Acute immune system herbs: echinacea (august folia, purpurea, spp); andrographis panniculata; bupleurum falcatum; commiphoria mol-mol (myrrh); baptisia tinctoria (wild indigo); holy basil (ocium sanctum); sambucus nigras (elder flower); ligustrum lucidum; lomatium dissectum; thyme (thymus vulgaris); cinnamon bark; and eupatorium perfoliatum (bone set).

*Anti-viral herbs:* St John's wort (hypericum perforatum); thuja occidentalis; garlic (allium sativum); onion (allium cepa); phyllanthus amurus; propolus; and olive leaf (olea europaea).

*Nutrients* such as: L-Lysine, Vitamin B5, biotin, Vitamin C, beta-carotenes, zinc gluconate, and bioflavonoids.

Acute immune herbs and nutrients may be of use in conditions like: Colds; flu; tonsillitis; bronchitis; herpes; measles; and chicken pox; for example!

*Chronic immune herbs:* astragalus membranaceus; eleuthrococcus senticosus (Siberian ginseng); uncaria tomentosa (cat's claw); hydrastis canadensis (golden seal); calendula officinalis; origanium oil; artemisia annua (Chinese wormwood); juglans nigra (black hulled walnut); pau d'arco (tabebuia avellanedae); barberry (berberis vulgaris); citrus seed extract (grapefruit) (citrus spp); noni (morinda citrifolia); withania somnifera (ashwaganda); shiitake (lentinula edodes); maitake (grifola frondoas); coriolus versicolour and cordycepsis sinesis (mushrooms); inostol hexaphosphate (IP6); di-methyl glysine (dmg); thymus gland extract; and antioxidants.

**Glyconutrients**: arabinogalactins (a soluble fibre extracted for the larch tree (larix decidua stem bark); colostrum (bovine); soya bean (glycine max dry seed); and transfer factor.

Chronic immune herbs and nutrients may be of use in conditions like: chronic fatigue syndrome; recurring fungal infections and parasite infestations: e.g. candida; salmonella; dysentery; microbiotic bacteria; toxoplasmosis; cytomegalovirus (cmv); epstein barre (glandular fever); ross river fever; influenza strains; parvovirus; gastro-intestinal and systemic infections; some sexually transmitted diseases; pelvic inflammatory diseases; and cancer support, for example.

**Genito/Urinary Herbs and Nutrients**: buchu (barosma betulina); arcytostaphyylos uva-ursi (bearberry); betula pendula (silver birch); crateava nurvala (cratevia); agropyron repens (couch grass); zea mays (corn silk); althea officinalis (marshmallow); eupatorium purpureum (gravel root); juniper (juniper communis); sage (salvia officinalis); lactobacilli; yarrow (achillea millefolium); d-mannose; and cranberry (vaccinium oxycoccus).


# Traditional Chinese Medicine

Traditional Chinese Medicine (TCM) is an ancient method of health care that combines the use of medicinal herbs, acupuncture, food therapy, massage, and therapeutic exercise. TCM has been practised for over three thousand years and today still one-quarter of the world population makes use of one or more of its therapies.

The approach to health and healing that TCM adopts differs from modern Western medicine and looks more so at the underlying cause of imbalances and patterns of disharmony in the body, and views each patient as being unique. The practice of TCM has evolved over thousands of years of observing and understanding the intricate works that go on in nature.

TCM recognises the human body as a reflection of the natural world – the part containing the whole. The flow of energy and fluids in the body are spoken in analogies with nature such as channels, rivers, seas, and reservoirs. A diagnosis might describe the body in terms of the elements – wind, heat, cold, dryness, and dampness.

This system of interrelating parts is kept harmonious by a system of dynamic balance between what is known as **yin** (the 'feminine' refers to the tissue of the organ) and **yang** (the 'masculine' refers to its activity) qualities.

Both are described as opposites and are interdependent with one another. Yin cannot exist without its opposite yang and vice versa. As in nature, the balance of the yin and yang constantly changes with the cycle of life because of both internal and external influences. TCM strives to maintain this see-sawing balance to prevent the manifestation of illness and dysfunction. Another fundamental concept to TCM is the belief in the life force or **qi**, (also referred to as 'Chi') that is central to the process of balance and is essential to all living things. Qi is inclusive of all energy that flows through the body but is not a solid substance. The manner in which this vital energy flows is via pathways called **meridians**.

These meridian channels flow along the surface of the body, and through the internal organs (similar to our body's complex nervous system); each of these 12 defined meridians are pressure points which when pressed or pinched (with needles) stimulate the flow of 'qi' and consequently strengthen or tonify the relevant organ/s associated with the blockage or stagnation causing the relative dysfunction or illness.

Like the principles of Ayurvedic medicine, TCM also believes in the important concept of the inter-relationship of the organs to each other and the five elements of nature. *The five phase theory* is a category system that matches the ten primary organs into five sections relevant to the five elements and respective yin and yang categories:

| Element | Yang Organ | Yin Organ |
|---------|-----------|-----------|
| Fire | Heart | Small intestine |
| Earth | Spleen | Stomach |
| Metal | Lungs | Large intestine |
| Water | Kidney | Bladder |
| Wood | Liver | Gall bladder |

All elements and organs synergistically interplay with each other. The yin organs are more substantial, solid, and passive in action; the yang organs are hollow and are more functional in action.

The practice of TCM involves varied diagnostic techniques that may differ from conventional medicine methods. The TCM practitioner may utilise various diagnostic techniques including observers and inspects the individual's complexion; general demeanour; body language; tongue; voice strength and tone; smelling various body excretions; the breath and/or body odour.

Palpation (feeling with the fingers) of the pulse at the radial arteries of both wrists (pulse diagnosis), the abdomen, and the meridian and/or acupuncture points. Pulse diagnosis examines the strength or weakness of the body 'qi' and 'blood' including the lymph and other bodily fluids. Pulse diagnosis can assist in assessing and determining how each organ and tissue is influenced via these factors.

Traditional Chinese Medicine (TCM) views infertility as one of seven different patterns of imbalance. Encompassing all the Western infertility diagnoses such as endometriosis and ovulatory dysfunction, these patterns are described in words such as 'damp heat', 'phlegm obstruction', 'liver qi stagnation' and 'blood stasis'. As different as these seven patterns are, they all involve some form of blockage.

One type of blockage is a physical obstruction of the blood and lymph as they move through the pathways of arteries and veins. The other is the energetic obstruction of 'qi' (the life force) as it moves through pathways of meridians.

Chinese medicine also classifies energy as yang and blood as yin. A person with excessive yang energy might be overweight, have an angry temperament, and high blood pressure. This type of individual may benefit from such foods that have a yin cooling effect such as asparagus; bananas; cucumbers; soy products (tofu); and watermelon.

The opposite yin energy person has a quite personality, who is listless or tires easily. Foods that this type of individual may benefit from include ones that have a yang warming effect such as beef; garlic; ginger; lamb; and pepper.

Neutral foods include black bean; cabbage; carrots; lemons; and rice and other grains.
These foods provide balance. To maintain health, one must consume the proper balance of these food groupings.

The infertility rate in China is only *3 per cent* in comparison to *over 15 per cent* in Western cultures; this fact reflects the effectiveness that TCM can have on enhancing fertility.

In TCM, the focus of treatment is not necessarily directly at the reproductive organs, but attention is directed towards the spleen, liver, and kidneys that are believed to govern over their functions. The spleen because of its influence on the immune system and blood flow to the uterus, the liver because of its role in hormone balance, removing damp heat as in water retention, tubal blockages and emotional activity, and the 'kidneys' because they're considered the body's source of sexual energy and treatments for irregular periods or ovulation dysfunction may involve directly treating the kidneys.

The kidneys are also believed to control the flow of the body's 'qi'. The reproductive system as such is recognised in TCM as secondary organs and is governed by the other primary organs and respective elements.

# TCM interpretation of the phases of a female's menstrual cycle

In TCM there are different energies that dominate each phase of the menstrual cycle:

**Phase 1:** *Kidney Yin (Ki Yi) and Blood* energies govern the follicular (proliferative), or hypothermal (low temperature) phase. Kidney Yin deficiency may present with symptoms such as: vaginal dryness and scant or missing cervical mucus. Oestrogen is a Yin energy hormone and should be dominant during this phase.

**Phase 2:** *Liver Qi (Lv Qi X) and Blood* movement control ovulation. At the peak of Yin energy, Liver Qi is triggered to begin the ovulation phase process transforming the Yin energy (oestrogen) to Yang energy (progesterone). Pain at ovulation may indicate blood stasis (BL X). Bloating may indicate Liver Qi Stagnation (Lv Qi X).

**Phase 3:** *Kidney Yang (Ki Yan-) and Spleen Qi (Sp-)* energies manage the luteal or hyperthermal (high temperature) phase. Yang energy dominates the luteal phase. If Kidney Yang and/or Spleen Qi is deficient then a 'luteal phase defect' may arise causing low progesterone production (short or ineffective luteal phase). Premenstrual spotting may indicate blood stasis, Qi deficiency. Severe breast tenderness may indicate Qi stagnation.

**Phase 4:** *Liver Qi (Lv Qi X)* helps the premenstrual transformation. If conception has not occurred Yang energies transform back into Yin energy. The corpus luteum then ceases its production of progesterone, the basal temperature falls and the menstrual period begins. If Qi and Blood are blocked and do not flow freely throughout the body, this can result in premenstrual symptoms (PMS) such as: irritability, period pain, headaches and bloating as examples.

**Phase 5:** *Blood* is allowed to flow. Menstruation is the time of rest for all energies.

## Male infertility from a TCM perspective, mainly falls under two broad categories:

1. Deficiency of Kidney (Ki Yi- or Ki Yan-) or the Spleen (Sp Qi-).
2. Excess of Stasis, stagnation, or damp heat (DH) in the pelvic organs.

Tonifying the kidneys, building the blood, clearing heat, and moving the Qi all have significant actions when improving sperm production and quality.

# Chinese Medicine Herbal Formulas for Reproductive Disorders

***Anemarrhena, Phellodendron & Rehmannia formula*** (Zhi Bai Di Huang Wan (Zhi Bai Ba Wei Wan, Chi Baku Ji O Gan): Yin tonifying formula. Action TCM: Moistens and tonifies the liver and kidney, clears heat and purges fire.

Modern applications in reproductive system include: Chronic urethritis/ nephritis; autonomic nervous system disorders; impotence; 'false' over-active libido; spermatorrhoea; climacteric disorders (post menopausal symptoms); and nocturnal emission. (Caution with oestrogen-sensitive disorders).

***Bupleurum & Chih-Shih (Zhi Shi) formula*** (Si Ni San, Shi Gyaku san): Harmonising formula (digestive, analgesic, and muscle relaxant). Modern applications to reproductive system include: autonomic nervous system disorders; neurosis; hysteria; depression; neurotic impotence; climacteric disorders; irregular menstruation; and premenstrual tension.

***Bupleurum & Paeonia formula*** (Jai Wei (dan Zhi) Xiao Yao San, Ka Mi Sho Yo San): Harmonising formula. Action TCM: Clears liver Qi stasis; strengthens spleen and tonifies blood; regulates menstruation; clears heat and cools blood. Gynaecology, psychology, and antidepressant: Modern applications to the reproductive system: chronic mastitis; chronic cystitis; chronic fatigue syndrome; emotional instability; neurosis; chronic endometritis; irregular menstruation; excessive menstrual flow; dysmenorrhoea; amenorrhoea; premenstrual tension; ovarian cysts; benign uterine tumours; endometriosis; and infertility.

Research has found that this formula can lower excessive oestrogen levels, therefore making it potentially beneficial for oestrogen/reproductive disorders such as breast and uterine cancer.

***Bupleurum & Tang Key (Dang Gui) formula*** (Xiao Yao San, Sho Yo San): Harmonising formula. (Obstetric and gynaecological). Action TCM: clears liver Qi stasis; strengthens the spleen; tonifies blood; and regulates menstruation. Modern applications to the reproductive system: autonomic nervous system; climacteric disorders; depression; stress; leucorrhoea; irregular menstruation; dysmenorrhoea; premenstrual tension; chronic mastitis; chronic cystitis; moodiness; and infertility.

***Cinnamon & Hoelen Combination*** (Gui Zhi Fu Ling Wan, Kei Shi Buku Ryo Gan): Blood moving formula (obstetric and gynaecology). Action TCM: Moves blood and transforms stagnation, reduces masses. Modern applications to the reproductive system: Poly cystic ovarian syndrome; endometriosis; ovaritis; menstrual irregularity; leucorrhoea; pelvic inflammatory disease (PID); prostatitis; benign prostatic hypertrophy; persistent dysfunctional uterine bleeding; dysmenorrhoea; amenorrhoea; uterine fibroids; ovarian cysts; dark clotted menstrual flow; and infertility.

**Ginseng & Astragalus Combination** (Tonifies spleen Qi and lifts prolapsed Yang). In Traditional Chinese botanical it is used as a nourishing tonic for both short and long term management of people with fatigue. Ginseng and astragalus combination is specifically valuable for male infertility due to oligospermia.

**Ginseng Nutritive Combination** (Ren Shen Yang Ying (Rong) Tang, Nin Jin Yo El To): Qi and Blood Tonifying formula (vital energy, enhance liver and circulation, strengthen digestion).
Actions TCM: tonifies Qi and blood; calms the Shen; expels cold; stops coughs. Modern applications to the reproductive system: post-partum disordersl post-haemorrhagel nocturnal emissions and impotence.

**Kidney Qi Pill** (Ji Sheng Shen Qi Wan): Studies that have been conducted with this TCM formulation have shown that sperm analysis after treatment improved sperm parameters in eighty-three of the eighty-seven cases, or 95 percent of the case subjects. By the end of the study, forty-nine of the men's wives (56.32 percent) were pregnant.

**Lotus Seed Combination** (Qing Xin Lian Zi, Sei Shin Ren Shi Yin): Qi and Yin Tonifying formula. (Diuretic and natural antibiotic); Action TCM: Invigorates spleen Qi and nourishes kidney Yin; clears heart fire; drains fluids. Modern applications to the reproductive system: autonomic nervous system disorders; climactic disorders; chronic cystitis; chronic gonorrhoea; leucorrhoea; prostatitis; impotence; spermatorrhoea; urinary retention; UTIs; and renal calculi.

**Morinda Combination** (Ba Ji Yin Yang Tang): Kidney yin and yang deficiency. Used for male reproductive disorders including: impotence; spermatorrhoea; low libido; general weakness; fatigue; and infertility. It has been used for women to prevent threatened miscarriages.
**NanBao:** Nanbao evolved from the highly guarded health and vitality formula that was prepared for the Chinese emperors, their wives, nobles and concubines for thousands of years. Nanbao is made from numerous herbs for easy absorption and assimilation. In Traditional Chinese Medicine terms Nanbao tonifies the Yang Qi, which essentially strengthens and improves circulation, helps relieve pain in the back and knees, enhances sex drive vitality and virility. It tones the blood circulation, thereby reducing numbness, pins and needles, and helps to relieve insomnia and headaches. This Chinese formula is one of the most used natural medicine supplements around the world, particularly in China and Japan.

**Paeonia & Liquorice Combination** (Shao Yao Gan Cao Tang, Shaku Yaku Kan Zo To): Harmonising formula. (Obstetric, gynaecology, and muscle relaxant). Action TCM: Harmonises the liver, resolves spasms and stops pain, tonifies the spleen. Modern applications to the reproductive system: Pain due to spasm; recurrent muscle cramps; dysmenorrhoea; polycystic ovarian syndrome; pelvic inflammatory disease; and infertility.

Studies have revealed the following actions:
  (1)  Peonia & liquorice combination enhances aromatase conversion of ovarian androgens into oestradiol.

  (2)  Oestradiol increases liver synthesis of sex hormone binding globulin (SHBG), which reduces the high level of free (active) testosterone associated with hirsutism.

  (3)  Decreases adrenergic stimulation of the hypothalamic GnRH output with a subsequent reduction in pituitary LH output and normalisation of the elevated LH: FSH ratio.

**Persica & Rhubarb Combination** (Tao He (Ren) Cheng Qi Tang, To Kaku Jo Ki To): Blood moving formula (anticoagulant, purgative).
Action TCM: Clear heat and purges, moves blood and disperses stagnation. Modern applications to the reproductive system: Dysmenorrhoea; amenorrhoea; irregular menstruation; post-partum vaginal discharge; pelvic haematocele; endometriosis; pelvic inflammatory disease; endometritis; intestinal adhesions; ovarian cysts; uterine bleeding; and infertility.

**Rehmannia Six formula** (Liu Wei Di Huang Wan, Roku Mi Ji Gan): Yin tonifying formula. Action TCM: Nourishing and enriches the liver, kidney yin (tonic, paediatric) clears deficient heat, drains damp. Modern applications to the reproductive system: autonomic nervous system disorders; impotence; spermatorrhoea; anovulation; amenorrhoea or scanty menstruation; post-menopause symptoms; and children who are slow to develop, either mentally or physically.

**Rehmannia Eight (hachimijigan) Combination** (Tonify Yin): This formula has been successfully used in China to treat hyperprolactinemia induced infertility and luteal phase defects, oligospermia, and prostatic hypertrophy (enlargement). Studies using hachimijiogan in men have shown improvements in sperm count, density, and motility.

**Tang Kuei (Dang-Gui) & Paeonia formula** (Dang Gui Shao Yao San, To Ki Shaku Yaku San): Blood tonic formula (gynaecological disorders). Action TCM: Tonifies and moves liver blood, aids the flow of liver Qi, strengthens the spleen and drains damp, regulates menstruation and stops pain. Modern applications to the reproductive system: irregular menstruation; habitual abortion (threatened miscarriage); functional menorrhagia; premenstrual tension; dysmenorrhoea; abdominal pains; oedema of pregnancy; floating kidneys; leucorrhoea; cold constitution; lumbago; post-partum weakness; and infertility.

It is used to balance luteal phase insufficiency and has been found in clinical studies that this formula improved plasm oestradiol and progesterone levels in the mid-luteal phase of the menstrual cycle, enhances follicular development, increasing fertility and normalising menstrual dysfunctions.

The formula contains: angelica sinensis (dang qui); paeonia alba (bai shao, white peony); ligusticum wallichi (chuan xiong cnidium); atractylodes macrocephala (bai zhu, atratylodes); poria cocos (fuling, hoelen); and alisma oriental (ze xie, alisma).

**Tang-Kuei (Dang-Gui) & Evodia Combination** (Wen Jing Tang, Un Kei To): Inner warming cold expelling formula. Action TCM: Tonic; tonifies blood quality; regulates menstruation; warms channels (menses); moves blood and transforms stagnation; invigorates Qi; and harmonises the stomach. Modern applications to the reproductive system: Taken when infertility is related to physical weakness, (chilling at the waist and feet, hot palms, dry lips); uterine bleeding; irregular menstruation; amenorrhoea; dysmenorrhoea; ovarian cysts; infertility; male infertility; climacteric disorders; autonomic nervous system disorders; leucorrhoea; habitual abortions (threatened miscarriage); and mild persistent uterine bleeding.

**Tang-Kuei (Dang-Gui) & Gardenia Combination** (Wen Qing Yin, Un Sei, In): Heat Clearing formula (Gynaecological and Skin disorders).
Action TCM: Clears heat and purges fire; anti-toxic; tonifies and moves stagnant blood; stops haemorrhage; antibiotic; and anticoagulant. Modern applications to the reproductive system: Post-partum and post-haemorrhage conditions; autonomic nervous system disorders; convalescence; irregular menstruation; midline pain in women; climactic disorders; paropsia; amenorrhoea; dysmenorrhoea; late menstruation; scanty menstruation; insufficient uterine development; ulcerated mucous membranes; metrorrhagia; menorrhagia; and chronic leucorrhoea.

**Tang-Kuei (Dang-Gui) & Ginseng Eight Combination** (Ba Zhen Tang, Hantchin To): Qi and Blood tonifying formula. Action TCM: Qi (spleen), Blood (liver), digestant, tonic supplement to blood and energy. Weakness during convalescence; no vigour; fatigue; anaemia; lumbago in women; menstrual irregularities; metrorrhagia; post-partum haemorrhage; autonomic nervous system disorders; midline pain in women; climactic disorders; paropsia; amenorrhoea; dysmenorrhoea; late menstruation; scanty menstruation; and insufficient uterine development.

**Tang-Kuei (Dang-Gui) Four Combination** (Si Wu Tang, Shi Motsu To): Blood tonifying formula (Blood tonic). Actions TCM: Regulates menstruation, tonifies and moves blood. Modern applications to the reproductive system: Malnutrition; autonomic nervous system; climactic disorders (menopause); mild anaemia; paropsia; menstrual disorders; amenorrhoea; infertility; insufficient uterine development; dysmenorrhoea; late menstruation; scanty menstruation; and pre and post-partum disorders.

**Wen Dan Tang** (Bamboo & Hoelen combination): Wen Dan Tang may be used for treating conditions such as: amenorrhea, anxiety, copious white / turbid leucorrhoea, infertility, insomnia, gastritis, obesity, and prolonged menstrual cycles when caused by TCM phlegm damp pattern.

***Zuo Gui Wan*** (Left Returning Formula): This formula is used for conditions such as: premature ejaculation; seminal emissions; infertility; amenorrhea; and dysfunctional uterine bleeding.

***Classic TCM formula for infertility with kidney yang:*** *Xian ling pi (yin yang huo)* Epimedium, + *ba ji tain* (Morinda) + *rou cong rong* (Cistanche) + *suo yang* (Cynomorium dongariorm). Prolonged menstrual cycle with scanty and light-coloured menstrual flow, or amenorrhea; low sex drive.

***Classic TCM formula for infertility with kidney yin:*** *Tu si zi* (Cuscuta), + *fu pen zi (*Rubus chingii) + *han lian cao* (Eclipta) + *nu zhen zi* (Ligustrum); Often shortened menstrual cycle scanty menstrual flow.

## Chinese Herb Combination to Support IVF

The uterus is a natural incubator which has to be kept at a constant temperature to facilitate the embryo implantation. Many of the fertility drugs used during IVF procedures such as Follicle Stimulating Hormone (FSH) can also produce some undesirable side effects of which excess lower abdomen fluid production is one. Excessive fluid accumulation in the abdomen can cause an increased cooling effect in the uterus. This excess fluid may be one of the primary reasons why many IVF procedures fail to take because it also cools the body's natural temperature.

Preparing several weeks prior to IVF/ICSI embryo transfers and several weeks after the implantation procedure by gently reducing excessive fluid build-up, may greatly help to improve the maintenance of correct body temperature and also enhance blood supply to nourish and oxygenate the uterine lining, therefore promoting a much more ideal environment for the embryo to implant and thrive.

Supporting the bodies stress responses during the IVF process may also increase the chances of a successful outcome. Excessive stress during medical-assisted fertility procedures can lead to unwanted body reaction such as excess muscular spasming (e.g. uterine wall), and inflammatory mediator response, which is not desirable for the chances of implantation success.

These are some of the more commonly used Chinese herbs used to support conception and IVF:

***Poria*** – A very effective mushroom extract that helps to drain the excess fluid caused by the hormones in the abdomen.

***Poria Core*** – This herb is useful to help support the body in relieving stress.

**Coicus Seed** – Another herb used to help eliminate excessive fluid, which in turn prevents the excess water from cooling the uterus keeping the uterus warm for implantation.

**Angelica sinensis (Dong Quai)** – This well-known female herb helps to warm the blood supply to the uterus, which in turn assists to prepare the uterus lining for implantation.

**Ligusticum** – This herb works well with Dong Quai to warm the uterus.

**Dipsacus** – Is also known to assist with warming the uterus and support implantation. Dipsacus also may help with bone formation, so it may be beneficial to use during the pregnancy for foetus skeletal development.
**Eucomia** – Supports the uterus to help prevent chances of miscarriage.

A TCM formula traditionally known as **Obtaining Birth Elixir** has a long and reputed history of use to enhance conception. A summary of the formula includes:

**Yi Mu Cao** – A uterine tonic that promotes blood flow into the pelvic area; it invigorates blood by reducing viscosity via the prostaglandins.

**Dang Gui, Bai Shao, Chai Hu and Xiang Fu** – Promote blood flow into the pelvic area, help regulate the menses, soothe the liver and nourish the blood. As well as resolve depression and soothe the emotions.

**Bai Zhu and Fu Ling** – Regulate the Spleen Energy and help in the promotion of blood and regulation of healthy digestive function.

## Australian Bush Essences and Bach Flower Remedies

Flower essences have a long history of assisting underlying emotional and psychological problems (particularly on a sub-conscious level) by gentle and positively influencing the mental/emotional body that in turn will positively influence the physical body.
Flower essences are used as catalysts to help unlock your full creative potential, attain emotional, spiritual, mental and physical balance, resolve negative beliefs and bring about a condition of harmony. Flower essences help to promote healing by releasing negative emotions and thought patterns.

Indigenous people have used flower essences all over the world for centuries. The Australian Aborigines have always used flower essences to restore emotional balance, as did the ancient Egyptians, and African tribes. They were also extremely popular in the Middle Ages.

These remedies are useful for clearing emotional blocks that may stop a person from getting in touch with their true self and life purpose. They help to give clarity to one's life purpose yet also offer courage and strength to follow one's goals and dreams. The following examples of flower essences are but only a few that may be used for reproductive disorders and individual constitution types.

Examples include:

**She Oak** - which helps to soothe the distress associated with infertility and is adopted in cases where infertility has no known origin.

**Turkey Bush** - is used in situations where creative blocks occur. Conception could be well regarded as the 'ultimate in creativity' and this flower essence is said to help release and get the creative juices flowing (literally) for both men and women.

**Old Man Banksia** - for those who have had many disappointments, feel very weary of trying, and are disheartened and frustrated.

**Sturt Pea** - helpful, especially when there has been a loss or miscarriage in the family. This may help to release you to the natural grieving process and to let go of the pain.

**Wisteria** - helps the person to become aware of their dual nature and become more balanced within themselves.

A useful pre-formulated product that I often use to help balance and harmonise the emotional cycle for women is called **Women Essence**™.

This formula contains the fluid extract essences from the Australian native flowers: *billy goat plum, bottlebrush, bush fuchsia, crowea, five corners, mulla mulla, old man banksia, peach-flowered tea tree, and she oak.*

I have found this product to be very successful for fertility and other female reproductive disorders when there is an origin that is significantly emotional based.

**Bach Remedies that may be considered**

**Agrimony** – for extreme nervousness and anxiety.

**Aspen** - the specific remedy for those who have vague unknown fears; who are afraid something terrible is going to happen but don't know what.

**Gentian** – helpful for those who are depressed, full of doubt, discouraged or disheartened

**Gorse** - can help when a person feels no more can be done for them; that their case is hopeless.

*Mimulus* - for fear of the known things.

*Rock rose* - for cases where there appears to be no hope, or when a person is very frightened. This could be used as a form of relaxation for women who have to undergo medical procedures but are frightened of yet another disappointment

*Rock water* – for tension, overanxiousness, or dissatisfaction with themselves.

*Vervain* – for melancholy depression.

*Walnut* - for protection against outside influences.

*Willow* – for resentment and irritability.

*Rescue remedy* – is a preformulated combination of bach remedies used for trauma and relieving distress.

## Aromatherapy for Men and Women

Aromatherapy is the practice of using pure essential oils extracted from flowers, leaves, stems, herbs, bark and wood of aromatic plants.

The practice of aromatherapy has been used by numerous ancient civilisations for their therapeutic qualities, to maintain health and to heal the body and mind. Aromatherapy combines our two most primitive senses, touch and smell. Touch, with our hands when applying or massaging into the body. Smell, by inhaling the scent of the essential oil.

The essential oils are believed to work in such a way that they maintain the balance of all the organs and systems of the body that are actively involved in fighting invading organisms and eliminating toxins, helping to keep us disease free, giving us health and well-being.

**The benefits of Aromatherapy may include**:
• Relief of pain
• Promoting tissue repair
• Enhancing the mind and spirit
• Stimulating immunity
• Restraining infection
• Enhancing and assisting pregnancy and childbirth.

There are a number of particular essential oils that are relevant to helping reproductive and infertility problems. Some of these may include:

• **Apricot Kernel** and **Sweet Almond** can be used as a carrier oils.

216

- *Clary Sage* – A tonic for the uterus (womb) and a hormone-balancer. Clary sage is a powerful muscle relaxant that can help with period pains. Has a particularly euphoric and tonic quality, working to promote well being and energy. NB: Not recommended to be used during the early stages of pregnancy.

- *Rose* – A tonic for the uterus, it calms PMT, regulates the menstrual cycle and promotes vaginal secretions. Promotes self-confidence and alleviates stress. Rose is said to increase semen production in men. Can help with sexual difficulties (such as impotence) since it has the power to release the 'happy' hormone dopamine. NB: Not to be used directly in pregnancy.

- *Ylang Ylang* – A hormone-balancer and uterus tonic; Ylang Ylang is an anti-depressant, aphrodisiac as well as an antiseptic.

- *Jasmine* – A hormone-balancer and uterine tonic. Jasmine has anti-depressant and nerve-calming properties and may also help men's sperm production. Not to be used in pregnancy, but recommended for childbirth.

- *Melissa (Lemon Balm)* – Regulates menstruation and is a uterus tonic. Also a tonic for the heart, calms breathing and uplifts the spirits, soothing the effects of shock and panic.

- *Geranium* – regulates the hormonal system. Can promote vaginal secretion and help with heavy periods. Is also a diuretic, helping poor circulation, is a tonic to the spirit and is said to have oestrogenic properties.

Other beneficial oils may include: basil; bergamot; chamomile; lavender; orange; lemon; lemon grass; jasmine; neroli; sandalwood; tangerine; and petigrain. All are particularly useful in helping relieve symptoms of stress.

### Aromatherapy remedies that may help reproductive conditions:

**Female conception**: Cinnamon; geranium; rose; sage; and lemon balm oils.

**Male conception**: Cinnamon; clary sage; jasmine; rose; sandalwood; and ylang ylang.

There are a numerous variety of essential oils that are contra-indicated to be used during pregnancy; seek advice from a qualified natural therapist specialising in this field for correct safety uses of these oils.

# Homeopathic Medicine

The practice of modern homeopathic medicine was formally founded by a German physician, Samuel Hahnemann. However, its roots can be traced back to Ancient Greek times. The basic principles of homeopathy are that the state of the human body is one of health and that we possess the natural ability to heal ourselves. The meaning of the word 'homeopathy' is derives from the Greek words *homoeo* (similar) and *pathos* (suffering). Hahnemann had developed a theory of the *Law of Similars* – 'Like Cures Like'.

What we know or describe as symptoms of disease are actually the body's efforts to protect itself against disease. Therefore, to affect a cure of the ailment, we should not suppress the symptoms, but rather seek to stimulate the body's innate natural healing processes. The suppression of symptoms can actually hamper the body's ability to cure itself if given the right conditions to do so.

The patient and not the illness, is the focus of homeopathic medicine. Homeopathy, like other holistic healing modalities, considers the state of the whole individual encompassing the physical, mental, and emotional. Homeopathy views illness as a result of an imbalance or change in the vital force energy patterns in the body.

The therapies used in homeopathy are based on specific energy or vibration patterns that they produce when introduced into the body. This resonance of energies between the remedy and individual activate the appropriate healing process. Not unlike trying to fine tune your TV reception into the right frequency to get a better picture.

The remedies used in homeopathy are derived from various natural sources such as animal, plant, and mineral, and are highly concentrated and minutely diluted to increase their potencies levels. The medicines are prescribed to match the specific symptoms. Homeopathic medicines are utilised worldwide and are a very safe and cost effective alternative therapy. The remedies are usually dispensed in liquid, pellet or tablet form.

The following are examples of homeopathic medicines used for both male and female reproductive disorders:

- *Agnus castus* - (female) sterility with sadness, leucorrhoea (white discharge); (male) impotence with no desire, and swollen testicles.
- *Aletris farinosa* - (female) tendency to abort, and uterine pain.
- *Apis* - (female) ovarian tumours (pain), and painful periods.
- *Argenicum metalicum* - (female) prolapse of uterus (pain); (male) pain in testicles, and seminal emissions.
- *Belladonna* - (female) dryness in vaginal, temperature too high; (male) testicles hot and drawn up and no interest in sex.
- *Borax* - (female) sterility with hot watery discharge, and herpes.

- **Bufo** - (female) epilepsy with period, ulceration of cervix, polyps; (male) impotence, involuntary emissions and spasms with coition.
- **Calcium Carbonate** - (female) sterility in the overweight, uterine polyps, (male) - weakness and irritability after coition.
- **Calendula -** (female) vaginal warts, uterine hypertrophy, heavy periods.
- **Conium maculation** - (female) painful periods, painful enlarged breasts, difficulty conceiving, inflammation of ovary; (male) increase desire, decreased power, feeble erection, and swollen hard testicles.
- **Eupion** - (female) disease in tubes, pain in right ovary, and backache.
- **Gelseminum** - (female) painful light period; (male) continual sweating in scrotum, and discharge corrosive.
- **Graphites** - (female) nausea/constipation with period, herpes; (male) ejaculation too soon, sexual debility, and herpes.
- **Hydrastis** - (female) cervical erosion, leucorrhoea (white discharge), itchy vulva; (male) yellow discharge.
- **Iodum** - (female) irregular periods, inflammation of ovary, lumps in breasts.
- **Lecithin** - (female) ovarian insufficiency (weakness in function); (male) no power, and feeble erection.
- **Lycopodium -** (female) coition painful, period late and lasts too long, pain in right ovary; (male) impotence, enlarged prostate, and psoriasis.
- **Medorrhinum** - (female) sterility, intense itch in vulva, genital warts, fishy odour, and offensive periods; (male) impotence enlarged prostate, and frequent painful urination.
- **Nuphur Luteum (Yellow Pond Lilly) 6x, 30x** - (male) used specifically for males with complete absence of sexual desire, impotence, spermatorrhea, and 'nervous weakness with marked symptoms in the sexual sphere'.
- **Onosmodium** - (female) uterine pain, no desire for sex, period early and lasts too long, yellow discharge, sore breasts; (male) impotence, deficient erection.
- **Oophorinum** - (female) ovarian cysts, acne, and hot flushes.
- **Palladium** - (female) prolapse and/retroversion of the uterus.
- **Phosphoric acid** - (male) sexual weakness, emissions at night and when passing stools, and herpes.
- **Phytolacca -** (female) mastitis, tumour of the glands, and ovarian pain; (male) pain in penis and/or testicles.
- **Platinum** - (female) - sterility with ovarian inflammation, itchy vulva, and sexual melancholia.
- **Plumbum** - (female) tendency to abort, and vagina hypersensitivity.
- **Pulsatilla** - (female) weeps easily, period erratic, tires easily; (male) inflammation or bruising to testis, prostatitis, and yellow discharge.
- **Sabina** - (female) threatened miscarriage, breakthrough bleeding at ovulation; (male) increased desire, and painful erection.
- **Thuja** - (female) vaginal warts, polyps, pain in left ovary; (male) pain in penis, warts, and enlarged prostate.
- **Viburnum opulus** - (female) frequent early miscarriage, heavy period, and congested ovaries.

Other beneficial homeopathic potency remedies may include:

Testosterone; aldosterone; thyroxinum 6x-12x; oestrogen 6x-12x; progesterone 6x-12x; hypophysis (pituitary extract) 12x; dhea; apol; oophorinum (ovary gland tissue) 6x-12x; orchitium (testicular extract) 6x-12x; follicle tissue; sepia; cantharis 4x; lycopium 6x; and caladium 6x.


# Benefits of Massage

Massage, which falls under the category of bodywork, involves the manipulation of muscles and other soft tissues. It is beneficial in treating a wide range of conditions and there is a huge variety of various styles and techniques available to choose from.

Some of the general effects that massage can have on the body may include:

- Increases metabolism
- Relaxes muscles
- Enhances removal of metabolic wastes
- Improves circulation of blood and lymph
- Relieves mental and physical fatigue
- Reduces pain
- Reduces tension and anxiety
- Calming to the nervous system
- Muscles and joints become more supple
- Improves skin tone.


### Swedish massage
Swedish massage is each conceived as having a specific therapeutic benefit. One of the primary goals of Swedish massage is to speed the venous blood return of unoxygenated and toxic blood from the extremities. Swedish massage shortens recovery time from muscular strain by flushing the tissues of lactic acid, uric acid, and other metabolic wastes. It increases circulation without increasing heart load. It stretches the ligaments and tendons keeping them supple and young. Swedish massage also stimulates the skin and nervous system and soothes the nerves themselves at the same time. It reduces stress, both emotional and physical, and is suggested in a regular program for stress management.


### Deep Tissue Massage
This approach is used to release chronic patterns of muscular tension using slow strokes, direct pressure, or friction. Often the movements are directed across the grain of the muscles (cross-fibre) using the fingers, thumbs, or elbows.

### Oriental Massage

Oriental Massage methods are based on the principles of Chinese medicine and the flow of energy or chi through the meridians. The geography of the acupuncture meridians is relied upon to determine points of applying the techniques and the ultimate goal is restoration of harmony or balance in the flow of chi. Strong pressure or very light pressure may be applied.

### Reflexology

Reflexology is an ancient practice of bodywork that applies stimulating massage and gentle pressure to the thousands of nerve endings and energy 'zones' in the sole of the feet. Each foot comprises 26 bones, 19 muscles, 107 ligaments and is required to support the full weight of the body. The sole of the feet in reflexology are represented as a map of the entire body.

Reflexology can help to:

- stimulate the flow of blood
- improve circulation
- increase energy levels and removes blockages
- releases tension and stress a balanced energy flow in the meridians
- decrease blood sugar levels
- to improve the health of the whole body and try to prevent the cause of disease.

Thumb pressure is applied to specific points that correspond somatotopically to specific areas or organs of the body such as the fallopian tubes, uterus, ovaries, prostate, and testis. Reflexology rids the body of toxins that have accumulated from chemicals in food, medication and pollution.

Reflexology works on the theory that ten zones of electrical energy extend throughout the body. By massaging points on the feet, hands and ears, it treats disease in the whole body. Endocrine and hormone imbalances can also be specifically treated for both sexes with reflexology techniques.

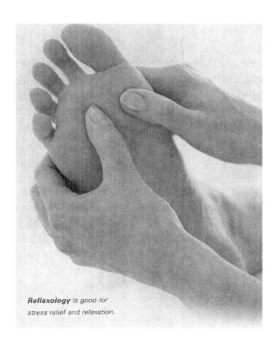

*Reflexology* is good for stress relief and relaxation.

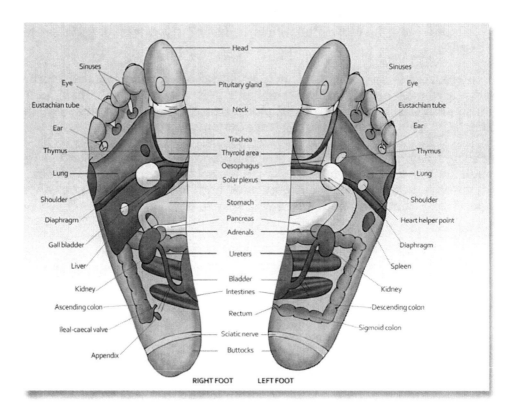

**Figure.15. Reflexology Feet Map**

### Reiki

Reiki is the Japanese word for *universal life force energy*. It is an ancient approach in which the practitioner is a kind of healer in the sense that he or she serves as a conduit for healing energy coming from the universe. The Reiki energy enters the practitioner through the top of the head and exits through the hands, being directed into the body or energy field of the recipient.

Reiki is another very subtle form of healing and may be done through clothing and without any physical contact between practitioner and client.

While all the above energetic methods appear to operate on different principles than most other varieties of massage therapy and bodywork, they nonetheless have an important and growing role.

### Shiatsu

Shiatsu is another form of massage technique the originated from China and then spread to countries such as Japan. Based on similar principles as acupuncture and traditional Chinese medicine, Shiatsu bodywork is used to locate any blockages in energy flow throughout the body and works to unblock these stagnations of energy flow to regain balance to achieve health and wellbeing.

Other forms of massage and body work include:
Body harmony; Body Talk; Bowen therapy; Chiropractic; Esalen massage; The Feldenkrais Method; NFT; Neuro linguistic programming (NLG); Neuro Muscular Massage; Osteopathy; Physiotherapy; Rolfing or Structural Integration; Sports Massage; and so on.


# Naturopathy

### 'Vis medicatrix naturae - the healing power of nature'

The Hippocratic School of Medicine (circa 400 BC) has moulded and influenced the basic principles of modern Naturopathic practices. Modern orthodox (techno/allopathy) medicine and Natural/Complementary Medicine both originated primarily from the same beginnings. Over the past centuries, the two systems of medicine have alternately diverged and converged, shaping each other, often in reaction. The Naturopathic model of medicine is philosophically 'Health-orientated' where Orthodox medicine is 'Disease-orientated'.

Naturopathy, or 'Nature Cure', is both a way of life and a concept of healing, employing various natural means of preventing and treating human disease. The fundamental philosophical cornerstone to the practice of Naturopathic Medicine is although the term naturopathic medicine was not used until the late nineteenth century its philosophical roots date back thousands of years drawing from the healing wisdom of many cultures. Hippocrates is considered to be the 'Father of a profound belief in the ability of the body to heal itself, given the proper opportunity to do so'.

The role of the naturopathic practitioner is to assist and facilitate this healing process by incorporating a variety of 'non-invasive, non-toxic, natural therapies' based on the patient's individual needs. Diet, lifestyle, work and personal history are all considered when determining a treatment regimen.

Naturopathic Medicine is not a single modality of health care, but rather a collective array of numerous, integrated complementary practices. Many of these modalities are discussed throughout this book such as clinical nutrition, diet therapy, herbal medicine, and homeopathy. Naturopaths may also utilise a variety of analysis tools to assist with diagnosis of dysfunction such as iridology (iris/scelera analysis); hair tissue mineral analysis; live blood analysis; and the application of various computer and electrodermal testing devices in modern practices.

Naturopathy comprises a common sense and 'vitalistic' approach to health, recognising the whole person and not just the physical symptoms of an illness. Treatment is directed at a structural, biochemical and mental/emotional level. The pursuit of optimal health, enhanced wellbeing and improved quality of life is the foundation of natural medicine. Naturopathic medicine does not focus on disease, but rather the underlying cause of disease. By addressing the origin of dysfunction with supportive treatment (rather than invasive or suppressive therapy) the body then has a more complete opportunity to correct and heal itself NATURALLY.

Life is viewed as more than just the sum of biochemical processes, and the body is believed to have an innate intelligence that is always striving for balance (perfection) and health. This healing energy is believed to pervade all living matter and is described in many ways such as the *Vital Life Force*, *Om*, *Prana* (Ayurvedic), *Chi or Qi*, (Traditional Chinese Medicine), and *Pneuma* (Greco-Roman constitutional 'Humoral' theory) to name a few!

Vitalism maintains that the symptoms accompanying disease are not directly caused by the morbific agent, e.g. bacteria; rather, they are the result of the organism's intrinsic response or reaction to the agent and the organism's attempt to defend and heal itself. Symptoms, then, are part of a constructive phenomenon that is the best 'choice' the organism can make, given the circumstances.

Health is viewed as more than just the absence of disease; it is considered to be a vital dynamic state which enables a person to thrive in, or adapt to, a wide range of environments and stresses. People who 'catch' every cold that comes by are not healthy when they are symptom free; they can be considered healthy only when they stop being overly susceptible to infection.

Health and disease can be looked at as points on a continuum, with death at one end and optimal function at the other. As the typical person goes through life, he or she drifts away from optimal function and moves relentlessly towards progressively greater dysfunction. Although such deterioration is endorsed by our society as a normal expectation of aging, it does not happen to animals in the wild, or to those few fortunate people who live in an optimal environment, i.e. no pollution, low stress, regular exercise and abundant natural, nutritious food. Death is indeed inevitable, but progressive disability is not.

Naturopaths are essentially preventative medicine specialists. Prevention of disease is encouraged through the elimination of toxins and by educating the individual on the principles of a natural diet and lifestyle. Most importantly, naturopathy empowers and motivates the patient to assume a more active and responsible role in his/her own health care. *This alone is powerful medicine.*

A revolution is occurring in health care. During the 1970s and 80s there has been an explosion in information in the science literature supporting and validating the use of natural medicines. Science and medicine now have in their possession the technology and understanding necessary to appreciate many aspects of Natural Medicine.

The 1970s and 80s were years of re-emergence for Naturopathic physicians. With the 1960s came a rebirth of awareness and interest into all things 'Natural'. A new generation arose that no longer accepted the status quo blindly. All aspects of modern society were scrutinised; among these the practice of modern medicine.

Even though something may be new, this does not always make it better! Thalidomide in Europe, DES-induced cancers, DDT, Viox and other drug-related tragedies have led the general public more and more to ask, not how effective a drug is, but how safe? With each new horror story of tragedies induced by drugs thought to be harmless for years, more people are seeking a safe alternative. Many of the advances in medicine in the future will be Naturopathic in philosophy. This illustrates the shift that is occurring in the medical paradigm. For example, through genetic engineering it is now feasible for many substances natural to the body to be produced in the laboratory. Although it must be emphasised that these substances should be reserved for end-stage disease and should in no way circumvent appropriate preventative measures, appropriate use of many of these substances could be consider Naturopathic in essence.

Examples of such substances are monoclonal antibodies directed against specific tumour antigens; various antiviral and immune-enhancing substances natural to the body in the treatment of acquired immunodeficiency syndrome (AIDS) such as interferon, interleukin, chymosin, etc; atrial natriuretic peptide in severe congestive heart disease; and human growth hormone in the treatment of growth hormone deficiency. The future for Naturopathic Medicine certainly looks very bright.

*Proverb – 'Give a man a fish you feed him for a day, teach a man to fish you feed him for a life time'.*

### Tai Chi

Tai Chi, known as 'meditation in motion' is an ancient Chinese technique similar to a 'soft and slow rhythmical flowing' form of martial art. Tai Chi releases the flow of energy throughout the body. When this energy becomes blocked, illness follows. The philosophical bases to Tai Chi are similar to other principles in traditional Chinese medicine practices. Tai Chi involves the study and practice of sequential movements to promote mediation, coordination, flexibility, and mind and body relaxation.

### Qi Gong

Qi Gong (pronounced chie-gong) is a slow-motion exercise with similarities to Tai Chi, though is an older technique. *Qi* means 'life force, energy,' and *gong* means 'work, a skill of practice'. Qi Gong concentrates on meditated breathing and movement disciplines to increase vital energy for emotional and physical health.

Qi exercises for the uterus:

- Lying on your back, raise and support the hips with a cushion and tense and relax the muscles of the pelvic floor, 100–300 times, as though you are trying to stop a bowel movement or urination. Do this 2-3 times a day.

- Lying on your back, relax every part of your body completely. Put your hands down beside your body, bend the knees and draw the knees up close to the buttocks. Lift your hips off the bed or floor while using your shoulders and feet for support and do this while inhaling; lower the hips while exhaling. Constrict the anus while breathing in; it has a pulling effect on the uterus. Relax the anus and the whole body while breathing out. Do this 10-30 times once a day.

- Lying on your stomach with the legs extending, stretched and crossed, constrict both the anus and vulva as hard as possible. Relax the muscles of the legs and pelvis completely. Do this 100 times a day.

### Yoga

Yoga is an ancient art of movement developed over five thousand years ago in India. Yoga involves exercises to stretch the muscles and joints to unify the consciousness to harmonies the mind, body and spirit. The art of yoga also teaches control techniques of breathing.

*Hatha* yoga is a term familiar to many who practise yoga, though it is not actually a particular style of yoga. Hatha is a Sanskrit word meaning 'wilful' and yoga is translated as 'union' or 'communion'. This is understood as meditation in action. Yoga is a common disciple that is taught in antenatal and active birthing classes. There are a number of different styles and adaptations that can be used, some of which are known as: Ananda; Ashtanga; Bikram; Kundalini; Tantra; Chakra; Raja; Sevananda; Tivamukti; Kripalu; Integral; and Phoenix rising yoga therapy. All the yoga postures help to remove obstructions from the body to enhance energy, well-being and achieve inner peace.

### Meditation

The mind and body relaxation method of meditation has been used by many cultures in some form or another for thousands of years. Of the many forms of meditation that are available, there are two common categories that they fall into: concentrative and mindfulness. Meditation usually involves sitting in a quite still position, observing your breathing pattern and controlling its rhythm.

The use of *mantra* such as concentrating on a light (e.g., flame) or sound pattern helps to calm the mind and unclutter negative thoughts and centre you in the present moment (not the past or future). Transcendental meditation (TM) is a very deep state of relaxation that has been scientifically studied for its health benefits, the findings include: it's effective at controlling anxiety; it enhances immune system function; reduces elevated blood pressure; successfully controls chronic pain tolerance; decreases the need for substance abuse; reduces daily reaction to stresses; and counteracts depression. The ultimate aim of meditation is to obtain spiritual enlightenment.

### Hypnotherapy

Hypnotherapy is a visualisation and imagery technique similar to meditation in many ways but is designed to unlock the un/subconscious mind guided by a therapist skilled in the art.

Hypnotherapy utilises deep relaxation methods to heighten the individual's receptiveness and awareness through verbal suggestion. The subconscious part of our mind has control of many involuntary body functions and in the case of infertility problems, when no identifiable physical cause can be found, some of the 'unexplained' causes for infertility may actually be directly linked to an imbalance of subconscious function, due to past deep-seated emotional trauma and so on.

The use of hypnotherapy may assist in unblocking and liberating the mind and body of unwanted emotional baggage that may be directly or indirectly affecting our abilities to manage stress. This imbalance may affect the regulation of the menstrual cycles; contribute to impotence problems; spasm to body tissues (e.g. impotent fallopian tubes); hinder the production of sperm; and alter correct nerve conduction and pain threshold levels.

### Colour Therapy and Chakras

The use of colour as a therapeutic tool has been used by many cultures for hundreds to thousands of years. Colours can have a profound and powerful healing effect on the body, mind and spirit. Colour communicates to us on both a conscious and subconscious level. Remember how you feel when you paint a different colour on your walls at home; the subtle changes in shade, intensity and blend within the various tones of these colours also summon differing responses from our emotions and physical body.

The live force that pervades all livings things is believed to flow throughout and around our body in spectrums of energy governed by colour, similar to that of a rainbow. There is believed to be specific point locations throughout the body called *'chakras'* that govern these energies. The right side of the body represents giving and is our masculine side. The left side represents our receiving and feminine side.

The colour **Yellow** is use to promote Happiness, Intellect and Memory. It is a vibrant, alive and energising colour. Yellow provokes the need to acquire knowledge; understanding; logic; practicality; analytical ability; and is related to our conscious left brain. Yellow is the energy colour of the digestive system. The chakra location for yellow is in the mid-torso or solar plexus region. It governs the pancreas, adrenals, stomach and spleen organs and glands. This chakra governs the way we feel about ourselves and the colour yellow promotes personal honour and self-confidence.

**Blue** is used to promote Calmness, Serenity and Inspiration. Blue embodies coolness, calmness, truth and peace. Blue provokes our right side of the conscious brain that controls self-expression; strength of will; reception to learning; fortitude to follow one's dream; loyalty; truthfulness; reliability; creativity; intuition; imagination; and fun. Blue is a female energy for communication, nurturing and capability. The chakra location for blue is in the throat region. The blue chakra governs the thyroid, parathyroids, the neck, throat, mouth, teeth and temporomandibular joints (TMJ).

**Green** is used to promote Love, Harmony, and Renewal. This colour is known as the 'balancer'. Green is a mixture of yellow and blue. Green combines both yin (female) and yang (male) opposite energies, a harmonious balance. Green is for inner knowing; giving and receiving love, acceptance and trust at a deeper level. The chakra location for green is in the chest, heart region. This chakra governs the thymus; heart circulation; immune system; the lungs; upper diaphragm; breasts; shoulders; upper back; and respiratory system. Turquoise is a mixture of blue and green and is for heartfelt, mass communication and boosts immune function.

**Red** is used to promote Vitality, Passion and Strength. It is very stimulating and vitalises the entire body, provokes action, and is linked to the reproductive system. Red could be described as the 'sexy' colour. Red is a male energy colour for power and creativity. The chakra location for red is in the lower pubic region and governs the coccyx and lower extremities such as legs and feet. It is referred to as the base chakra.

**Orange** is used to promote Spirituality, Energy and Abundance. Orange also radiates feeling of warmth, intimacy and tolerance. It increases personal courage and enhances mental and physical energy.

The chakra location for orange is in the navel or umbilical region. It is called the sacral chakra and restores emotional balance and is associated with the reproductive organs.

Buddhist monks and Hare Krishnas wear orange robes to support emotional response to their spiritual disciplines. This chakra covers the lower bowel, bladder, uterus, kidneys, and ovaries. It may be worth your while to try wearing orange-coloured underpants and see what happens – you never know!

**Scarlet** is used to promote Arousal and Sexual stimulation, very handy when trying to make babies. This colour may stimulate body hormones and blood and would be useful for infertility, impotence and frigidity problems.

**Magenta** is used to promote Universal Love, Divine Understanding and Joy. It is believed that the aura of a pregnant woman radiates the colour magenta. Magenta is good for evoking energy and is a revitaliser to the body's ethereal field.

**Violet** is used to promote True Devotion and Spirituality. It is also useful in improving one's level of inspiration (to see the larger picture), inner wisdom, and open one's heart to spirituality. Violet is the tone for service. The chakra location for violet is on top of the scalp region – the crown chakra – and governs divine enlightenment/cosmic consciousness. This chakra is said to be activated when all other chakra centres are refined and fully balanced. The crown chakra governs the nervous and skeletal systems, the pituitary gland, and the brain.

**Indigo** is another purple-blue colour like violet though a little darker; the darker the tone the more serious the message. Purple-based colours combine both red and blue, and are balancing and appealing for both males and females.

The chakra location for Indigo is in the centre of the forehead or 'third eye' zone, between the eyebrows. Purples are a magic colour and are for the higher inner self awareness, both spiritual and psychic. The third eye chakra governs the pineal gland, the eyes, ears, and nose. Indigo is associated with the mind; patience, intelligence, intuition, the ability to live in the now, seek information and openness to the ideas of others.

**Gold** is used to promote Divine Wisdom, Forgiveness and Love. Gold helps to assist with the deepest healing level – the Soul.

**White** is used to promote Purity, Innocence and Trust, and combines all colours.

**Pink** is used to promote Unconditional Love. It is used to stimulate the feelings of romance, creative imagination, and peace.

**Black** is used to promote Power, Success and Drive. Black can enhance self-confidence, strength and is used with much success in business.

### Mind/Body Medicine

Mind/Body medicine may soon revolutionise modern health care. Scientists that practise psychoneuroimmunology (PNI) have begun to explore and understand the complex interconnections between mind and body.

The mind and body are inseparable; modern medicine defines disease on purely a physical level. There is a direct relationship that exists between the mind/consciousness, the brain/nervous system and the immune system. The various changes in our day-to-day lives cause stress and emotional reactions. Our innate personality types can also predispose our bodies to specific physical ailments due to the way we feel and consciously and unconsciously interpret information from our internal and external environments. Mood, attitude, and belief can affect virtually every chronic illness. Fear, cynicism, as well as feelings of hopelessness and helplessness, can have a detrimental effect on health. Whereas feelings of happiness, joy, love, courage, humour, faith, sense of control, hopefulness and optimism can all directly or indirectly affect our wellness.

The subconscious (the body's auto pilot) and conscious (the body's manual control) minds are powerful bridges to the rest of the body's functions and control. The subconscious is not unlike a complex data base in a very advanced computer. Like a computer (at present) the subconscious mind cannot discriminate between right and wrong (whereas the conscious mind does; it processes and interprets information – *cogito, ergo sum* 'I think, therefore I am')!

The subconscious is the storage system part of the mind (like a hard drive of a computer) that files away the information of the collective day-to-day experiences of our life. When these files are disorganised or stored away incorrectly, then we start to run into trouble (not unlike when an important file gets misplaced in the workplace!).

Like a computer, the subconscious mind is constantly being programmed and reprogrammed depending on what information we choose to feed into this program. If our experiences are positive ones than we program positive subconscious memories that will lead to positive outputs; if our experiences are negative then we program negative memory patterns and get subsequent (or consequent) negative outputs. 'You reap what you sow'!

For example, you have been trying to conceive a baby for some time, and with each passing monthly cycle, you become more and more emotional disheartened and anxious. In a sense, the negative information that is being programmed into your subconscious will ultimately cause subtle changes to the physiology of the body.

The longer and more severe the negative information is being programmed into the mind, the more severe the physiological response will be. As Einstein once said *'with every action will come an equal and opposite reaction'.*

These negative thought patterns can become an *X-factor* in unexplained fertility; the subconscious will continually replay that same program or scenario outcome over and over until it is reprogrammed, like a cracked record with a glitch in it. To delete these glitches, the mind needs to experience positive information to rewrite a new 'positive' program to change the outcome to a positive one. These will then affect control and function over our mental and physical wellbeing.

A creative mind visualisation technique that could be very useful for fertility is one that involves vividly imagining the biological processes that occur step by step in the fertilisation and conception of baby making. Visualise your baby growing, the embryo attaching itself to your uterine wall and forming the protective placenta that keeps it safe and nourished. Inspiration may come from, say, viewing filmed documentaries on conception so you can see the results of a positive outcome. Repeat these images in your own mind, to help retrain your body's own physiology to also achieve the same positive outcome. This similar technique is adapted by elite athletes mentally visualising the outcome of their event; thoughts provoke feelings, and feelings provoke action.

In quantum physics there is a principle called the *'law of attraction',* the secret to attracting what you want. The greatest individuals throughout history have learnt how to utilise this law, manifesting thought into reality. In health you may hear of people who are facing death from a terminal disease such as cancer, where modern medicine can no longer help. A person paralysed from an injury is told they will never walk again. Through the power of positive thinking and the unwavering belief that they will be well, their affliction miraculously disappears, unexplained by medical science. You hear about these things happening all the time. You ask the right questions, the universe will provide the right answers.

There are many techniques that are available to assist you in re-balancing this mind-body connection. Examples of these include: biofeedback; counselling; meditation; visual imagery; positive reinforcing affirmations; neuro-linguistic programming (nlp); body talk; flower essence remedies; kinesiology; positive self-dialogue; pellowah healing; psychology; psychotherapy; and life coaching; and so on.

# Chapter 9

# *Stress and Fertility*

## *'Who took the jam out of your donut'?*

The definition of stress is anything that requires us to adapt and make changes to our habits, routines, thought processes, and lifestyles. It is also anything that requires the delicate systems of the body to adapt to new chemicals and processes from environmental pollution, drugs and other external toxins, plus internal toxicity resulting from poor diet, dysbiosis or ill health, as well as an increase in stress hormones such as cortical and adrenalin.

A certain amount of stress or pressure in life is necessary to drive, motivate and stimulate a positive adaptation. It is defined as a person's response to their environment and is measured in terms of arousal or stimulation. Every individual has their own homeostatic level of stress at which they function optimally. When stress is intense or unresolved it has a negative impact physiologically and emotionally.

The brain is the first part of the body to respond to stress; it does this in two ways. Firstly by stimulating a release of the stress hormones adrenaline and noradrenaline resulting in an increase in heart rate, blood pressure, breathing and blood flow to the muscles and brain. During chronic stress this allows bacteria, viruses or tumours to flourish and makes blood more prone to clotting.

The second response is the release of cortisol and other steroids, which in excess promote the accumulation of abdominal fat, suppress immunity, shrink brain cells and impair memory. Stress has also been attributed to increased depression; phobias; chemical dependency; heart disease; cancer; migraines; irritable bowel syndrome (IBS); ulcers; insomnia; gastric reflux; sexual dysfunction; and infertility.

**There are three phases of stress:**

*Phase 1* – **Alarm phase**: When a stressful event occurs, this is the time of increased adrenaline, reflexes and resistance. This is the fright-flight-fight response.

**Phase 2 – Resistance phase**: Repeated or chronic stress results in the need to develop 'mental and physical coping' strategies to manage or 'resist' the continued stress.

**Phase 3 – Exhaustion phase**: If the stress or strain goes beyond the resistance phase, organ damage, immune suppression and other ill effects such as inability to function socially and mentally occurs. This often is described as *'adrenal exhaustion'*. Some examples of exhaustion phase may include conditions such as: Chronic fatigue syndrome and nervous breakdown.

## Stress and DHEA

DHEA or *Dehydroepiandrosterone* is a naturally occurring hormone in the body that has much claim as an antidote to the diseases of aging and as a whole-body rejuvenator. It is the most abundant hormone or steroid found in the bloodstream. DHEA works synergistically with other naturally occurring hormones such as melatonin and human growth hormone (HGH). DHEA is an essential building block for sex and other hormones such as oestrogen and testosterone.

DHEA is made from cholesterol in the adrenal glands (above the kidneys). Initially pregnenolone is manufactured from cholesterol, and from *Pregnenolone*, progesterone and DHEA are produced.

Progesterone goes on to produce cortisol, aldosterone, oestrogen and testosterone. Aldosterone is important in the balance of electrolytes and minerals in the body.

Cortisol is released by adrenals as a response to stress. Cortisol in normal levels is vital for our daily functions. In times of stress our body provides glucose as the primary source of energy. If cortisol is constantly at a high level, it affects our amount of glucose from all stores in the body. When the glucose stores are depleted then it turns to your muscles to break down protein to produce energy. This results in ongoing loss of muscle bulk and development of flabby muscles.

### The Effect of Stress on our Bodies
Stress is part of our day-to-day life and is inevitable. Stressors on our bodies come in many forms:

1   Physical
2   Emotional
3   Chemical
4   Electromagnetic

Stress generates many free radicals, which in turn will cause oxidative stress, and the aftermath will be degenerative disease. Our body responds to acute stress by stimulating the sympathetic system, which releases norepinephrine (adrenalin precursor), which in turn together with stress stimulates the hypothalamus to secrete ACTH (adrenocorticotropic hormone) to stimulate the adrenals in order to make cortisol and DHEA.

Excessive stress levels during the time of conception can affect the male's pituitary gland function thereby inhibiting the action of sperm being mixed with the seminal fluids leading to little or no sperm in the semen.

Stress can also cause chemical alterations in the female body contributing to conditions such as amenorrhoea (absence of menstrual periods), delayed or irregular ovulation, and even anovulation (where no ovulation takes place during that cycle).

The hypothalamus gland is particularly affected during responses to stress on the body. This gland has many vital functions, some of which are appetite regulation, temperature control and emotional responses. This stress reaction in turn disrupts pituitary gland activity that may cause an elevation of hormones like prolactin.

The female reproductive system may respond by altering various vaginal and uterine secretions. These secretions can hinder the release of enzymes necessary for the sperm to penetrate the ovum's outer surfaces.

This process is known as 'Capacitation'. Furthermore, stress can also affect the progression and transport of the sperm and ovum through the fallopian tube on its way to the uterine lining for implantation. The hypothalamus-pituitary axis interplays with other glands and organs such as the adrenals. When the adrenal gland activity is excessive, such as during nervous tension, hormones like aldosterone are released in larger than normal quantities.

Various nutrients are then compromised from being absorbed properly or are excreted more rapidly than usual, thus contributing to a vicious cycle of further inappropriate physical and chemical reactions if the stress reaction is not brought into balance effectively.

### Natural Methods to Enhance DHEA and Stress Control

- Do regular exercise.
- Stress management – e.g. have clear, well-defined goals. Work out where you want to be and what you need to do to get there. Ensure your goals are **S.M.A.R.T.** S – Specific, M - measurable, A – achievable, R – realistic, and T – timed.
- Develop effective coping strategies – e.g. Quit addictive substances/ behaviours, and learn to improve communication skills.
- Live for today – as opposed to dwelling in the past or worrying about the future; learn from your experiences.
- Get adequate sleep.
- Learn relaxation, breathing and meditation techniques. Master your mind or your mind will master you!

- Manage your weight.
- Nutrients that benefit adaption to stress may include: Vitamins A; Vitamin B complex (especially Vitamin B5 and B6); choline; Vitamin C; Vitamin E; trace element zinc; chromium; and minerals such as magnesium.
- Amino Acid Tyrosine, 5- Hydroxy-Tryptophan (5HT), L-Tryptophan, Acetyl-L-Carnitine, and Phosphtidylserine (PS)
- Methyl Sulfony/methane (MSM) and Beta 1; 3 glucan (from Ip6 (Inositol Hexophosphate; S-adenosyl methionine (Same); Reishii, Shitake and Maitake mushrooms; and homeopathic DHEA or Pregnenolone.
- Adrenal/adaptogenic herbs: liquorice; ginsengs (Siberian, panax, codonopsis, maca, withania, tienchi); astragalus; rhodiola root; schizandra; and wild yam.
- Calming herbs: chamomile; hops; kava kava; skullcap; lavender; lemon balm; magnolia; oats; passionflower; valerian; St John's wort; and zizyphus.
- Aromatherapy scents: lavender and natural vanilla essence are examples of oils that can induce relaxation to reduce stress levels.

Our body tries to stay in a state of balance so called *homeostasis*. However, as the stress becomes chronic the body goes through adaptation and exhaustion stages.

When stress is chronic and at the stage of adaptation, there is excess secretion of ACTH and cortisol, but DHEA levels are stable. Adaptation brings along some ill effects including abnormal blood sugar, the beginning of osteoporosis, and an increase in body fat deposition, salt and water retention and lower immune system. At the exhaustion stage there are constant high levels of cortisol, but on the other hand DHEA is decreased and insulin becomes erratic. Your immune system is now quite weak hence becoming prone to infection. You are in danger of developing coronary heart disease, diabetes, stroke, cancer, chronic fatigue syndrome and other degenerative diseases. One of the most valuable assets a person can have in life is the ability to be relaxed, poised, and centred. This 'centring' or concentration can bring even the most difficult of tasks within your capabilities.

If you have been attempting to fall pregnant and things are just not happening, *change your routine,* TAKE A LONG WELL-DESERVED HOLIDAY. If I had a dollar for each time a couple changed their daily routine and relaxed their minds and a pregnancy soon occurred thereafter, I would be able to afford to kick back myself to sip cocktails on the sunny beaches of Tahiti (dream on)!

### *Oral DHEA Supplementation may have the following benefits:*

1. Reduces platelet aggregation (mildly), which means thinning the blood, hence reducing the incidence of heart attack and stroke.
2. Lipolysis or the burning of fat and increasing muscle bulk.

3. Improving libido and sexual vitality in both men and women (particularly if DHEA levels are low).
4. Helps in menopause and prevents osteoporosis.
5. Lowers LDL cholesterol, which is the bad cholesterol, and therefore assists in the prevention of atherosclerosis and coronary heart disease.
6. Helps in Alzheimer's disease; some cancers (non-hormone dependent); diabetes; hypertension; obesity; adrenal insufficiency; auto-immune diseases such as lupus (SLE); rheumatoid arthritis; psoriasis; and enhancing athletic performance.
7. Enhances immune system function, and has been used in HIV and AIDS treatment.
8. A potent antioxidant and nerve rejuvenator.

DHEA is *not* recommended for individuals with prostate, breast, and ovarian or uterine cancers, as they are hormone dependent. Minimal acne and mild facial hair growth have been reported in some older females using DHEA therapy.

Prior to taking supplemental DHEA, one should have a salivary or blood test associated with serum cortisol levels. At the age of 30, both men and women produce roughly 30–50mg of pregnenolone daily and from mid 40s declines.

Blood tests of less than 180ng/dl (nanogram per decilitre) in women, and 220ng/dl in men, may require replacement therapy. Blood levels of DHEA should be checked regularly to gauge the therapeutic levels. DHEA is believed to reach its highest peak at the age of 25 (this may also contribute to one of the reasons why we may cope with stress better at that age). DHEA declines as we age and reaches its lowest level by mid 50s. Supplemental doses of DHEA range from 4 to 15mg daily.

## Problems with the Pill

### Is it a blessing or a curse – the so-called medical miracle?
### Has the public been told the real truth?

If your endocrine system was to be symbolised as a 'chicken egg' and the contraceptive pill as an 'egg beater' – what do you think may happen when they are put together...?

The orally active synthetic hormones such as the oral contraceptive pill – OCP – were introduced to the world population in the 1960s. Since that time, the contraceptive pill has been at the centre of much controversy and debate between various moral, religious and scientific groups. The Pill, it seems, has had a double-edged-sword effect on modern civilisation. On one hand it has liberated aspects of sexual freedom and given greater control over our reproductive destiny, but on the other hand we are now bearing witness, decades later, to the aftermath of consequences that synthetic hormones are having on our reproductive and general health. The Contraceptive Pill that was to deliver our salvation may also bring about our demise.

Almost 90 per cent of women have taken hormones (about 200 million women around the world), either for period, hormonal problems or contraception, before they have had their first pregnancy. These hormones can be up to 5000 times more powerful than naturally occurring hormones. One third of ethynylestradiol is not metabolised in the body and is excreted unchanged and subsequently enters the sewers and recirculates.

Although the amount of ethynylestradiol in our water supply is small, it adds to other sources of oestrogens such as mycotoxins, chlorinated pesticides and organo-phosphates thus contributing to a compounding, accumulative effect on our bodies. These oestrogenic contaminants may be a major factor in the declining male sperm counts, increased incidence of undescended testes, testicular and prostate cancer.

The level of oestrogen in the foetus can influence brain development. Oestrogen tends to feminise the brain, while testosterone masculinises the brain. Exogenous (foreign) hormones directly lower nutrients such as zinc and raise copper levels in blood serum. They also lower the body's levels of B vitamins (Vitamin B6 in particular) and folic acid. Both omega 6 and 3 essential fatty acids are often deficient in users of the Pill. Fifty per cent of women who have taken the Pill for more than 5 years have shown reduced pancreatic exocrine function, therefore leading to poor digestive activity.

Recent studies into the effect that synthetic hormones have on the body revealed some concerning statistics: 1 in 4 women have a life-time risk of developing breast cancer; many of these are oestrogen sensitive, therefore oestrogens may be a cause or could aggravate the disease. Higher rates of in-situ cervical cancer were linked to women who started using the Pill at a young age. One in 5 women have a 'positive' result in their Pap smear test (which ironically means NOT good)!

It is a known fact that oestrogen stimulates viral replication. Breast, cervical, liver and melanoma cancers all have possible viral aetiology. These forms of cancers are increasing in prevalence. Foreign oestrogens may contribute to immune suppression by inducing the production of defective T-helper immune cells, while stimulating suppressor immune cell activity.

These oestrogen hormones develop and dilate blood vessels that can potentially encourage the spread of infection and cancers. Most long-term studies show increases in bacterial, fungal and viral infections (impaired immunity); blood clots; diabetes; strokes; cardiovascular disease; cervicitis; breast cancer; cervical cancer; infertility; serious heavy menstrual bleeding; also endometriosis; and pelvic inflammatory disease. A soaring increased ratio of hysterectomies are most common in women who have taken the Pill.

**The effects of the Contraceptive Pill may deplete or interfere with the metabolism of the nutritional status in the body:**

Vitamin B1, (thiamine) Vitamin B2 (riboflavin), Vitamin B (pyridoxine) Vitamin B12 (cobalamin) bioflavonoid, iron, Vitamin K, selenium and biotin (helps to prevent candida albicans overgrowth in the gut) and Vitamin C can be lowered by up to 30 per cent. It is necessary for sex hormone production, though taking reasonably high levels of Vitamin C while on the Pill can potentiate the oestrogen concentration leading to possible side effects.

*Vitamin E:* which helps to normalise oestrogen levels, can be lowered by approximately 20 per cent in blood plasma results. Blood lipids may increase the bad form of cholesterol, triglycerides and low-density lipids, thus contributing to risk of heart disease.

*Prostaglandins:* Certain prostaglandins are decreased that are required for clot formation, pain tolerance and hormone production.

*Vitamin A:* can be increased in the blood and can take several months to normalise after coming off the Pill.

*Selenium levels:* can be reduced on the Pill. Its anti-oxidant action is important to protect the foetus for developing various deformities.

*Folic Acid:* The Pill decreases its levels, therefore contributing to potential congenital abnormalities, poor cell division and cellular abnormalities particularly of the cervix.

*Copper/Zinc:* Zinc levels are significantly lowered whereas copper absorption increases. The ratio imbalance of these nutrients can impact on numerous aspects of reproductive, foetal and pregnancy health.

*Magnesium and Potassium*: may be compromised by the Pill, which can affect fertile mucus formation.

*Calcium*: absorption maybe increased which can be an actual benefit.

The Oral Contraceptive Pill is usually manufactured in various ratios of oestrogen and progesterone.

The mini-Pill, however, is usually only synthetic progesterone based, but also has its problems. It can affect changes in the cervical mucus and endometrium, which disrupts the egg and/or sperm passage in the fallopian tube. The mini-Pill does not necessarily suppress ovulation; therefore, ectopic pregnancies can be more likely.

Synthetic progesterone is also linked to affecting hypothalamus activity and may have a masculinising effect on a female infant.

Many female health problems and symptoms occur due to hormone imbalances, typically oestrogen dominance. Oestrogen dominance or progesterone deficiency occurs in women where there is a high oestrogen ratio.

*Symptoms of this hormone imbalance are many and include:*

- Tenderness and fibrocystic breasts;
- Tendency for increased body fat;
- Increased blood pressure, salt and fluid retention;
- Thyroid hormone imbalances;
- Decreased sex drive; changes in sense of smell;
- Decreased blood sugar control;
- Zinc depletion and copper retention which can result in mood swings, depression and violent outbursts;
- Increased risk of endometrial, breast and ovarian cancers;
- Impaired liver and gall bladder function; appetite changes;
- Increases in incidence and growth of fibroids, leading to hysterectomy;
- Hair loss and growth of facial hair; impaired immunity;
- Migraines; weight gain; skin discolouration; increased tendency to thrush;
- Miscarriages; fluid retention; impaired fertility; depression;
- Pre menstrual symptoms; increased incidence of ocular disorders;
- Increased blood clotting (2 to 8-fold increase in risk of thrombosis); Increased risk of heart attack (3 to 6-fold according to age).

The normalising of this hormonal ratio is the prime objective in nutritional treatment.

Vitamin B6 and methionine normalise this ratio as methionine detoxifies oestrogen through methylation and reduces oestrogen excess. Excretion of oestrogen metabolises via the bowel is improved with a high fibre diet and vitamin C.

The effects of the Pill appear to continue for a relatively long term after the pills use has stopped. Because the Pill scrambles brain–ovary communication channels, unscrambling them doesn't always happen quickly. Most women need 2 to 3 months at least to return to a normal cycle. A study found that nearly 25 per cent of women could not fall pregnant for at least 13 months after stopping. Certain volatile fatty acids called *copulins* are secreted in the vagina and are believed to play a role in stimulating male sexual interest and behaviour. Women who take the Pill, however, may not secrete copulins.

### Depo – Provera
This method of birth control is administered via injection (usually in the arm or buttock) by your doctor every 3 months. Like the mini-pill, it contains progestin, which helps to stop monthly ovulation, thickens cervical mucus, and prevents implantation of fertilised eggs in the uterus.

With the use of Depo-Provera the women is likely to stop her monthly period cycle altogether. After Depo-Provera is stopped it may also take several months to more than a year before ovulation may re-commence. This drug has long–acting effects. The longer that you are on this drug, the longer it may take before ovulation may begin again.

### Implanon
This method of contraception works via the implantation of a single plastic rod shaped similar to the size of a match. The slow release form of progestin is usually place under the bicep area in the arm and can be felt to touch under the skin. Like the mini-pill, it thickens cervical mucus, slowing down sperm and interfering with implantation of the egg, but it is active for up to 3 years. After removal or stoppage of use of the implant there may be a noticeable delay in ovulation with this device also.

### Evra
Evra is a self-administered patch that's usually worn on the hip and changed weekly for 3 weeks, then not worn on the fourth week. It releases a daily dose of oestrogen and progesterone, similar to the combined pill.

Newer aerosol versions are in the works to replace to old-fashioned oral pill version. These new ways of administering these drugs into the body are best absorbed through the skin to minimise high doses like in the oral pill and are said to maintain better blood levels of the drugs.

Newer versions of the copper IUDs (Intra-Uterine Device) are also available; the older original types of IUDs were linked to causing some horrendous problems to the reproductive system in the past such as pelvic inflammatory disease and severe tubal blockages.

### Nuva Ring
The latest innovation in contraception devices, the Nuva ring is a flexible plastic ring with a diameter of about two inches. The ring is inserted into the vagina and slowly releases low doses of oestrogen and progestin hormones that prevent the ovaries from producing mature eggs. The device is used for three weeks (21 days) and the removed for seven days' break to allow the body to have its menstrual cycle. The Nuva ring is then replaced the following month after menstruation is completed if contraception is desired to continue.

### Foreign oestrogen's effect on males
Although many synthetic oestrogens like DES are now outlawed, many livestock and poultry are still hormonally manipulated, especially dairy cows. Cow's milk contains substantial amounts of oestrogen due to modern farming techniques. The rise in consumption of dairy products since the 1940s inversely parallels the drop in male sperm counts. Avoidance or at the very least minimal consumption of hormone-fed animal products and milk products may be important for males who have low sperm production and testosterone levels.

This accumulative pooling effect of these foreign oestrogenic factors may also greatly impact during foetal development. Animal-based studies have shown that these oestrogens inhibit the multiplication of the sperm-producing cells of the testes – the Sertoli cells. The number of the Sertoli cells is directly proportional to the amount of sperm that can be produced.

Sertoli cells formation occurs primarily during foetal life and before puberty. It is controlled by follicle-stimulating hormone (FSH). Oestrogens administered early in life inhibit FSH secretion, resulting in a reduction of the number of Sertoli cells, and, in adult life, reduced sperm production.

Mothers-to-be may be able to minimise the oestrogen exposure to the developing foetus by improving fibre intake, decreasing saturated fats and consuming moderate amounts of foods such as legume beans, nuts, seeds and soy-based foods containing isoflavonoids (phytoestrogens). Isoflavonoids bind to oestrogen receptors and exert a very mild oestrogenic action that actually has an anti-oestrogenic effect, as it prevents the binding of the body's own oestrogen (that is much more potent) to the receptor.

Phyto oestrogen/Phyto sterols (plants compounds similar in structure to human hormones) may also reduce the effects of oestrogens on the body by also stimulating the production of sex hormone-binding globulin (SHBG), so the oestrogen is bound and subsequently becomes less potent.

Other foods that would also be of benefit include: cruciferous vegetables that contain phyto chemicals *Indole 3 Carbinol (I3C)* and *Diindolymethane (DIM)* that may also block and balance oestrogen activity in the body and are also beneficial to assist with the treatment protocols of hormone dependant cancers.

These substances are highly available in foods such as: broccoli; cauliflower; bok choy; watercress; cabbage; turnips; rosemary; and brussels sprouts. Supplemental therapeutic dosages of I3C and DIM should really be avoided during pregnancy, though consuming the foods that contain these phytochemicals in small quantities may be very beneficial.

### Saliva Testing

Saliva hormone testing, together with symptom analysis, is the best way to diagnose oestrogen dominance. Conventional blood tests for hormones will not detect oestrogen dominance, because blood tests measure equal amounts of hormone, including up to 90 per cent of hormone that is stored.

Saliva tests, on the other hand, measure the fat-soluble portion of oestrogen and progesterone that the body is actually experiencing. Levels of hormone in saliva vary from day to day, and this is a common criticism of saliva testing. The reality is, however, that hormones do vary naturally from day to day. It is sensible, therefore, to choose a testing method that can detect that variation. Saliva tests are a convenient way to collect a sample at home during the days and times in which hormone imbalance is suspected.

Saliva tests are also the only way in which oestrogen dominance - a low ratio between progesterone to oestrogen – can be accurately detected. In addition to oestrogen and progesterone, saliva can also be tested for levels of testosterone, melatonin, cortisol and DHEA.

### Bio-identical Hormones

Bio-identical hormones are hormones that are exactly identical to human hormones at a molecular level. The difference between bio-identical hormones and conventional pharmaceutical hormones cannot be emphasised enough. In order to be patented, the pharmaceutical hormones were designed to be slightly different from human hormones, and that slight difference is very significant.

These molecules have some similar effects to human hormones, but also have some very different and sinister effects, such as cancer. An example is the horse oestrogen, *Equilin*, which is found in *Premarin* and *Premia* and other conjugated oestrogens. It is eight times more potent than human oestrogen.

The greater the difference in the structure of the molecule from human oestrogen, the greater the problems become. Ethinylestradiol, a common ingredient in birth control pills, is 1000 times more potent than human oestrogen. Stronger oestrogens mean a greater risk for potential breast cancer, and more side effects such as bloating, water retention and depression.

The difference between progesterone and its substitutes is even more profound. Progesterone is a hormone involved in many aspects of health. Its substitutes – progestins marked as Provera, Primolut and many contraceptive pills – are known to cause weight gain, blood clots, anxiety and breast cancer. *Progestins* are NOT human progesterone, even though many doctors do not understand the distinction. Consider this: progesterone is essential for foetal growth; indeed that is one of its main purposes. Bio–identical progesterone is used clinically to prevent early miscarriage. Progestins, on the other hand, can never be given during pregnancy because they may cause abortion and birth defects.

### Benefits of Natural Progesterone

Progesterone is a hormone produced by the ovaries, placenta and nervous tissue. It is named for its role in promoting gestation, but its complete role is much larger than that.

Progesterone receptors are found on almost every tissue in the body, and progesterone's main role is to balance the metabolism-suppressing effects of oestrogen. Progesterone increases metabolism, burns fat, relieves depression and anxiety, acts as a natural diuretic, normalises blood clotting, stimulates new bone formation, and stabilises blood sugar. It is also strongly protective against the cancer-promoting effects of oestrogen.

Progesterone is the relaxing, grounding, vital hormone that our bodies are designed to receive in a constant monthly supply. In addition, progesterone is produced in large amounts during pregnancy, up to 20 times non-pregnant levels. Progesterone is the reason that pregnancy is protective against breast cancer.

Many women are deficient in progesterone. This is because successful ovulation is required for the ovary to produce progesterone, and, in our modern world, women as young as 30 do not ovulate regularly.

For many women, ovulation is blocked by environmental oestrogen mimics, such as organochlorine pollution, plastics and pesticides, and by chronically high insulin from a diet too high in sugar and refined flour. High insulin also causes the ovaries to produce testosterone, which is a primary cause of Poly Cystic Ovary Syndrome (PCOS).

The progesterone that women do manage to produce is frequently depleted by stress, which causes progesterone to be converted to the stress hormone cortisol. On top of this, progesterone deficiency is worsened further by the contraceptive pill, which inhibits ovulation and blocks progesterone from its receptors.

# Chapter 10

# *Menstrual & Female Reproductive Disorders*

**'The usual suspects – when things go wrong'**

Menstrual disorders are all too common. Essentially, female menstrual and reproductive disorders arise as a consequence of disturbances in hormone production, elimination and metabolism. Hormones that underlie these disorders include gonadal hormones (e.g. oestrogen, progesterone, testosterone); insulin; thyroid hormones; and even stress hormones (e.g. cortisol). Disturbances in the balance of these hormones are the result of endogenous and exogenous factors such as environmental toxins, inflammation, stress, poor diet and lack of exercise.

It is estimated that as many as 90 per cent of women of reproductive age experience some menstrual and/or hormonal disorder that affects them on a regular basis. This includes conditions such as premenstrual syndrome (PMS), dysmenorrhoea, endometriosis, uterine fibroids, and polycystic ovarian syndrome (PCOS). More than half of all women experience regular period pain, and about three quarters have PMS symptoms. A woman's health is the barometer of her diet, lifestyle and environment – the female body is highly responsive to these influences and female reproductive health is grounded in the quality of a woman's nutrition and the purity of her internal and external environment.

The first consideration with your doctor, natural therapist or specialist practitioner should always be to exclude any pathology or disease process that may be the causative factor. Any bleeding between periods (metrorrhagia) should be investigated for possible cancer, fibroids, cervical lesions, or other pathology prior to attempting the general therapeutic recommendations. Most menstrual problems can be caused by hormonal imbalances and a 24-hour urine sample may be used as a simple method of evaluating oestrogen levels. Evidence of ovulation may also be found by keeping a morning temperature chart. This will aid evaluation and help direct therapy.

Probably the most effective way to upset the entire hormonal balance is to take contraceptive pills. This convinces the body that it is pregnant. After stopping the pill many women fail to regain normal periods for varying periods of months to several years. Amenorrhea following use of the contraceptive pill is very common.

Other hormonal disorders involving the pituitary, adrenals, or thyroid may also produce amenorrhea or abnormal bleeding cycles. This may be physiological, as with hypothyroidism due to iodine deficiency; or psychological, affecting first the hypothalamus then pituitary, thyroid, and ovaries. Stress or the contraceptive pill may also profoundly affect the adrenal glands, which produce 20 per cent of the total oestrogen output. These glands are very sensitive to changes in blood sugar levels, so that hypoglycaemia may depress adrenal function over time.

Extreme diets, such as strict fruitarianism, very low protein diets, or repeated strict weight-loss regimens, often cause amenorrhea. On these restricted diets, the levels of circulating hormones fall until a normal menstrual cycle is no longer possible and pregnancy unlikely.

Anorexia nervosa – this disorder is a psychological problem leading to extreme weight loss and amenorrhea. The strong remarks above are not meant for sufferers of this disorder, who need psychological counselling to cope with their problem, which often results from an inability to adjust to sexual maturity.

Another major cause of menstrual abnormality is poor body mechanics. In the woman with normal posture, with strong abdominal muscles and pelvic supports, the female organs are suspended unencumbered within the pelvis. If, however, the abdominal muscles are weakened, or there is an excess lordotic curve in the low back, the abdominal contents prolapse and put pressure on the pelvic organs. This may result from simple lack of demanding exercises, spinal lesions causing an increase in the lumbar curve, or something as common as habitual wearing of high-heeled shoes, which increases the lumbar curve. Constipation and loaded bowel syndrome may also cause intestinal prolapse.

Failure to do sufficient prenatal and especially postnatal exercises may lead to weakening of the supporting ligaments of the female organs. This is a common finding in menstrual disorders. The resultant prolapse interferes with normal blood and lymph flow, resulting in congestion and reduction in local tissue vitality.

Diet may play a major role in menstrual problems. As previously mentioned, a protein-deficient diet causes amenorrhea and infertility. Hypoglycaemia, nutritional anaemia, iodine deficiency, and hypothyroidism are some of the more widely accepted nutritional causes of menstrual disorders. Vitamin B complex deficiency and calcium deficiency are also now being recognised. Certainly calcium deficiency related to cramps is fairly well proven. Vitamin B6 deficiency is also associated with the premenstrual tension syndrome of irritability, cramps, fluid retention and acne flare.

Stress and psychological problems may profoundly affect menstrual flow. It is not uncommon for amenorrhea to follow a severe psychological and physical trauma. Fear of pregnancy may also be a common factor in menstrual disorders of all kinds. Less obvious psychological problems may also be the cause and should be sought through careful questioning.

An interesting type of amenorrhea has recently been coined 'marathoner's amenorrhea' found exclusively among those females who regularly run long distances. Certain levels of body fat and cholesterol are needed for proper hormone production, and when these levels are reduced, hormone production is impaired including those involved in the menstrual cycle.

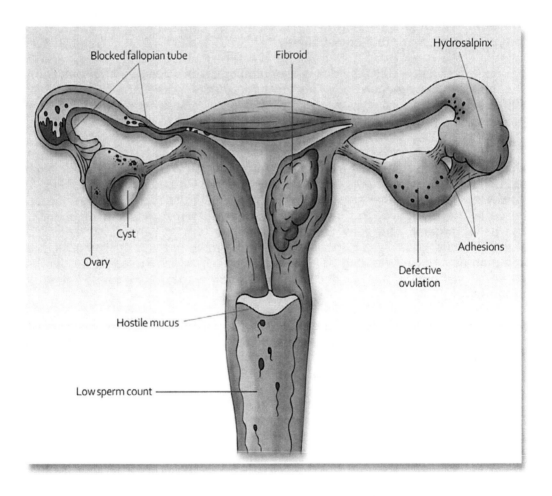

*Figure.16. Abnormal female reproductive system – causes of female infertility*

## Therapeutic agents

### Vitamins and minerals

As with many problems with one's health, the usefulness or otherwise of specific supplements and botanicals will depend on the individual specific history, and the presenting signs and symptoms.

The following are listed without prioritising, and selection might best be undertaken in consultation with your naturopathic physician. Dosages of nutrients and herbal medicines are only recommended as a general guide.

*\* If you require additional information regarding any specific individual nutrient and/or botanical agent then please refer to the respective chapters on Clinical Nutrition and Herbal Medicine. The herbs and nutrients in this section shall be referred by their common names.*

- *Vitamin A*: 10,000-25,000 IU 1-2 times daily.

- *Vitamin B complex*: 50mg 1-3 times daily. Intramuscular injection may be useful.

- *Vitamin B6*: for premenstrual tension and acne; 100mg 3-4 times daily, initially then twice daily.

- *Folic acid*: 25-50mg daily-especially with abnormal PAP smears.

- *Vitamin C plus bioflavonoid*: for excess bleeding. 1000-2000mg 2 or more times per day, up to bowel tolerance.

- *Vitamin D*: 400-1000 IU daily. Increases calcium absorption along with acidic environment (hydrochloric acid, Vitamin C, cider vinegar, lemon juice etc.). Take care in prescribing Vitamin D; it is often taken in excess in the diet, and can have toxic effects. A prescription for plenty of sunshine is safer.

- *Vitamin E*: 400 IU 1-2 times daily.

- *Vitamin K*: for excess bleeding: antihemorrhagic, clotting factors (alfalfa, seaweed, spinach, cabbage and other vitamin K foods).

- *Calcium* levels are lowest just before menstruation begins. Low calcium may be related to menstrual tension syndrome, along with vitamin B6. Calcium is especially useful with cramps and heavy blood loss. 1-2 tablets per hour are taken in acute cases. 1000-2500mg daily as regular dose. Higher doses in individual cases.

- *Iron*: even one heavy period may use up the entire month's supply of iron. Heavy blood loss always requires iron. 25-50mg daily.

- *Magnesium*: 200mg 2-3 times daily, or 1mg for every 2mg of calcium.

- *Zinc*: 25mg 1-2 times daily.

### Others

- Brewer's yeast
- Lecithin
- Choline/inositol
- Garlic
- Kelp
- Alfalfa
- Essential fatty acids (GLA, evening primrose oil)
- EPA (eicosapentaenoic acid): 3-10g daily
- Chlorophyll: 2-3 tbs. 4-6 times daily
- Protein supplements
- Tryptophan (with doctors prescription)
- Raw adrenal tablets
- Desiccated thyroid extract.

# Amenorrhea and Oligomenorrhea

## Amenorrhea

Absence or suppression of menstruation. It is referred to as primary amenorrhea if you have never had a period and are over the age of 15. Secondary if you have had a previously regular cycle such as before pregnancies, lactation or menopause.

This condition accounts for 20 per cent of all female infertility. It may be caused by a blockage of the reproductive system, i.e. a lack of ovulation due to underlying problems; anatomical defects of the uterus or outflow tract; hyper-prolactinaemia (high prolactin levels); malnutrition; hypothyalmic-pituitary dysfunction; extreme weight loss; excess strenuous exercise; severe stress; drug abuse; autoimmune endocrine disease; exteme obesity; hyper-androgenism; anabolic steroid use; breast-feeding; premature ovarian failure; intracranical tumour; GnRH deficiency; imperforated hymen; pseudo-hermaphroditism (high LH: defective testosterone synthesis); and numerous other causal factors.

Prior to undergoing treatment for this condition it is recommended that a pregnancy test be performed to rule out an undiagnosed pregnancy first. Best to be safe than sorry!

### Medical treatments
Oestrogen replacement therapy; combined oral contraceptive (oestrogen and progesterone); medroxyprogesterone; conjugated oestrogens; alterative oestrogen replacement; selective oestrogen receptor modulators (SERMs) e.g. raloxifene; pulsatile GnRH; long-acting GnRH analogues; and dopamine agonists (if hyperprolctinaemia is the cause).

**Oligomenorrhea**

Infrequent or scanty menstruation.

**Causes:** Pregnancy, *always check first by having a pregnancy test done*; ovarian cysts; PCOS; hypothalamus/pituitary/ovarian dysfunction; sclerosing of endometrium; low body fat (under 10 per cent); excessive body fat (over 35 per cent); high anxiety/stress/shock; low oestrogen (common); 'cold state'; blood stasis; anovulation; excessively elevated prolactin levels (possible induced via certain drug use); premature menopause; dysfunctional thyroid; extreme exercise regimes (marathona 'amenorrhea'); congenital defects; blockage of the cervix/uterus/vagina; pseudocyesis 'phantom pregnancy'; Cushing's syndrome; congenital adrenal hyperplasia; premature ovarian failure; prolactinoma; Asherman's syndrome; and cervical stenosis.

If you have had a previously regular menstrual cycle, but the period has been absent for more than six months. Cause other than pregnancy, lactation or menopause. Late onset of period if has secondary sex characteristics. Medical evaluation is needed if late onset with no secondary sex characteristics.

**Botanicals:** (Main) if you have never experienced a period over the age of 15. Emmenagogues to promote menstrual flow:
- Rue (ruta graveotons); blue cohosh; mugwort; mother wort (mild); tansy.
- Dong quai: hormone balancer, blood tonic and emmenagogue
- False unicorn root: if there is low oestrogen
- Panax ginseng: adaptogenic
- Ginger: circulatory stimulant, especially if a 'cold state' (where heat relieves).
- Chaste tree (Vitex): best taken at 7.00am and 4.00pm to help promote ovulation
- Reproductive tonic and endocrine herbs: bladderwrack (kelp), blue flag, cramp bark, damiana, golden seal, liquorice, and squaw vine.
- If low body weight: rhemannia (cured), and withania.

TCM Herbal formulas: Ba Zhen Wan (Ginseng & Danggui Eight Combination), Shi Quan Da Bu Wan (Ginseng & Danggui Ten Combination), Shi Xiao Wan (Pteropus & Salvia formula), Jai Wei Xiao Yao San (Bupleurum & Peonia formula).

**Homeopathy:** Ferrum 30C, Lycopodium 30C, and Calcarea 30C.
Sepia 30C – is possibly the most commonly used homeopathic medicine for infertility in women. *Sepia* has been particularly helpful in 'post-pill' infertility (trouble conceiving after being on the contraceptive pill). However, it may also be effective in other circumstances. The normal dose that may be recommended is 30C of Sepia, taken at two pills weekly for two to three months. Oophorinum folliculinum (human ovary/ovarian follicle) - may be recommended to assist ovulation stimulation. Aristolochia – may be used when periods are light and/or irregular.

**Botanicals:** (Secondary)
- Angelica (blood stasis)
- Black cohosh: ovarian pain and cramps
- Blazing star: for low ovarian function, hypo-estrogenism, 10-30 drops tincture 3 times daily
- Elecampane
- Liquorice root tea: tonic
- Life root: uterine tonic, increases local circulation. 10-30 drops tincture 2-4 times daily.
- Mother's wort: gentle emmenagogue/Nervine.
- Mugwort: gentle emmenagogue
- Peonia
- Pennyroyal: strong infusion, 3-4 times daily
- Pulsatilla: 10 drops 3 times daily; especially if due to stress, apprehension, or other emotional suppression (blood stasis), (cold state feeble pulse)
- Tansy - emmenagogue
- If due to low body fat – Dong Quai, withania & rhemmania (cured).
- Nervous system herbs: withania, valerian, and oats
- Emmenagogues – to promote bleed flow: sandalwood, wormwood, prickly ash.

**Aromatherapy** oil remedies may include: Chamomile; clary sage; fennel; hyssop; juniper; pennyroyal; basil; lavender; marjoram; mugwort; lemon balm; peppermint; rose; rosemary; and sage.

**Homeopathic remedies:** treatment selection will vary depending on specific underlying cause: agnus castus 6x, calcarea carbonica 6x, pulsatilla 3x, sepia 1x, graphites 3x, cimicifuga racemosa 6x and kali carbonicum 6x.

**Acupuncture/Acupressure Points:** GB 21 (shoulder well) this point is located at the highest point of the trapezius muscle, located towards the back, between the neck and the shoulder and just above the shoulder blade (note: not be stimulated during pregnancy), other points may include: Lv 3, LI 4, Sp 6, and Sp 10.

## Dysmenorrhea

Painful or difficult menstrual periods; cramp-like pains or steady dull ache 24-48 hours prior to menstruation persisting for variable periods of time. Pain results from myometrial uterine contractions stimulated by increased prostaglandin production in secretory endometrium. Up to 40 per cent of female adults have some degree of menstrual pain.

- Painful or difficult menstruation, often in younger reproductive years (15-25 years of age).
- Typically pain is central, but can be to one side, suspect adhesions or ovarian involvement, if to one side (secondary dysmenorrhea)
- Congestive dysmenorrhea – discomfort, or heavy aching feeling before period.

250

- Spasmodic dysmenorrhea cramping before bleeding starts, difficult flow.
- Pain can be due to ischaemia – lack of blood supply to endometrium – congestive dysmenorrhea.
- Pain can be due to 'bad' prostaglandin accumulation – usually only occurs in ovulatory phases where eggs are produced, when no eggs are produced, e.g. anovulation, menses usually lighter or 'spotting' normal – no pain.
- Constipation can increase absorption of oestrogens and contribute to dysmenorrhea. Improving soluble fibre intake in diet can benefit.
- Liver hypofunction may also contribute to poor elimination/breakdown of oestrogens.
- Too strong contraction of the cervix – period is blocked and causes greater pain. Muscle relaxants would benefit in this case. Inflammatory menstrual problems may also have irritable bowel syndrome (IBS).
- If pain starts *before* bleeding then vital force low – need to stimulate (Siberian ginseng) example.
- If pain *during* bleeding then generally due to blood stasis (congestive).
- If pain *after* bleeding then vital force low – need to build and strengthen.
- If pain *late* in the cycle – possible endometriosis.
- Ovarian pain (also called *Mittelschmerz* in German, meaning 'pain in the middle') usually occurs during the mid-cycle, often affecting one side. Ovarian pain may be caused be ovarian cyst rupturing, or excessive fluid release at ovulation from the follicle/corpus luteum cavity.

**Major causative factors of dysmenorrhoea may include:** Inflammation; endometriosis; narrow cervical os; cervical stenosis; extra-uterine pregnancy; endometrial poly; fibroids; uterine/pelvic infection; pelvic inflammatory disease (PID); intrauterine device (IUD); abdominal surgery; and sexually transmitted diseases.

### *Botanicals – Main*
Antispasmodic herbs:
Black cohosh – especially if pain comes before bleeding, with bloating and swollen breasts, ovaries and radiating down the legs
Black Haw: uterine spasmolytis
Blue cohosh: pain in cervix
Cramp bark: spasmolytic, uterine sedative
Dong quai: uterine decongestant, tonic, and circulatory stimulant
Ginger: circulatory stimulant
Wild yam root: cramps, ovarian neuralgia
Corydalis and Pulsatilla: analgesic, spasmolytic.
TCM Herbal formulas:
Tao Hong Si Wu Wan (Persica, Carthamus & Danggui combination) used with pattern of blood stagnation.
Xiao Yao San (Bupleurum & Dang Gui formula) and Zhe Chong Yin (Cinnamon & Persica Combination) used with patterns if Qi stagnation.
Wen Jing Tang (Dang Gui & Evodia combination) and Dang Gui Shao Yao San (Dang Gui & Peony combination) used with patterns of cold obstructing the uterus.

Ba Zhen Tang (Dang Gui & Ginseng Eight combination) used with Qi and Blood
vacuity pattern.

### Botanicals - Secondary

Angelica sinensis or Dong Quai: Blood stasis (dark)

Black haw: anti-spasmodic, useful with menstrual cramps. 15-30 drops tincture
3 times daily.

Chamomile tea: mild calmative.

Cayenne (capsicum spp)

Dan shen (saliva miltiorrhiza)

False unicorn root: a uterine tonic used in ovarian dysmenorrhea.

Ginger root: (anti inflammatory, circulatory stimulant).

Jamaican dogwood: anodyne pain relief, good for headaches also.

Lady's slipper: for hysteria

Life root: uterine tonic, useful in atonic conditions. 15-30 drops tincture 3
times daily

Mother's wort, mugwort

Paeonia: uterine decongestant

Pulsatilla: analgesic, particularly ovarian pains

Poke root: lymphatic, use with caution

White willow bark: natural aspirin. Help with pain relief, analgesic, anti-
inflammatory (also white poplar and meadow sweet)

Wood betony: anodyne pain relief, also good for headache

Californian poppy: pain relief

Vitex Agnus Castus: if also have other PMS symptoms (but is best not used for
dysmenorrhoea alone).

Red raspberry: uterine astringent

Squaw vine: used in dysmenorrhea especially of menarche (delayed period)

Valerian: sedative, anti spasmodic.

**Nutrition:** magnesium; calcium; potassium; evening primrose oil; Vitamins C
and E; Vitamins A and B complex (esp. niacin and B6).

**Homeopathic remedies**: apis 6x; arnica 6x; bellis perennis 3x; chamomilla
6x; gelsemium 6x; magnesia phoshorica 3x; and viburnum opulus 3x. Other
homeopathic remedies may include: pulsatilla; cactus grandiflorus; and kalium
carbonicum.

**Massage:** If tactile therapies aggravate the condition it may indicate blood
stasis; if it improves – Qi obstruction. Rub aromatherapy/essential oils over
abdominal area. These may include clary sage; geranium; rose; lemon grass;
warmed sesame seed oil; bentonite clay warmed and rubbed and wrapped over
the torso. There are also numerous Acupuncture points that can also be used
to allay period pains.

**Acupuncture/Acupressure Points:** LI 4, Lv 3, Sp 6, Sp 8, UB 32, UB 34,
Ren 4, K 5, St 28, St 29 and Liver 5.

**Medical:** There is a range of treatments depending upon the levels of dysmenorrhea. Anodyne/pain killers such as: aspirin; Panadol (paracetamol); Nurofen (ibuprophen); Mersyndol/forte (paracetamol/codeine phosphate/doxylamine succinate). Prostaglandin-inhibiting drugs such as Ponstan (mefenamic acid), Naprogesic, and Act 3 are some of the first considered treatment medication. These drugs are not without side effects, which predominantly involve the gastro-digestive system. If pain is severe drugs such as Duphaston may be considered.

Pathology tests may include: white blood cell (WBC) count – high levels of WBC in the blood serum can indicate leukocytosis dur to infection or cancer. Erythrocyte sedimentation rate (ESR) – elevated ESR in women under 50 years of age is considered indicative of inflammatory disease, infection and/or pregnancy. Cervical/vaginal swab cultures are taken to rule out localised infections such as: bacterial; candidiasis; protozoal; and viral.

## Menorrhagia

Menstruation is extremely heavy (haemorrhage) or prolonged menses. The menstrual cycle may be normal. Menorrhagia can be caused by: uterine fibroids (if very large may require surgical removal); endometrial polyps; endometriosis; adenomyosis; pelvic inflammatory disease; miscarriage; abnormal thyroid function; hormonal imbalances; tubal ligation; inter-uterine devices (IUD); and von Willebrand's disease (a congenital blood clotting disorder).

The prime cause of functional menorrhagia is due to an excessive release of arachidonic acid by the endometrium as a result of increased production of prostaglandins of the E2 series. Contributing factors that may associate with this condition are iron and Vitamin A deficiencies, hypothyroidism, and congenital deficiencies of clotting factors. A woman's body on average loses 40 per cent more calcium in menstrual bleeding than normal, so heavy periods can deplete her reserves very quickly; this may affect fertility, particularly if heavy bleeding has been going on for a long time.

Menorrhagia due to anovulation accounts for 70 per cent of dysfunctional uterine bleeding. It is a result of unopposed oestrogen due to progesterone deficiency. Bleeding is often prolonged and/or profuse, with pain and clotting. It may occur every 2-3 weeks for 7-plus days, possible resulting in anaemia (iron deficiency).

Menorrhagia due to luteal phase defects can result from increased oestrogen-to-progesterone ratios. There is often a shorter cycle of 23-26 days, spot bleeding for 3-6 days before the menses properly begins, and usually heavy periods for the first 2-3 days. Menorrhagia due to prolonged luteal phase may be a result of perimenopausal failure of hormone feedback mechanisms, leading to a relatively high progesterone-to-oestrogen ratio, with the possibility of raised androgen levels. Bleeding is usually scanty and prolonged.

Menorrhagia due to ovarian atrophy results from low levels of both progesterone and oestrogen. Bleeding is irregular, with the cycle so variable as to be non-existent.

### Medical Investigations
Medically functional menorrhagia may be investigated using vaginal ultrasound, hysteroscopy or diagnostic D&C procedures. Blood pathology tests may include: Iron studies to assess for iron deficiency; in general, serum ferritin is the preferred; hormone function blood test – FSH, LH, prolactin, oestradiol (E2), progesterone (P4); adrenal hormones e.g. cortisol; and blood coagulation factors.

### Medical Treatments
Progesterone-releasing IUDs have been used such as levonorgestrel to treat abnormal functional bleeding. Prostaglandin inhibitors such as Naprogestic and Ponstan have been used as have progesterone medications like Norethisterone, Provera or Primolut in the second half or continually through the menstrual cycle. Short term use of GnRH atonists such as Zoladex and Synarel have also been utilised medically if other methods have proven ineffective.

A definitive treatment for menorrhagia is to perform hysterectomy (removal of the uterus); dilation and curettage, and transvaginal endometrial resection are alternatives; endometrial ablation (destruction) by the use of applied heat (thermo-ablation) or other methods. Small fibroids may be dealt with by local removal (myomectomy).

### Herbal Medicine
Take herbs 7 days before due date of period and for first 4 days of period.

### Botanicals – Main
- Black haw: astringent, haemostatic
- Blue cohosh: uterine tonic and if cause is pelvic congestion
- Cranesbill: astringent
- Shepherd's purse: uterine anti-hemorrhagic
- Bethroot (trillium eractum): anti-hemorrhagic
- False unicorn root (helonias luteum): uterine tonic
- Ladies mantle: uterine anti-haemorrhagic
- Horsetail: anti-haemorrhagic
- Raspberry leaf: uterine anti-haemorrhagic, uterine tonic
- Squaw vine: uterine tonic
- Witch hazel: astringent
- Yarrow: anti-haemorrhagic, normalises circulation.

### Homeopathic remedies: Borax 30C, China 30C, and Belladonna 30C.

### Botanicals – Secondary
- Avens (Geum urbanum)
- Amaranth: astringent 15-25 drops tincture 3-4 times daily

- Angelica sinensis, Dong Quai: uterine tonic
- Black haw: haemostatic and astringent
- Black horehound (ballota nigra)
- Burnet root – is used in TCM
- Cinnamon: use infusion, 1 cup 2-3 times daily
- Cramp bark or high bush cranberry
- Geranium (Geranium maculatum): 15-20 drops tincture
- Golden seal: Mucous membrane tropo- restorative
- Horsetail (equisetum arvense)
- Lesser periwinkle: haemostatic and astringent
- Life root: uterine tonic, useful in atonic conditions. 15-30 drops tincture 3-4 times daily
- Lady's mantle: haemostatic, astringent
- Panax noto ginseng (tenchi ginseng)
- Rhemannia (cured)
- Red raspberry: uterine tonic
- Solomon's seal
- Squaw vine
- Strawberry leaf tea
- White oak bark: astringent
- Yarrow: anti-haemorrhagic

If the cause is due to under active thyroid consider: kelp; blue flag; and poke root (use with caution).

Liver problems may also be involved: dandelion root and St Mary's thistle are good examples of liver tonic herbs. Liver tonics may help to improve oestrogen break-down and elimination.

Over-stimulation of the uterine lining from oestrogen may cause heavy menstrual loss with pain.

If the condition is due to pelvic congestion: cayenne, ginger, and ginkgo, and other body-work techniques may be recommended.

***TCM herbs and formulas to stop bleeding***: Bulrush; cattail pollen (Pu Huang); Agrimonia (Xian He Cao); Pseudogingeng (San Qi); Japonicus (Japanese thistle, Da Ji); and Artemisia (Ai Ye).

Xiong Gui Jiao Ai Tang (Dang Gui and gelatin combination), and Zhi Bai Di Huang Wan (anemarrhena, phellodendron & rehmannia combination) used with blood heat pattern.

Gui Pi Tang (Ginseng & Longan combination) used with Qi vacuity pattern.

Si Wu Tang (Dang Gui Four combination) used with blood stasis pattern.

***Acupuncture/Acupressure points***: Spleen 1, Conception Vessel 4, Liver 1, Liver 3, Ki 8, Sp 8, and Du 20 may also help to settle excessive bleeding.

**Blood builders**: organic iron or chelate form; dong quai; nettles; withania; astragalus; codonopsis; panax ginseng; Vitamin B12; Vitamin C; bioflavonoids, alfalfa (Vitamin K); and parsley are all beneficial to prevent anaemia and some help to reduce excess bleeding.

Other nutrients include: Vitamin A and iodine; evening primrose oil (DHA/EFA); flavonoids (quercetin); silica; lysine; proline; Vitamin E, and Vitamin K.

**Homeopathic remedies**: ambrosia 3x; apis 3x; belladonna 3x; calcium carbonate 3x; chamomile 3x; crocus 3x; hamamelis virginica 3x; ipecacuanha 3x; kali carbonica 3x; kali nitricum 3x; magnesia muriatica 3x; sepia 3x; thlaspi bursa pastoris 3x; trillium pendulum 3x; and sabina 3x.

Other homeopathic remedies to consider reducing heavy menstrual periods may include: phosphorus; calcarea phosporia; carborundum; and natrum muriaticum.

**Aromatherapy** oils for heavy periods: Cypress and Rose.


## Naturopathic Interpretation of Menstrual Loss

### Colour and consistency

* Note – These associated signs are not a representation of medical diagnosis or pathology. Further investigation may be required to access underlying cause.

### Bright red blood
Bright blood is generally seen to be an indication that the period is normal, although fiery-looking and very bright blood may be an indication of excessive heat possibly associated with local infection or constitutional type (choleric).

Herbal medicines that exert Cooling or Astringent actions may be considered. In TCM, If the blood is bright red and profuse, with a shorter than 28-day cycle then herbs that cool the blood such as red peony (Chi Shoa) and moutan (Mu Dan Pi) may be considered to use throughout the cycle.

### Dark, brown or thick blood
Dark blood that appears brown, thick and looks like old blood is believed to be a sign of sluggish menstrual flow. Very dark red blood loss is considered to be quite normal and may indicate good blood quality. The dark, brownish sluggish blood may be an indication of poor uterine tone. Herbal medicines that exert uterine tonic, emmenagogue and/or spasmolytic actions may be recommended. In TCM, if the blood is scant and brownish in colour this is recognised as a blood deficiency or blood stasis pattern.

TCM herbs that may be used include: Dong Quai and formulas like Four Substances Decoction with Safflower and Peach Pit (Tao Hong Si Wu Tang) to tonify and invigorate the blood. The applications of warmed castor-oil packs to the lower abdomen after menstruation and before ovulation may also be beneficial.

### Thin, pale or watery blood

The type of blood loss may be an indication of poor blood quality. Pale-ish blood loss may be associated with deregulation of hormone balance – particularly when the woman is eating poorly, exercising excessively, and is tired and weak. Watery blood loss is common after surgical procedures of the uterus; these may include curettes (D&C) and terminations. Herbal medicines that enrich the blood and exert hormone regulation actions may be utilised. In TCM, if the blood is pink and watery this may be recognised as a Spleen Qi deficiency. TCM herbs that may be used include: ginseng (Ren Shen), astragalus (Huang Qi), and atractylodes (Bai Zhu).

If the uterine lining is too thin (less than 7 millimetres on ultrasound) and/or the menstrual blood is very scant, light and less than 3 days, then uterine-building herbs may be considered. Some of these include: artemisia (Ai Ye); leonurus (Yi Mu Cao); placenta (Zi He Che); red raspberry leaf; and four-substance decoction (Si Wu Tang).

### Menstrual Blood Clots

Clots may be an indication of excessive blood flow and are formed when the anti-clotting factors that are normally present in the menstrual blood are not keeping the blood in a fluid state due to the volume of blood loss. Herbal medicines that may be used include uterine tonics, emmenagogues or astringents. In TCM, blood flow that is heavy, dark and appears clotty, and is accompanied by pain, is recognised as a blood stasis condition. TCM herbs that may be used include: Peach kernel (Tao Ren); safflower (Hong Hua); frankincense (Ru Xiang); and achyranthes (Huai Niu Xi). The use of sanitary napkins (pads) would be recommended to use instead of tampons for this type of bleeding.

## Metrorrhagia

Bleeding between periods and irregular flow at a time other than the menstrual period usually mid-cycle. Also referred to as inter-menstrual or threshold bleeding. Bleeding commonly occurs at ovulation, though may happen at any time during the cycle.

Many conditions may cause Metrorrhagia; hormonal factors and cervical lesions are the most common. Uterine cancer should be investigated and ruled out also as it may also cause this type of bleeding. Other possible common causes of Metrorrhagia include: Endometrial hyperplasia; polyps; cervical eversion/ectropion; ovarian cysts; contraception drugs; malnutrition; excessive low body weight; placental malfunction during pregnancy; hydatidiform mole; ectopic pregnancy; and embryo implantation bleeds.

It is best to get a medical diagnosis with this condition, as it can indicate serious problems, which should be excluded before herbal treatment is commenced. Treatment is the same as for Menorrhagia, with herbs taken for the whole of the cycle, and with less emphasis on astringents.

### Botanicals
- Pulsatilla
- Blue cohosh
- Chaste tree: best taken at 7.00am and 4.00pm.
- False unicorn root

**Homeopathy**: Agnus 6C.

### Polymenorrhagia

Polymenorrhagia is a short cycle with heavy menstrual bleeding patterns.

**Causes**: commonly due to unopposed oestrogen stimulation caused by tumours or diseased state, causing hypertrophy of endometrial tissue and increased sloughing of tissue.

### Herbal Medicines
- Vitex
- Blue cohosh
- Lady's mantel
- Shepherd's purse
- Raspberry leaf
- False unicorn root (only if pathology of ovaries present)
- Withania
- Panax
- Horsetail

### Prolongation of period

Prolonged bleeding, often with intermittent scanty loss, not necessarily heavy.

For example the bleed seems like it goes for two weeks or more and then stops for a bit at the beginning, then starts bleeding again for another 4 to 5 days.

**Causes**: corpus luteum not bleeding down as it should. Low oestrogen and progesterone trigger menses as normal as corpus luteum degenerates, but it maintains its presence in the ovum, thus inhibiting new follicle growth and oestrogen production, which 'stops' menses. Treatment by promotion of corpus luteum function earlier will promote LH with Vitex to break down the corpus luteum better.

False unicorn root may be used in the first half of the cycle and Vitex during the second half of the cycle, as well as uterine anti-haemorrhagics such as: shepherd's purse; lady's mantle; beth root; and raspberry leaf.

### Polymenorrhea

Polymenorrhea is defined as a short menstrual cycle, bleeding normal, but cycle is less than 24 days. The cause is possibly due to hypothalamin-pituitary or ovarian dysfunction leading to an inadequate luteal phase of the menstrual cycle, causing the corpus luteum to break down too quickly – low oestrogen and progesterone trigger menses.

### *Herbal medicines:*
Vitex (main herb) promotes luteinising hormone (LH). Oestrogen and progesterone rising quickly together inhibit LH and lead to corpus luteum breakdown.
***Nervine tonics***: withania; oats; panax; verbena; and damiana.

***Sedatives***: St John's wort; valeriana; and skullcap.


# Premenstrual Syndrome (PMT/S)

### *'The grumpy monthly - the bitch is back'*

Premenstrual tension or syndrome (PMT or PMS) is a condition that has symptoms that occur just prior to and in some cases during menstruation: abdominal distension; depression; irritability; enema; sore breasts; nausea.

The syndrome has been recognised for centuries as a 'witch cycle'. In traditional Chinese medicine it is called *Dragon's Thunder*. Sufferers of PMS can experience a vast diversity in the variety of symptoms that can be involved in this condition in the week or fortnight prior to menstruation. Generally these symptoms can be divided into five (5) main subgroups that may also overlap one another, each with distinctive characteristics and hormonal links.

The onset usually occurs 4–10 days prior to menstruation and ends abruptly after the onset of menses flow. Approximately 75 per cent of women experience PMS to some degree. PMS should not be confused with dysmenorrhoea, which refers to pain or cramps during menstruation. Blood hormone pathology of sex hormones may present as being normal; this may suggest that many of the underlying causes of PMS link to an abnormal response of central neurotransmitters and receptor function to these transmitters is not functioning properly (e.g. GABA abnormalities).

The cyclical characteristics may include:

1. **PMT-P or PMT-Pain:** Crampy pain and reduced pain threshold characterises this group.

2. **PMT-A or PMT-Anxiety:** Symptoms of nervous tension, anxiety, mood swings, and irritability characterise this group. Raised oestrogen, and low progesterone levels.

3. **PMT-C or PMT-Craving:** This group shows symptoms of increased appetite; sweet craving; headaches; fatigue; acne flares; dizziness; or fainting and heart pounding. Biochemically, they seem to have an exaggerated insulin response to carbohydrates as well as decreased synthesis of prostaglandin PGE1. Magnesium deficiency may also be present. Increased carbohydrate tolerance, low progesterone, and increased PGE1 levels.

4. **PMT-D or PMT-Depression:** Depression, crying forgetfulness, confusion, and insomnia may characterise this group. Biochemically, this group has low oestrogen-to-progesterone ratio and elevated adrenal androgens. They may also appear to have higher body lead burden than normal individuals. Low blood estrogen; increased progesterone and increased adrenal function.

5. **PMT-H or PMT-Hyper-hydration:** Fluid retention, weight gain, swelling of extremities, breast tenderness and abdominal bloating characterise this group. Elevated oestrogen levels can draw water particles to it, thus contributing to oedema swelling. Increased aldosterone.

**Premenstrual Dysphoric Disorder (PMDD) – SUPER PMS**
*PMS on the roids – Men be afraid, be very afraid...you can run but you can't hide...?*

Super PMS is a severe, disabling form of PMS. In PMDD, the main symptoms are mood disorders such as depression, tension, and persistent anger or irritability. Women with PMDD usually also have physical symptoms, such as headaches; joint and muscle pain; lack of energy; bloating; and breast tenderness.

The majority of symptoms that are associated with PMT are due to hormone and nutritional imbalances. The female hormone oestrogen has been found to be elevated in the late luteal phase of the menstrual cycle, reaching its maximal point 1-5 days before menses. By contrast, progesterone in PMT shows a reduction in the mid-luteal phase, reaching its lowest relative deficiency 5-10 days before menstruation. Other studies have implicated increased levels of follicle-stimulating hormone (FSH), aldosterone, and prolactin.

Elevated oestrogen-to-progesterone ratios have been shown to contribute to premenstrual anxiety, irritability, and depression. Elevated oestrogen is known to interact with brain enzymes to cause an elevation of adrenalin, which is known to trigger anxiety; with noradrenalin, known to promote hostility and irritability; with serotonin, which helps cause nervous tension, fluid retention, and the inability to concentrate. Dopamine, which is believed to balance the effects of these three amines by enhancing relaxation and mental alertness, is found to be at reduced levels. Studies have shown that the highest number of accidents, suicide attempts, and violent crimes committed by women occur in the premenstrual period 4–7 days prior to menstruation.

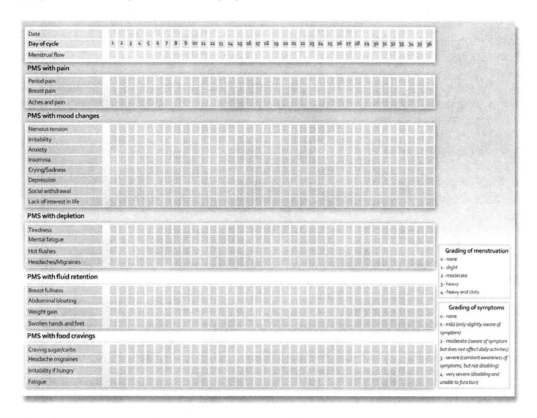

*PMS diary chart of signs and symptoms*

The symptoms of PMT show a striking similarity to those associated with the loss of activity in the thyroid gland. Giving thyroid hormone replacement has been found to relieve many PMT symptoms. Some of the features of PMT are also similar to the effects that are produced by injection of Prolactin.

Dopamine has been shown to decrease Prolactin secretion; the amino acid DL-Phenylalanine and Tyrosine are both a precursor nutrient to thyroid hormones or dopamine that may be of benefit in lowering excessive secretions of this hormone. Decreased synthesis of the transmitter serotonin during the luteal phase (post-ovulation stage) of the menstrual cycle suggests an important role of this neuroendocrine mechanism in PMS.

The oral contraceptive pill users have been shown to have a significant increase in plasma tyrosine trans-aminase activity and a significant fall in plasma tyrosine levels in mid-cycle and luteal phases. This reduced availability of tyrosine to the brain may result in lowered brain or adrenaline levels. Symptoms that may occur due to this imbalance include: altered moods; poor coping ability; and disturbances in appetite.

It is known that ovarian hormones influence calcium, magnesium, and Vitamin D metabolism. Oestrogen regulates calcium metabolism, intestinal calcium absorption and parathyroid gene expression and secretion, triggering fluctuations across the menstrual cycle. Hypo or hypercalcemia (low or high blood calcium levels) share many of the symptoms associated with PMT. Evidence indicates that luteal phase symptomology may also be linked to an underlying calcium deregulation problem such as hyper-parathyroidism and Vitamin D deficiencies.

### Natural treatments:

### 1 PMS-A (anxiety)
Herbs - wood betony (betonica); passionflower; polygala; lavender; lime tree; lady's slipper; valerian; zizyphus; skullcap; californian poppy; kava kava; vitex agnus castus; chamomile; ginger; and withania.

Nutrients – magnesium; calcium; Vitamin B6 and methionine (normalise oestrogen : progesterone ratio); and flax (linseed) oil may help with reducing panic attacks.

### 2 PMS-C (cravings)
Herbs - gymnema silvestra; cinnamon; goat's rue; bilberry; fenugreek; jambul; blue flag; brindleberry; codonopsis; stevia; globe artichoke; fringe tree; liquorice; slippery elm; and mother wort.

Nutrients - dha/epa; biotin; chromium; manganese; vanadium (trace amounts); zinc; lipoic acid, magnesium; Vitamin B1; B3; n-acytel-cysteine; and l-carnitine.

### 3 PMS-D (depression)
Herbs - blue cohosh; withania; St John's wort (not to be used with other ssri medication); panax ginseng; false unicorn root; damiana; oat seed; lavender; lemon balm (melissa); ginkgo biloba; morinda (noni); rosemary; and vervain.

Nutrients – Tyrosine; 5–hydroxy–tryptophan (5HT) (at night); S-adenosyl-methionine (Same); magnesium; potassium; and Vitamin B complex.

### 4 PMS-H (hyper-hydration)
Herbs - Dandelion leaf; celery seed; cnicus benedictus (blessed thistle); corn silk; horse chestnut; clivers; poke root (caution); parsley; butcher's broom;

*vitex agnus castus* (for breast pain and swelling); birch leaf; and ginkgo biloba may also be effective.

Nutrients – Magnesium; Vitamin B6 (regulates aldosterone, thereby promotes diuresis); Vitamin E (reduces breast soreness). Avoid excess salt intake and methylxanthines (in coffee).

## 5  PMS-P (pain) (e.g. cramp pain)

Herbs – corydalis; ginger; asia sarum; cramp bark; black haw; wild yam (extract and creams); dong quai; lady's mantle; pulsatilla; bethroot; blue cohosh; black cohosh; morinda; motherwort; shepherd's purse; false unicorn root; peppermint; squaw vine; raspberry leaf; jamaican dogwood; californian poppy; vitex; peonia; golden seal; valerian; white willow bark; feverfew; chamomile; and wood betony.

**Nutrients** – Magnesium; Essential Fatty Acids (evening primrose oil); bromelain; and Vitamin E.

## Main Nutrients used generally for PMS

Vitamin B complex 50mg 2-3 times daily

Vitamin B6 – up to 250mg twice daily (short time)

Vitamin E 400 IU 2-3 times daily

Vitamin C 1000mg-2000mg 2-3 times daily

Vitamin A 10,000 IU- up to 100,000 (for several days) (caution with elevated doses) prior to menstrual cycle

Calcium 1,000mg –1500mg daily (best with Vitamin D 200IU-400IU)

Magnesium 500mg 2-3 times daily (balance with calcium 2:1 ratio calcium to magnesium)

Zinc 25mg – 50mg daily

Evening Primrose Oil (GLA) 1000mg 3 times daily

Selenium - 50-200 ug daily.

Wild yam or natural progesterone creams applied and rubbed into various skin areas may reduce PMS symptoms, to be applied during the second half of the menstrual cycle post-ovulation until menses onset.

## Medical treatments

To improve hormone profile: Contraceptive pill; GnRH agonists; Danazol; oestradiol patches or implants; progestens; or progesterone.

To help regulate prostaglandin dysfunction: Ponstan (mefenamic acid); Naprogesic; Naprosyn; and Anaprox (naproxen sodium).

For PMS (D) with severe depression: Psychotropic medication such as anti-depressants. Selective serotonin reuptake inhibitors (SSRIs) may be considered for short-term trial.

For PMS Hyperhydration (fluid retention): Medicinal strength diuretics may be recommended.

### Etiological considerations

Improper diet deficient in B6; folic acid; B2; B complex; calcium; iron; Vitamin K; protein; junk foods (refined foods, coffee, tea, soda, excess salt and excess meat which contains high phosphorus levels causing calcium deficiency) results in nutritional deficiencies.

1. Extreme diets: fruitarians (who only eat fruit foods); protein deficiency; excess dieting; anorexia; low /no fat; low cholesterol levels.
2. Hypoglycaemia
3. Methylxanthines (coffee, tea chocolate, and cola): these are associated with dysmenorrhea and premenstrual syndrome.
4. Stress/psychological - Anxiety; depression; fear of pregnancy or of maturity; sudden shock; sexual problems.
5. Hormonal - Oestrogen therapy; contraceptive pill.
6. Pathology – Cancer; endometriosis; fibroids; misplaced womb; salpingitis; cervical lesion.
7. Other diseases – endocrine disorders (pituitary; thyroid, ovary, liver); hypertension; diabetes; blood disorders (including anaemia); kidney disease; syphilis; scurvy.

### General

Dong quai can be used in nearly all menstrual problems (caution during extremely heavy menstrual bleeding).

### TCM herbal Formulas used for PMS:

Xiao Yao San (Bupleurum & Dang Gui formula) used with pattern of Liver qi stagnation. Chai Hu Shu Gan Tang (Bupleurum & Cyperus combination) used with patterns of Liver qi stagnation with blood stasis.

Other formulas that may also be considered include: Jai Wei Xiao Yao San (Bupleurum & Peony formula), Bu Zhong Yi Qi Tang (Ginseng & Astragalus combination), Gui Pi Tang (Ginseng & Longan combination), Qi Ju Di Huang Wan (Lycium, Chrysanthemum & Rehmannia formula) and Wen Dan Tang (Bamboo & Hoelen combination).

### Acupuncture points that are useful in PMS:

- **Kidney 27** – these two points are located in the hollow just below your collar bone, in line with the outer edge of your neck.

- **Stomach 18** – is located under the breast area, approximately 4 thumb widths from the mid-line (sternum), between the 5th and 6th ribs, below the nipple. Others may include: Heart 7, Liver 3, Colon 4, Bladder 10, Tai Yang and Gall Bladder 1. For headaches points: LI 4, St 36, and GB 20.

### Essential oils to consider using for PMS include: bergamot; chamomile; clary sage lavender; geranium; neroli; orange blossom; rose; and ylang ylang. They can either be applied to the body with carrier base oil, put in a soothing bath or in an oil burner to savour the aroma.

*Homeopathic remedies* for PMS: Aletris farinose 3x, Calcarea carbonica 3x, Natrum muriaticum 6x, Sepia 3x, Magnesia carbonicum or phosphate 6x, and Nux vomica 3x. Other homeopathic remedies may include: Pulsatilla and Lachesis.

**Bleeding from a poorly stimulated endometrium (oestrogen deficiency)**
*Symptoms*: bleeding is cyclical and irregular – 'threshold bleeding'; often occurs near menopause, may be profuse, (e.g. bleeding mid-cycle). Break-through bleeding is sometimes caused by a decreased sensitivity to FSH and LH. Low levels of oestrogen produce a slight shedding of the uterus lining. Decreased FSH and LH utilisation reduces the chances of ovulation. Without ovulation, inadequate progesterone is produced to sustain the uterine lining and bleeding occurs. At the other end of the scale excessive oestrogen can also stimulate too much uterine lining to be produced, thus leading to bleeding.

*Cause*: low oestrogen.

*Herbal medicines*:
* False unicorn root
* Peonia
* Wild yam
* Black cohosh
* Dong quai
* Ladies' mantle
* Yarrow

**Cystic Hyperplasia of the Endometrium**

*Symptoms:* – often amenorrheal (absent bleeding) for 6-8 weeks, followed by a cyclical and profuse bleeding, difficult to distinguish from poor oestrogen stimulation of the endometrium, though the cause is different.

*Cause:* oestrogen is unopposed by progesterone, resulting in marked endometrial proliferation (cystic hyperplasia).

*Herbal Medicines:*
Vitex (supports progesterone)
Blue cohosh (supports progesterone)
Anti-haemorrhagic such as: Lady's mantle, shepherd's purse, and yarrow (to settle excessive bleeding).

# Cervical dysplasia

Cervical dysplasia is a condition when the atypical epithelial cells on the uterine cervix develop abnormally and may progress into cancerous cells. In the USA, cervical cancer is the second leading cause of death of females surpassed only by breast cancer. One of the first signs of cervical cancer is vaginal bleeding between periods, after intercourse, or after menopause. There may also be an increase in vaginal discharge.

| | |
|---|---|
| **Stage 1** | – *Dysplasia with low or high risk* |
| | – *Low – abnormal cells, but no cancer risk* |
| | – *High – abnormal cells, 10 per cent will prove to be cancerous* |
| **Stage 2** | – *carcinoma in situ (confined) 15 to 30 per cent proven to have invaded surrounding tissue  (moderate)* |
| **Stage 3** | – *Cancer – 50 per cent proven to have invaded surrounding tissue (very high). Survival time after 5 years is 50 per cent (if untreated).* |

Causes of cervical dysplasia may include STDs (sexually transmitted diseases), due to human papilloma virus (HPV) (venereal warts), and has shown to be a major precursor of cancer as it brings about changes to tissue.

There is increased risk with sexual exposure to men with HVP, or sexual exposure to men with exposure to women with cervical intraepithelial neoplasia – first stage cancer (CIN). Increased risk associated with early intercourse, multiple partners, cervical erosion (ulcerations) from trauma such as childbirth or infection increase risk.

Co-factors that may also be contributing factors to this condition are: smoking; long-term use of the oral contraceptive pill; chronic cervicitis; herpes simplex virus (HSV) infection, immune compromised; and carcinogens.

Prognosis is very good with early treatment; if the condition is left too long a hysterectomy may be required. Regular, conversional pap smear testing is how the condition is monitored. A biopsy may be recommended if the cell results are abnormal to monitor the progression of the condition.

The *Thin Prep* is a newer method that is proving very successful at identifying even the earliest pre-cancer changes in cervical cells.

A new vaccine called Gardasil has been developed in Australia that is proving almost 100 per cent effective in preventing cervical cancer from forming. The vaccine works on stopping HPV from occurring and its application is also be used for males. This revolutionary breakthrough may be the stepping stone to eradicating cervical cancer in the future.

### Supportive natural treatments may include:

### Herbal medicines:
Poke root (phytolacca) and Calendula for lymphatic system support.
Panax ginseng, Siberian ginseng and withania for adaptogen support.
St Mary's thistle, chaparral, and turmeric for anti-oxidant support.
Echinacea, picrorrhiza, and Pau d'arco for immunostimulant support.

Douche (vaginal wash) containing: calendula, goldenseal, chickweed, turmeric.

*Nutritional support:*
Folic acid has been shown to reverse early-stage cervical dysplasia and reduce risk of cancer of the cervix. Indole-3-Carbinol (I3C) may be helpful in increasing oestrogen metabolism reducing cervical intraepithelial neoplasia, inhibiting tumour growth.
Evening Primrose Oil: anti-inflammatory.

*Medical*:
A new nano-golden bullet cancer treatment is in development that involves injecting into the blood stream microscopic glass spheres (140 millionths of a millimetre across), coated in gold. The nano-spheres particles circulate through the body and 'fall' through holes in leaky blood vessels in the tumour (cancer). The spheres 'light up' under low energy infra-red light, pinpointing the location of the cancer. A more powerful beam is then used converting light into heat, and destroying the tumour.

Unlike conventional cancer treatments, the golden-bullet approach uses no toxic chemicals and no radiation, reducing the risk of unpleasant side effects. Cancer scientists predict that this new technology may have wide applications in numerous types of cancers such as: cervix, breast, brain, skin, and neck. It may also prove to be much cheaper than existing treatments.

## Cervical erosion

Cervical erosion is ulceration of the surface epithelium of the cervix resulting from trauma such as childbirth, infection, or an outgrowth of uterine lining. A discharge may be present. This condition is more common when women have been using the oral contraceptive pill on a regular basis.

Diagnosis is during a pap smear. This condition may predispose the women to future cervical cancer if not treated promptly.

*Herbal treatments may include*: Douching with astringent and anti-microbial herbs using equal parts of e.g. calendula; golden seal; raspberry leaf; Echinacea; slippery elm (30 grams to 500ml) with a teaspoon of cider vinegar and 5 per cent tea tree oil. Vitamin E cream may be applied to the cervix.

Herbs to support hormones: Vitex agnus castus and false unicorn root.

# Leucorrhoea/Vaginitis/Pelvic Inflammatory Disease (PID)

### Leucorrhoea
Leucorrhoea is a condition when there is vaginal discharge but there is no infection on its own.

## Vaginitis

Vaginitis is a condition involving inflammation and/or infection with possible concurrent inflammation of the vulva. There are three types of vaginitis including:

1. *Atrophic* – Due to hormone deficiency (e.g. oestrogens), affects up to 40% of menopausal women.
2. *Irritant* – Caused by physical, chemical agent or allergic reaction e.g. soap.
3. *Infectious* – e.g. chlamydia.

The condition can be caused by a reaction to an external agent – spermicides, deodorants, even sperm. If the condition is caused via a suspected infection, or if there is a change in normal vaginal smell, a vaginal culture swab may be required to diagnose the type of culprit bug.

If there is a white discharge this is regarded as a 'cold' condition; if there is a yellow discharge this is a 'hot' condition.

Vaginitis may be due to an overgrowth of flora such as thrush or due to the introduction of an infectious organism during intercourse, for example.

## Gardnerella vaginalis (Hemophilus) or Bacterial vaginitis

This disorder causes 40–50 per cent of cases of STDs and is commonly involved in non-specific vaginitis, characterised by a fishy (unpleasant) odour and a white to off-white (greyish) colour, and watery discharge. Gardnerella is found in 20 per cent of women; though it is normally present in small quantities, it can overgrow the healthy lactobacilli bacteria in the vagina. Vaginal fluid acidity is normally decreased. Males usually have no symptoms. Other bacteria such as ureaplasma urealyticum and mycoplasma hominis can behave in similar ways to gardnerella. The incubation period is bacterial vaginitis is: 3 to 5 days.

***Medical treatments for bacterial vaginitis:*** most commonly involve using antibiotic medications such as: Metronidazole (Flagyl). Homeopathic remedies may include Borax veneta.

## Trichomoniasis

Trichomoniasis causes 30 per cent of cases of STDs and is a species of protozoan or anaerobic parasite. This microbe may have no distinct odour, though is characteristic of causing a greenish-yellow frothy discharge. Trichomoniasis may cause irritated genital membranes, severe itching, burning with urination and pain during intercourse. Males may be asymptomatic and must be treated to avoid spreading the microbe. This micro-organism is commonly associated with thrush (Candida). Trichomoniasis prefers to grow in a pH environment between 5.5 and 5.8; the hormone progesterone increases vaginal pH levels. Incubation period of Trichomoniasis is 3 to 20 days.

***Medical treatments for Trichomoniasis***: Metronidazole (Flagyl).

## Chlamydia trachomonis

This is estimated to affect approximately 40 per cent of women. This infection can be transmitted or contracted during anal, oral or vaginal sex with an infected partner. Chlamydia accounts for the bulk of the epidemic of STDs and in the USA alone 4 million new cases are diagnosed each year, of which is estimated to cause sterility in fifty thousand of those people.

Symptoms of chlamydia include difficult or burning with urination; genital inflammation; pain with intercourse; itching; and vaginal or urethral discharge. Though, many may also be asymptomatic and it affects both men and women. Males who contract chlamydia can develop prostatitis and inflammation of the seminal vesicles causing symptoms such as pain and swelling in the testicles, pain when urinating, and a watery discharge from the penis.

Babies born to mothers with chlamydia can suffer conjunctivitis (an infection of the eyes) and pneumonia; both mother and child will require to be treated with antibiotic therapy in this situation. A complication of chlamydia trachomatis is a condition called Fitz-Hugh-Curtis Syndrome, which is an infection and inflammation of tissue around the liver. Possible signs and symptoms may include: upper abdominal pain which is usually worse when lying down or turning; vaginal discharge; vulval itch; and pain on passing urine.

The incubation period of chlamydia is between 7 to 21 days.

***Medical treatments for Chlamydia***: Some of the types of antibiotics that may be used kill off chlamydia include: azithromycin, tetracycline and doxycycline (Vibramycin). A vaccine and a topical preparation are also in the works that can help to prevent contracting chlamydia. Using condoms during intercourse with spermicides such as Nonoxynol-9 can also protect against transmission. Chlamydia has also been linked to a type of arthritis found in young women.

## Candida Albicans

Also known as Candidiasis, Dysbiosis or Thrush; this is a fungal (yeast) organism that occurs naturally in the gut, skin and vaginal areas of the body. Candida is usually kept in check by 'friendly' bacteria (normal flora) that reside in the gut; however, when these good bacteria become compromised the candida organism then proliferates (a battle of good versus evil). Candida overgrowth is a very common condition.

***Factors that may contribute to candida overgrowth***:

- Poor digestive enzyme production and nutrition absorption
- High dietary consumption of yeast and refined sugar containing foods
- Broad-spectrum antibiotic use
- Hormone treatments such as the contraceptive pill and steroids
- Disease or illnesses (immune-compromised conditions such as AIDS and diabetes)
- Chronic stress and adrenal dysfunction
- Gastrointestinal dysfunction

- Thrush: excessive humidity and hot weather; synthetic underclothing e.g. pantyhose, intercourse with an infected partner, and hormone imbalances.

***Symptoms and characteristics of candida dysbiosis may include****:*
Vaginal thrush discharge (white cheesy plaque around the vulva and perineum with possible 'yeasty' odour); itching and/or vaginitis (burning, irritating sensation and reddening around the vaginal and rectum areas); food cravings especially for sugars; abdominal bloating and flatulence; bowel habits have changed; irritable bowel syndrome (IBS); increased allergies; mood swings; and alcohol intolerance. Males may have a discharge for the penis.

The incubation period of Candida is one to two days.

Candida can affect fertility by interfering with the sperm transporting to the egg, making it difficult for conception to take place. The yeast infection can contribute to an inflammatory and heightened immune response into the reproductive region, therefore compromising conception success.

***Natural treatments for candidiasis*** may include: caprylic acid (octanoic acid); biotin; lactobacillus species; bifidus; garlic; barberry; calendula; citrus seed extract; Echinacea; par d'arco; golden seal; cinnamon bark oil; savory oil; colostrums; wild indigo; tea tree (not internally); and neem (not to be used prior to or during pregnancy). Soluble fibres such as slippery elm and digestive enzymes supplementation may also be useful to combat candida overgrowths.

***Homeopathic remedies may include***: Isopathy; Helonias; Kreosotum; Pulsatilla; Sepia; and Thuja.

***Douche for vaginal thrush may include herbs:*** Golden seal; white pony lily; uva ursi; witch hazel; calendula; white vinegar (approx 2 tablespoons); tea tree oil (approx 4 drops) mixed into 1 litre (=2 pints) of warm, purified water. (Don't use douches during pregnancy).

Reduce foods that may feed that fungus: Decrease all refined carbohydrates especially sugar; lollies (sweets); soft drinks; white flour; breads; white rice; pasta; miso soup; soy sauce; vinegar; dried fruit; dry roasted peanuts; alcohol beverages; all yeast; and fermented foods.

Increase foods such as: acidophilus yogurt, garlic and cranberry (juice).
Wear underclothing that is of natural fibre and always air through.

***Medical treatments*** may include drugs in tablet or powder form; creams and suppositories such as: Canesten, Nystatin, Monistat, Femstat, Gyne-lotrimin, and Diflucan. Triazole anti-fungals such as: Itraconazole or Imidazole anti-fungal cream/pessaries such as Clotrimazole.

**Gonorrhoea (Neisseria gonorrhoeae)**

A gonococci bacterium that often causes no symptoms in women; though, if it does cause symptoms they may include for women frequent and painful urination; vaginal discharge; abnormal menstrual bleeding; acute inflammation in the pelvic region; and anal itching. Men with gonorrhoea usually do suffer from symptoms that may include a pus, mucousy yellow discharge from the penis, with slow, difficult and painful urination (I've heard it explained eloquently as feeling like 'pissing razor-blades').

Symptoms may appear between 2 to 21 days after initial contact with the infection. If it is not treated, the microbe can move into the bloodstream and travel to the bones, joints, tendons, and other tissues, causing a systemic illness that may cause aching, mild fever, inflamed joints and at time skin lesions.

*Medical treatments for Gonorrhoea:*

Broad spectrum antibiotics such as: Tetracycline and injectable drugs like spectinomycin hydrochloride and penicillin-related medication ampicillin.

**Herpes virus**

Herpes simplex is a recurrent virus infection of the skin or mucous membranes characterised by single or multiple clusters of small vesicle eruptions (ulcers) on an erythematous base frequently occurring about the mouth, lips, genitals or eyes. The incubation period is 2 to 21 days and the breakout lasts initially 2 to 4 weeks; recurrent attacks approximately 5 to 10 days.

Herpes simplex type 1 (HSV-1) and type 2 (HSV-2) cause both cold sores and genital herpes. Genital herpes is the most prevalent sexually transmitted disease and the risk of clinical herpes infection after sexual contact with an individual with active lesions is estimated to be 75 per cent. Outbreaks may follow minor infection, trauma, stress – emotional, dietary, and environmental – and after sun exposure. Immuno-suppressed individuals are more prone to develop a chronic, persistent infection.

A mild tingling, itching or burning sensation may be experienced just prior the outbreak. When the outbreak has occurred they present like tiny fluid-filled blisters that are high infectious. Other symptoms that may accompany this condition are urethral discharge; painful urination; fever; malaise; neuritis (nerve pain in the 2nd and 3rd sacral dermatomes – down the back of the legs); headaches; and mild flu-like symptoms.

After a few days the blisters may erupt with pus and form painful ulcerations. HSV-1 (cold sore type) and HSV-2 (genital type) can form in either location (I don't need to draw you a picture how that may happen, just think about it for a minute!). The incubation period for genital herpes is 2 to 4 days.

***Natural treatments for Herpes include:***

***Herbal medicines:*** St John's wort; astragalus; cat's claw; golden seal; lemon balm (if used early – internally and externally); charraral; liquorice; garlic; olive leaf; spirulina; tea tree (topically); echinacea; myrrh; and red clover.

***Nutrients:*** try amino acid L-Lysine – 1,200mg daily, (a diet high in arginine and low in lysine has been shown to facilitate herpes infection); acidophilus; beta 1,3-D-glucan; reishi, shiitake and maitake mushrooms; inositol hexaphosphate (Ip6); Co enzyme Q 10; Vitamin A; Vitamin B complex; Vitamin B12 injection; Vitamin C; bioflavonoids; bromelain; selenium; Di-methyl glycine (DMG); DMSO; Vitamin E; lecithin; essential fatty acids; and zinc.

Avoid all chocolate, peanuts and almonds as they are high in arginine. Though, arginine is an important nutrient for sperm production and males that suffer from herpes and have low sperm counts may need to control infection by other means, if arginine is a required nutrient.
Apply ice to the lesion during the very early (prodrome) phase can abort outbreak.

Avoid excessive stress and sun exposure.

***Medical treatments:*** Medical drugs and creams such as: Acyclovir (Zovirax), Choraphor, Valacyclovir (Valtrex), Famciclovir (Famvir), and Isotretinoin have been used with some success for herpes.

### Venereal warts
Small wart growths that are caused by human papilloma virus (HPV). There are approximately 60 known types of HPV. These warts can develop singularly or in clusters. There are three main types that are usually involved: Common warts, plantar warts, and genital warts (condyloma acuminata).

Genital warts are usually soft, moist growths that may be found in or around the anus, groin, scrotum, penis, urethra and vagina. These types of warts may appear pinkish or red in colour and resemble tiny cauliflower heads. Genital warts are high contagious and transmittable. The incubation period of HPV can be between 1 to 6 months after initial infection. Condyloma acuminata incubation period is seven to ten days.

Genital warts appear to contribute to changes in the cervix that may be a precursor to cervical dysplasia and squamous cell carcinoma of the cervix.

The virus can be self-limiting or very aggressive, especially in pregnancy. Exposure to warts during birth may lead to future laryngeal papilloma in young children. Males can be usually asymptomatic. Pap smears should be performed every 6 months after contacting the virus to observe any cervical cell changes. The *Vira Pap* is a specific test for venereal wart.

***Natural treatments for venereal warts include***:
Require Immune stimulant, anti-viral, lymphatic and tonic herbs.

*Thuja* is the specific herbal remedy against HPV. Also consider poke root; andrographis; astragalus; Echinacea; garlic; myrrh; oil of clove; lemongrass; peppermint; picrorrhiza; reishi and shiitake mushrooms.

Applied topically to the wart: aloe vera gel; black walnut; carica papaya (paw paw leaves); chelidonium juice from the fresh plant; chickweed; golden seal; thuja essential oil; dandelion leaf juice; tea tree; pau d'arco; and wintergreen. Also castor oil and baking soda pasted on the wart may also be useful.
***Nutrients***: Vitamin B Complex; Vitamin C; bioflavonoids; sulphur-containing amino acid such as L-cysteine; methylsulfonylmethane (MSM); Vitamin A, Vitamin E; and zinc.

## Medical treatments:
Medical treatments of warts are normally lanced (cut-off), lasered, or frozen off with liquid nitrogen (cryotherapy). Take-home topical applications: Podofilix and Imiquimod. Medical drugs such as: Bleomycin (Blenoxane), Canthardin, Podophyllin, Trichloracetic acid (TCA), and Interferon alpha injections (but have numerous side effects) have been used with success to get rid of the warts.

New vaccinations are now available to prevent HPV infection. The vaccine needs to be administered during childhood or prior to becoming sexually active to be effective. HPV is highly present in women who develop cervical dysplasia, which can progress to cervical cancer if untreated. Early vaccination to HPV may help to prevent future generations of women developing these potentially serious conditions.

## Other forms of sexually transmitted diseases may include:

- Acquired immune deficiency syndrome (AIDS); Hepatitis B and C; chancroid (haemophilus ducreyi) bacteria; crabs (public lice phthirus pubis – pubic pediculosis); dcabies
- Lymphogranuloma venereum (LGV), T-mycoplasm, granuloma inguinale, trichomoniasis (trichomanas vaginalis) and dyphilis (treponema pallium).
- Vaginitis in younger girls may be due to decreased hygiene and be caused via E-coli, streptococcus and staphylococcus infections. The vulva may be appearing inflamed with increased local redness with gardnerella, trichomonas, and yeast infections; candida typically is known as one of the worst irritants. Leucorrhoea is usually due to infection of the mucous membranes of the urinary tract, not just the vagina as in vaginitis.

Symptoms may be present continuously or just during menstrual period time. If you are having intercourse during this time (though, you may be too sore to even try), condoms are recommended to be used to avoid spreading the infection. Trichomonas is particularly contagious.

The normal vaginal pH (acidity) is 4.5 or lower due to the formation of lactic acid from lactobacilli. This interaction between the micro-organism and the normal flora inhibit the potential overgrowth of the organisms. Approximately 5 to 10 different organisms can often be cultured from a women's vagina with no abnormal discharge. The most prevalent of these microbes may include corynebacterium, lactobacilli, and streptococci.

## Vaginismus
Is a condition that causes the pelvic floor muscles to go into spasm before or during intercourse that can lead to sexual problems in females, and an inability to achieve penetration can cause painful intercourse called dyspareunia. The condition is an unconscious reaction and can be linked to possible psychological factors such as anxiety.

## Vulvar vestibulitis
Is a condition that involves severe unexplained burning pain of the vulva, labia, and sometimes the vagina. Women should avoid wearing tight underwear; activities such as bicycle riding; reduce foods high in oxalates such as caffeine, chocolate, tomatoes, peanuts, and sardines. Supplementing calcium citrate has some benefits in vulvar vestibulitis. Medical treatment may be similar to that of HPV; the application of heat seems to soothe the symptoms.

# Pelvic Inflammatory Disease (PID)

Pelvic Inflammatory Disease can include infections of the fallopian tube (salpingitis); ovaries; uterus (endometritis); pelvic peritoneum (peritonitis); and/or broad ligaments. It is more typical to affect women under the age of 25, though is uncommon before the commencement of menstruation, during pregnancy and after menopause. During a medical physical internal examination there may be severe pain on moving the cervix area.

The condition may also present with elevated temperature; abnormal uterine discharge, with or without bleeding; pain with intercourse; excessive vaginal bleeding during and also not during period time; nausea; and vomiting.

If the condition goes untreated approximately 1 in 4 women may become infertile or have an increased risk of ectopic pregnancy occurring due to scarring of the tubes or adhesions as a result of the chronic inflammation. Conditions such as Irritable Bowel Syndrome (IBS) may mimic many of the PID signs and symptoms as should be ruled out. Treatment may require the uses of antibiotics, and further medical investigations and pathology may be warranted to eliminate any other serious condition.

### Herbal Medicines that may be considered for PID:
- Immunostimulants and anti-microbials such as: andrographis; cat's claw; barberry; Echinacea; cranesbill; garlic; golden seal; thuja (also for

274

adhesions); pau d' arco; picororhiza; red clover; wild indigo (baptisia); and myrrh.

- Lymphatic herbs: Calendula and poke root.
- Tonic herbs used in chronic disorders such as: astragalus; dong quai; Siberian ginseng; suma; and withania.
- Uterine Tonics: Beth root; blue cohosh; false unicorn root; true unicorn root; and raspberry leaf.
- White pond lily (nymphaea odorata) and yarrow (achillea millefolium) used internally and externally in decrease vaginal discharges.
- TCM Herbal formula: Wen Jing Tang (Danggui & Evodia combination), Bei Xie Fen Qing Yin (Tokoro combination), Leucorrhea pills (Yu Dai Wan), Zhi Bai Ba Wei Wan (Anamarrhena, Phelledendron, & Rehmannia combination).
- For vaginitis and leucchoea: Wan Dai Tang (Atractylodes & Dioscerea combination).

**Nutrients:**
- Recolonise vaginal environment with lactobacillus acidophilus. Acidophilus cultured yogurts and probiotic supplements, slippery elm would be extremely beneficial. Acidophilus can be used and inserted in pessary form also to balance the vaginal cultural environment.
- Garlic: is one of the best-known anti-fungal and anti-microbial foods effective against thrush.
- Increase the consumption of cranberry juice that contains hippuric acid as it acidifies the urine and decreases the risk of infection. Cranberry is also high in Vitamin C and bioflavonoids that are also very helpful because of their effects of enhancing immune activity and healing.
- Vitamin E: has also shown to help resist chlamydia infection.
- Evening primrose oil: can help to reduce inflammation.
- Zinc: can help to improve the health of the general reproductive system and to enhance immune function to fight against the infective microbes and boost wound healing.
- Colloidal Silver: taken internally and also can be washed or douched at the site of the infection is an invaluable and safe antiseptic agent to fight off the micro overgrowth (known to be effective against approximately 350 pathogens) and soothes the inflammation.
- Apple cider vinegar, iodine and/or tea tree oil douches.
- Avoid or decrease saturated fats, sugar, yeast and processed foods in diet.

**Homeopathic remedies** for vaginal discharge may include: Calcarea carbonica 3x, kali carbonicum 3x, thuja occidentalis 3x, cocculus indicus, eupion 3x, pulsatilla 6x, and sepia 6x.

# Cystitis (Bladder Infection) and Urinary Tract Infections

Cystitis can affect both men and women. If the infection is in the bladder it is called *cystitis*, in the urethra is *urethritis* and in the kidney *pyelonephritis*. It is estimated that 85 per cent of urinary tract infections (UTIs) are caused by a bacteria escherichia coli (E-coli). Chlamydia can also cause bladder problems. If males contract bladder infection it is considered to be a more serious problem, and cause prostatitis.

Characteristic to bladder infections is the increased urgency or desire the empty the bladder (urinate). The urine may often appear cloudy in colour, have a strong, unpleasant odour and may also contain blood. Women are more common to contract an ascending infection due to the shortness of the urethra in comparison to males.

### *Natural treatments for cystitis and UTIs:*
- Herbs such as: Birch leaf – a natural diuretic and reduces pain associated with bladder infection. Others may include: Dandelion leaf; hydrangea; buchu - good for getting rid of both acid- and alkaline-dependent micro-organisms; Bilberry; corn silk; uva ursi (bearberry); marshmallow root; and goldenseal.
- TCM herbal formula: Wu Ling San (Hoelen Five formula).
- Cranberry and blueberry juice prevent microbes from adhering to the bladder lining.
- D-Mannose is one of the more effective natural treatments of UTIs particularly when caused by E.coli. This naturally occurring simple sugar (not cane sugar) works by sticking to the E.coli bacteria present on the surface of the cells of the bladder lining. D-mannose is both a preventative and a treatment for E.coli UTIs.
- Aloe vera juice contains mannose that also prevents bacterial adhesion to mucous membranes and reduces symptoms.
- Drink plenty of water daily, especially during an acute attack to help flush out the infection. Try to consume 3 litres daily.
- Try to consume more alkalising foods in diet.
- Increase foods such as garlic, celery, and parsley in the diet.
- Avoid citrus fruits such as oranges; alcohol; caffeine; carbonated drinks; and refined processed food.
- Remember to keep the genital and anal areas hygienically clean and dry. Wear natural fibre underclothing.
- Increase your consumption of acidophilus probiotics and/or use also as a douche locally.
- If a women is suffering an infection then use sanitary pads rather than tampons that may contain the infection.

# Tubal Obstruction

A very common cause of female infertility is the blocked or partially obstructed fallopian tubes.

Blockages of the fallopian tubes can be caused by appendicitis, endometriosis, peritonitis, (inflammation of the membrane of the abdominal cavity), and Pelvic Inflammatory Diseases (PID). The tubes may also be blocked due excessive mucous production.

Scar tissue and adhesion can also be a result if left untreated and can obstruct embryo implantation. Scar tissue and adhesions are usually a consequence of previous pelvic infections; ectopic pregnancies – when a pregnancy occurs in the fallopian tubes – are at a much greater risk due to this condition and are potentially very dangerous, if not life threatening, if not detected early as the tube can rupture – the pregnancy is unlikely to be viable in this case.

If the tubes remain blocked, the ovum when released can be obstructed as it tries to travel through the tube to reach the sperm and vice versa.

Medically, this blockage may be diagnosed via a dye flush through the tubes during a laparoscopy procedure or a *hysterosalpingogram*. Blockages can also affect the tubes' patience, i.e. the tubes may begin to pulsate in an inappropriate spasmodic manner. The cilia that line the inside of the tubes work by washing the sperm and egg together. Their function can also be affected or they may be even damaged because of the condition. Chronic stress is also commonly linked to tubal obstruction.

## *Natural Treatments for Tubal Obstructions*
- Blockages can usually be treated successfully with a combination of strict dietary regimens, nutritional support including plenty of Vitamin C; Vitamin A; Vitamin E; bioflavonoid; magnesium; silica; selenium; potassium chloride (PC); proline; lysine; and other antioxidants.
- Herbal remedies such as: calendula; clivers; golden seal; golden rod; horse chestnut; horsetail; horseradish; garlic; and fenugreek may be used to remove congestion.
- In TCM, Chinese herbs such as: platycodon (Jie Geng), tribulus (Bai Ji Li) and astragalus (Huang Qi) may also have application for tubal obstruction.
- Vigorous hydrotherapy e.g. swimming, and hot and cold sitz baths are effective in removing internal inflammation and congestion.
- If the tubes remain blocked after all other treatment options have been considered then conception may be possible in this case only through medically assisted technology that can bypass this blockage such as in IVF.
- Micro surgery to clear the blockage has also shown to be quite successful.

**Tubal Ligation**

Tubal ligation is a female surgical sterilisation procedure involving having the fallopian tubes tied. A tubal reversal or *tubal reanastomosis* involves a microsurgical procedure to undo the blockage. Many factors may need to be considered before undergoing this reversal procedure.

- Tubal reanastomosis is a very expensive procedure
- If the woman is over 40, IVF through egg retrieval may be recommended
- Does the partner have any sperm problems? If so IVF or ICSI may also be a better option
- Tubal reversals also have increased risks of scar tissue forming, infection and ectopic pregnancies occurring.
- Success may depend on what method of tubal blockage was performed. These may include: clamping with clips or ring reversal is much more successful. Cauterisation or have large sections of the tube removed the success rate if much lower. If the surgeon feels that there is sufficient tube remaining and the fimbriated end of the tube (where the end enters from the ovary) is functioning correctly then the success rate of reversal is similar to that of IVF procedures.

# Uterine Myoma – Fibroids and Endometrial Polyps

Uterine fibroids (also called *leiomyomas* or *myomas*) are benign (non-cancerous) growths (tumours) that can form on the interior muscular wall (the *myometrium*) as well as the exterior of the uterus. Fibroids are abnormal muscle cells and depending on their position within the uterus determines what they are called: submucosal (protrudes into the cavity of the uterus), intramural (within the uterus), or subserous (forms outside the uterus, subserous fibroids are usually small and don't normally interfere with fertility).

There may be more than one fibroid present, and are usually detected during a medical pelvic examination. Myomas that are attached via a stalk in the uterus are referred to as *pedunculated*.

Approximately 20 to 30 per cent of all women are estimated to develop fibroids predominantly during their late thirties and early forties, and then shrink (atrophy) after menopause. One of the possible culprits to their formation is suggested to be caused by excessive oestrogen during this stage; there also appears to be some link to a genetic predisposition for fibroids to develop as well. Many women with fibroids have been found to have elevated levels of human growth hormone. During pregnancy fibroids are also known to potentially increase in size.

About half the women who have fibroid tumours are free of symptoms. Others may have abnormally heavy or frequent menstrual periods.

Some of the associated signs and symptoms include: anaemia (due to heavy bleeding); fatigue; weakness; bloating; cramping; increased vaginal discharge; clotting; pain and/or bleeding with intercourse; and break-through bleeding at times other than during the period.

Fibroids can potentially affect the progression of sperm entering, or movement through the uterus.

If an ovum is fertilised, having fibroids may also hinder correct implantation to the uterine lining. When fibroids grow larger than 6 to 7 centimetres in size this may cause a diversion in blood flow and potentially cause hormonal changes. If an embryo happens to implant onto the uterine lining, the changes that may be caused by the fibroid can potential hinder the proper formation and attachment of the placenta, and restrict adequate blood, oxygen and nutrient supply to the uterus, thus affecting the viability of the forming embryo. Many women that I have spoken with who have had troubles conceiving say that they suffer from *poor circulation*, cool hands and feet. An extremely large number of these women were also diagnosed with fibroids and/or endometriosis; possibly a significant link?

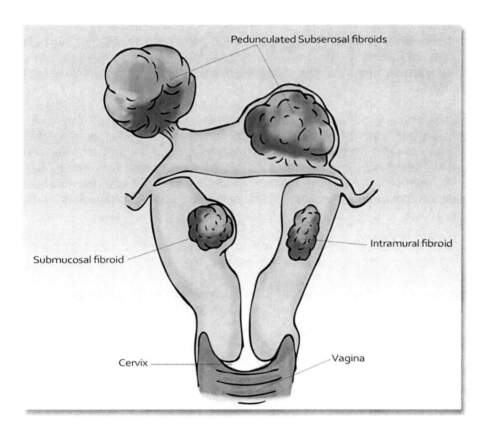

**Figure.17. Various types of fibroids**

279

## Medical Treatments for Fibroids

One of the first medical lines of treatment may involve the recommendation of oral contraceptive pills (OCPs), either combination pills or progesterone-only, in an effort to manage symptoms. OCPs may actually increase fibroid size, but often decreases the menstrual flow and aids relief of pelvic pain. Gonadotropin-releasing hormone analogues (GnRH analogues) may be used for short periods to decrease oestrogen levels to reduce fibroids. Non-steroidal anti-inflammatory agents such as ibuprofen have shown to relieve pelvic pain.

Depending on the actual location of the fibroid/s it can also exert pressure upon the bladder and bowel, cause pain in the legs, back, and pelvis, and is able to also cause a blockage to the urethra contributing to potential kidney obstruction. Extremely large fibroids may require surgical intervention; a large percentage (over 30 per cent of woman in the USA alone) have hysterectomies (surgical removal of the uterus) performed on them due to these growths.

An alternative procedure that may be used for women of child-bearing age is a *myomectomy*. This procedure is a more exact and technically complicated surgery; the recovery time is much greater than with the hysterectomy. But this type of surgery may help to preserve the uterus and give you a chance if you are attempting conception.

With the myomectomy surgical intervention this may not be a total solution to rid the body from fibroids. There is still a 50 per cent chance that fibroids may grow back in future. Other procedures that may be used are: *Laparoscopic myolysis; laparotomy; uterine fibroid embolisation (EM); and hysteroscopic resection.*

The embolisation procedure involves medication to be infused into the blood vessels that feed the fibroid tumour. This causes tiny blood clots or 'embolisms' that starve the fibroids from its nutrient supply. This in turn leads to the tumour eventually disintegrating and dies off. This procedure does appear to cause a high scar-tissue formation. Medical investigations to diagnose the presence of fibroids may include: Ultrasound scan and/or Magnetic Resonance Imaging (MRI).

If you are trying to fall pregnant it would be advisable to discuss this with your specialist prior to undergoing this procedure.

Prescription medications such as *Lucrin* may be used to suppress ovarian function, and decrease some fibroid growths via decreasing oestrogen production.

Other medications that may be used to encourage tumour disintegration or shrinkage include: danzol (Danocrine), leuprolide acetate (also used to treat endometriosis), and LHRH.

Many of these medications also have various side effects, many of which mimic menopausal-like symptoms such as: hot flushing; dry vagina; temporary menstruation stoppage; and possible cholesterol elevation (Danocrine).

**Natural treatments that can be used for fibroids include:**
Mainly used to help controls symptoms as well as shrink small to medium fibroids.

**Herbal Medicines:**
- Vitex agnus castus: to reduce excess oestrogen (main herb used).
- Cheladonium and thuja: are specific remedies to reduce abnormal growths
- Calendular and echinacea: lymphatic herbs and accelerate healing.
- Corydalis: reduces bleed stasis and has pain relieve properties.
- Dong Quai: reduces blood stasis and anti-platelet properties, to be used with anti-haemorrhagic herbs such as shepard's purse, yarrow, horsetail, lady's mantle, cranesbill, beth root, periwinkle and panax noto-ginseng (Tienchi) to stop excessive bleeding (Noto-ginseng should not be used during pregnancy).
- Hydrastis Canadensis (golden seal): restores mucous membranes.
- Poke root (phytolacca decandra): is indicated for firm, hard swellings.
- Raspberry leaf (Rubus idaeus): is a classic uterine tonic, usually for fibroids.
- Black haw (viburnum prunifolium): can be used in combination with other herbs to help restrain excess bleed flow due to fibroids, polyps, and carcinomas.
- Blue cohosh (Caulophyllum) and false unicorn root (Helonias): even though they are more commonly known to be oestrogenic herbs, they are also good uterine tonic and may be considered in treatment protocols.
- Cinnamon: has been used in traditional American Indian medicine for fibroid bleeding.
- Damiana (Turnera diffusa): Reduce size of fibroid
- Dan Shen (Salvia miltirrhiza): used to treat congealed blood; dark, red clots during menses; and pelvic congestion.
- Liver tonic herbs: Dandelion root; St Mary's thistle; scutellaria (Chinese skullcap); and turmeric. Green tea; blue flag; bayberry; violet leaves; red clover; and burdock may also be used.
- TCM herbal formulas: Nei Xiao Luo Li Wan (Fritillaria & Figwort Combination), Gui Zhi Fu Ling Wan (Cinnamon & Hoelen combination).

**Nutrients that can be used for fibroids are:**
- Co enzyme Q 10: as it promote immune function and tissue oxygenation.
- Iron: if excessive bleeding is prevent and/or anaemia is indicated.
- L-Lysine and L-Proline (amino acids): as they are important substances needed for connective tissue repair.

- L-Arginine: is known to retard tumour growth.
- Shiitake and maitake mushroom extracts: Are believed to have a strengthening affect on the body and can inhibit certain tumour growth.
- Vitamin A (with other carotenoids): Promotes tissue repair.
- Vitamin C (with bioflavonoids): Promote tissue healing.
- Vitamin E: is believed to reduce fibroid size.
- Zinc (with copper): are also used in tissue healing and repair.
- Magnesium, pure fish oil, evening primrose oil, potassium chloride, and potassium sulphate are also important nutrients.
- Indole-3-carbinol: Increases the detoxification mechanisms of oestrogen that contribute to fibroid growth.

Other: Bentonite clay: pasted on the pelvis area, during menstrual week.
Increase foods such as fresh vegetables – broccoli, cabbage, cauliflower and other brassicas; include moderate amounts of alfalfa and soy products (e.g. tofu).
Avoid foods that are high in saturated fats such as meat and dairy products. (Many also contain excessive hormones such as oestrogens). Avoid excessive coffee intake and talcum powder use of the perineal area.

Homeopathic remedies: Thlaspi 6C, Phosphorus 6C, Fraxinus 6C, and Silicea 6C.

## Ovarian Cysts

These are swellings in the ovary that are closed epithelial sacs containing fluid or semi-solid substances. Occasionally, the cysts are actually tumours (cancerous) in the ovaries. Symptoms of ovarian tumours usually do not present until tumour is well advanced. Some ladies may experience no symptoms; others may suffer from intermittent pain and swelling particularly during menstruation, intercourse and ovulation.

Thyroid dysfunction has been linked to ovarian cyst disease and if the cyst grows too large it can affect fertility by blocking the egg's ability to transport through the fallopian tube to fertilise with the sperm or even stop ovulation occurring.

Diagnosis of cysts is usually investigated via: pelvic sonogram, magnetic resonance image (MRI) scanner, or a computerised topography scan (CT). If any of these investigations have shown evidence of potential cyst formation, a laparoscopy may be performed to confirm these earlier finding.

*Follicular cysts* are the most common and develop due to overproduction of Luteinising Hormone (LH) to stimulate ovulation or disorders of the hypothalamic-pituitary-ovarian axis.

*Corpus Luteal Cysts* usually come and go with the menstrual cycle (cyclical). Corpus cysts are functional and can secrete hormones. Luteal cysts may interfere with progesterone production and can delay the onset of menstruation, or can cause an alteration in blood loss during the period.

**Endometrial cysts** can grow to the size of footballs with 'normal' menses during growth. Cysts can also be caused by endometriosis when they are filled with blood. The pain may be severe is they bleed, twist or rupture.

Ovarian cystic disease can be associated with thyroid dysfunctions. Diagnosis of these cysts is usually done via medical laparoscopy, palpation or ultrasound.

**Dermoids cysts** are another variety of growth that can contain tissue debris, such as hair, teeth, and eyeballs (Doesn't that sound wonderful!).

**Functional cysts:** are most often benign and may disappear on their own.

**Adenomas cysts:** are usually solid, long-lasting, and are potentially cancerous growths that almost always require to be removed surgically.

**Meigs Syndrome:** (Demons-Meigs syndrome) is a condition the has a fibrous growth within an ovary that causes abnormal levels of sex hormones to be produced, also fluid retention can cause abdominal swelling. This condition requires surgical removal of tumour. Infertility is a complication of the syndrome.

### Cyst problems
Torsion of ovarian cysts can be associated with severe pain. Torsion is when the ovary containing the cyst twists and cuts off its own blood supply, causing death of the ovarian tissue.

When cyst grow too large (over 5 cm), they can rupture at any time causing adhesions and pain. Blood-filled cysts usually associated with endometriosis tend to grow with each period cycle and are prone to rupture even when relatively small. Particularly large cysts can cause damage to ovarian tissue and prevent the ovaries' capacity to ovulate and produce hormones.

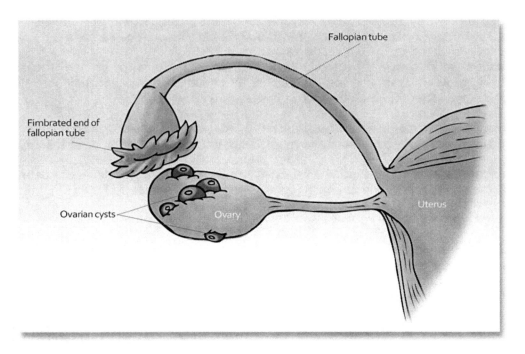

*Illustration of Ovarian Cysts*

**Medical treatments for ovarian cysts** may include being on a contraception pill for a period of time to help shrink or dissolve the cyst.

Prior to commencing treatment malignancy needs to be ruled out before proceeding. An ovarian cystectomy may be required to surgically remove the cyst/s, which is similar but slightly more complex than a laparoscopic procedure.

## Natural treatments for ovarian cysts

**Herbal medicines**: Follicular cysts: Vitex (chaste tree) and caulophyllum thalactroides (blue cohosh) can reduce cyst size and formation.

**TCM Herbal formulas**: Gui Zhi Fu Ling Wan (Cinnamon & Hoelen combination), Zhe Chong Yin (Cinnamon & Persica combination) and Tao Hong Si Wu Tang (Persica, Carthamus and Dang Gui combination).

**Luteal Cysts**: Phyto-oestrogenic herbs such as: False unicorn root (chamaelirium luteum), and peony (paeonia lactiflora) can reduce cyst size and formation.

**Herbs to promote cyst degeneration**: thuja; chelidonium; poke root; red clover; Echinacea; calendula; blue flag; fenugreek; golden seal; and violet leaves.

**For Blood and qi stagnation**: Salvia miltiorrhiza (Dan Shen); corydalis; prickly ash; cayenne; and dong quai.

**Ovarian Pain**: anemone pulsatilla; cramp bark; wild yam; black haw; squaw vine; and ginger.

**Nutrients** such as: Vitamin E; and B complex Vitamins can also be useful.

**Homeopathic remedies**: Apis 6C, Lachesis 6C and Iodum 6C.

# Cystic Mastitis (Benign Breast Lumps, fibrocystic breasts)

Cystic mastitis is a non-cancerous condition that is often associated with premenstrual syndrome (PMS) and ovarian cysts. It is characterised by the presents of cysts, or lumps, in the breast tissue.

This condition also goes by the names fibrocystic changes, chronic cystic mastitis, and mammary dysphasia. This condition is caused by the monthly changes in oestrogen and progesterone and low iodine status – hypothyroidism – is associated with this condition. Excess oestrogen hastens the development of this dysplasia when iodine is inadequate in the diet.

Breast lumps affect more than half of all women of child-bearing age, most commonly between the ages thirty and fifty. Symptoms of this condition may include breast tenderness and lumpiness and are most predominant prior to menstruation.
The increased incidence of breast cysts is also believed to be link to an infrequent in bowel movements (e.g. constipation). Medically, fluid aspiration procedures using a fine needle may be performed to remove fluid from the cysts. Normally, fluid from the breast tissue is collected and transported out of the tissue via the lymphatic system. When the lymphatic system becomes stagnant and congested, the fluid accumulates in the breast tissues and eventually develops fibrous tissue around this area and thickens forming the cyst/s. The breasts often swell near menstruation time and feel full, have increased sensitivity, and may have a dull ache or feel burning as a result of the increase in pressure.

Medically, the drug *Danazol* (Danocrine) has been use to shrink breast cysts, via decreasing oestrogen output, though this drug also has some very unpleasant side effects and should be only used after other measures have been unsuccessful.

**Natural Treatments for Breast Lumps**

*Herbal Medicines*
- Echinacea angustifolia and clivers (Gallium aparine): is mild lymphatic and immune stimulating in action that can reduce infection of the breast.

- Picrorrhiza kurra: for infections.
- Red Clover: Improves lymphatic drainage and contains phyto-oestrogens.
- Poke root (not during pregnancy), blue flag, violet leaves, sage, yarrow, marshmallow leaves, cream or poultice: rubbed into the breast tissue, break down hard glandular swelling and reduces inflammation and soreness.
- Black Cohosh (cimicifuga rasemosa): useful for mastitis with breast pain.
- Kudzu (Pueraria lobata): keeps oestrogen from activating cysts, kudzu is abundant in isoflavones to reduce the production of 'bad' oestrogens.
- Green tea: reduces growth of existing cysts and formation of new cysts.
- Polygonum cuspidatum root (Japanese knotweed): contains the phytoestogen resevertrol, and is a potent chemopreventive agent, reservertrol acts as an SERMs, regulating oestrogen receptor activity amphoterically, exerting a oestrogen balancing/ detoxifying action.
- Flax seed (Linum usitissimum): is the richest food source of ligans, one of the three major classes of phyto-eostrogens. Flaxseed is also beneficial in balancing oestrogen status.
- Rosemary leaf (Rosmarinus officinalis): can assist in modulation of phase 1 cytochrome P450 enzymes which may reduce the production of bad oestrogens.
- Vitex: balances oestrogen and progesterone production; limits testosterone production.
- Soy isoflavone concentration: may benefit by keeping oestrogen from activating cysts.
- Indole-3-carbinol (I3C) or Diindolylmethane (DIM): help to eliminate estrogens from activating cysts. Foods such as cabbage, cauliflower, brussels sprouts and broccoli contain I-3-C. (Not to be used in therapeutic doses during pregnancy)!
- Liver herbs: Dandelion leaf/root, greater chelidine, and St Mary's thistle.
- St John's Wort ointment and steamed cabbage leaves over the breast area.

**Other herbs** may include: Dong quai; kelp (high iodine content); golden seal; mullein; pau d'arco; peonia; red clover; squaw vine; wild yam; ginger; turmeric; celery seed; dandelion root and leaves; and parsley.

**TCM herbal formulas**: Jai Wei Xiao Yao San (Bupleurum and Peony formula) and cinnamon and hoelen combination (Gui Zhi Fu Ling Tang).

### Nutrition:

Increase intake of vegetable and fruit juices such as celery and cranberry. Eat more raw foods including nuts, seeds, grains, and iodine-containing foods. Make sure that your diet contains adequate soluble fibre, avoid getting constipation.

Food contain germanium can help to improve tissue oxygenation such as garlic, shiitake mushrooms, and onions. Oily cold-water fish may help to regulate prostaglandins.

Decrease saturated fats, chocolate, sugar, alcohol, refined foods. Reduce intake of tea, coffee, and caffeinated drinks as they contain 'methyl xanthines' which can promote fluid retention and abnormal cellular growth.

Exposure to cigarette smoke has also been linked to this condition.

Lugol's iodine solution can be acquired from the chemist or drug store. This solution is painted on the vaginal area and is said to reduce most minor breast lumps in many cases within several days of use.

Other beneficial nutrients may include: Vitamin A; Vitamin E; B complex vitamins especially Vitamin B6; evening primrose oil (EPO); and carotenoids such as beta-carotene; Vitamin C with bioflavonoids; Vitamin D3; zinc; tyrosine; co-enzyme Q 10; indole-3-carbinol (I3C), diindolylmethane (DIM); Iodine; selenium; and bromelain. Comfrey cream (only used externally), Vitamin E cream, lemon juice compress, and bentonite clay: rubbed into or applied to the breast tissue can help to sooth discomfort and break up hard tissue swelling.

# Endometriosis

### 'Not going with the flow'
The endometrium is the inner layer of the wall of the womb (uterus), which changes in structure and thickness during the menstrual cycle. These changes allow the wall to become receptive to the fertilised egg (ovum) for a very brief time. If an egg is not fertilised or implanted into the endometrium, the result is the monthly bleeding, or period.

Endometriosis is a condition in which the uterine lining (endometrium) breaks (sloughs) off and enters the abdominal cavity, where it grows in an abnormal situation, such as attached to the ovaries, fallopian tubes, or behind the uterus itself (endometrial tissue can potentially end up in any location in the body). Blood-filled cysts may form on the ovaries.

Since this migration is part of the endometrium, it builds up each month and then bleeds as usual (like normal inner uterine endometrial tissue), although the blood is unable to leave the body with the menstrual flow.

This condition usually causes pain, which may worsen before, during, or after menstruation. It may not be the bleeding which causes the pain, but a chemical reaction in the endometrial 'implants' that irritate the lining of the pelvis. There may also be lower backache, pain on intercourse, or, sometimes, no symptoms at all. In severe cases, the scarring, distortion of tissue, of formation of adhesions where the endometrium has attached (possibly to the intestines or other organs) can cause infertility.

287

Endometriosis can also lead to infertility in less severe cases, where the reasons are not so obvious, through these may be to do with an effect on the sperm.

Endometriosis affects 10–20 per cent of all women during their reproductive life, with a peak incidence at 25–35 years. The traditional diagnostic profile of endometriosis is secondary dysmenorrhoea (painful periods) usually worse on day 2 or 3 of menstrual cycle, 30%); dyspareunia (30%) painful intercourse; pain on defecation and/or urination; bleeding from rectum and/or urinary tract (from endometrial tissue); infertility (50% of infertile women will have some degree of endometriosis); fixed retroverted uterus; and tender nodules in the pouch of Douglas/retro-vaginal septum. Non-specific pelvic pain occurs in about 15 per cent of patients.

Menorrhagia with possible ovarian dysfunction is found in 15 per cent and Polycystic Ovarian Syndrome in 35 per cent of ladies with endometriosis. Some women may be asymptomatic but the condition can still progress.

Altogether, 40 per cent of women suffering from this condition will have fertility problems, and 30 per cent of female infertility is due to it.

Endometriosis is believed to be the current number 1# (one) gynaecological cause of female infertility. The cause of this condition is not totally clear, though several factors that may be involved including:

Hormonal imbalance (overproduction and/or poor clearance of oestrogen); genetic factors - endometriosis does run in families; menstrual tissue flowing back (retrograde) into the fallopian tube (several suspect causes of this could be from the use of IUD devices, insertable tampons, cervical narrowing, and the contraceptive pill); poor circulation/lymphatic drainage; links between candidas (vaginal thrush); overuse of antibiotics; allergies; inflammation (imbalance of 'bad' prostaglandins); and other immunological dysfunctions (increased macrophage, lymphokine activity; decreased T-and natural killer (NK)-cell responsiveness) are all contributing factors. Ironically, pregnancy may even alleviate symptoms and delay recurrence; endometriosis typically stops altogether after menopause.

Despite disagreement over the cause of endometriosis, more is known today about this condition than ever before. Research has shown that exposure to environmental polychlorinated biphenyls (PCBs) and dioxin, types of hazardous waste material, can spontaneously cause endometriosis. This may contribute to the rise in this condition in recent years.

Endometriosis may also have an auto-immune component to the condition, immune macrophages normally should clean up this endometrial tissue; endometrial lesion implants can become self-fuelling by abnormally biosynthesising its own oestrogen supply. Defective immune responses cause inflammation that prevents the endometrial tissue from being currently dealt with.

Women who have also developed this condition appear to have a greater history of more vaginal yeast infection, hay fever, eczema, and food sensitivities. It is estimated that 5 to 7 million American and Canadian women alone, at any given time, suffer from endometriosis.

Normally, the most dominant hormone during the first half of the menses cycle is oestrogen with progesterone the dominant hormone in the latter part of the cycle. Therefore, women with short cycle length have increased exposure to higher circulating oestrogen levels to the protective progesterone.

Dysmenorrhoea leads to greater uterine contractability and could predispose to greater tubal reflux of menses and hence endometriosis Researchers have shown that earlier onset menstruation, obesity, being tall in height, poor cell-mediated immunity and ovulation dysfunction are all associated with an increased incidence of this disease.

Women with endometriosis generally don't have higher-than-normal circulating oestrogen sensitivity. Another factor with endometriosis is that women living in countries with a higher incidence of this condition are observed to have excessive saturated fat intake in comparison to the ratio of Essential Fatty Acids (EFAs).

This imbalance may increase target organ receptors to have a greater affinity to steroidal molecules such as oestrogen. Hypothyroidism may also increase oestrogen receptor density.

The presence of endometrial tissue and other matter such as damaged blood cells within the peritoneal cavity will signal an activated inflammatory response by the body's immune modulator cells. The cells involved may include mononuclear phagocytes, macrophages that will generate oxidant stress that will give rise to the formation of lipid peroxides and the generation of growth factors and cytokines will contribute to the symptoms of endometriosis. The pain is associated with an imbalance of prostaglandins.

In Chinese medicine endometriosis is classified as a stagnant blood condition, which can be caused by poor diet and consuming excessive, cold and greasy foods, and inactivity. The adhesions that can form from endometriosis can potentially restrict release of the oocyte and can block the lumen of the fallopian tube increasing the possibility of ectopic pregnancy.

The imbalance of prostaglandins in the peritoneal fluid may prevent ovulation by contributing to luteal phase defects, causing failure of correct follicle rupture and disturb the ovum transport through the fallopian tubes. The rate of spontaneous miscarriage is increased in endometriosis, which may be due to the elevation of inflammatory 'bad' prostaglandins, and/or cell-mediated immune dysregulation that may be having an inappropriate response to the embryo.

The endometriosis that is associated with infertility is located very superficially in the peritoneal cavity, just on the peritoneal surface, the serosa. This is different to the endometriosis that causes pain, which is more likely to be several millimetres deep, growing into the underlying tissue. Superficial endometriosis has glands that secrete mucus, just like the endometrium in the uterus secretes mucus in the second half of the menstrual cycle. This mucus, if it were to specially adhere to the fimbrial ends of the tubes (responsible for attracting the mucus surrounding eggs called the cumulus), could stop the egg from entering the tube, with the egg more likely either to remain within the follicle or to float into oblivion in the inner abyss of the abdomen.

The presence of endometrial overproduction in the uterus, particularly in the presence of any degree of endometrial hyperplasia, is harmful to implantation, and can complicate some ovulation disorders, especially PCOD, in which oestrogen is over-produced. The endometrium must be fully got rid of before starting a medically assisted conception cycle such as IVF, either with a full two weeks' course of progesterone to bring on proper menstruation or with a curettage (D&C).

Medically, endometriosis is diagnosed by laparoscopy (keyhole telescope inserted into the abdominal cavity near the navel area as the entry point), and treated with drugs which suppress ovulation and possible menstruation (not what you really want if trying to fall pregnant!), or with laser surgery, where de-bulking of the unwanted endometrial tissue mass is removed. Though, the benefits of this procedure may only be temporary, as the 'underlying cause' of the problem has not been fully addressed.

Many women find that the endometriosis is already forming back within a few months after the surgery; many also experience additional problems of further scar tissue and adhesion developing after these procedures. This may suggest that if conception has not been reached in the early stages of this condition, before multiple procedures are performed, then conception percentages may decrease with each intervention. Some of the medical drugs used are based on male hormones, and can increase male characteristics in females.

New diagnostic tests are currently under development to detect endometriosis reducing the need for the current invasive procedures like laparoscopy. A 'protein finger print' procedure similar to the Pap smear may be available in the near future.

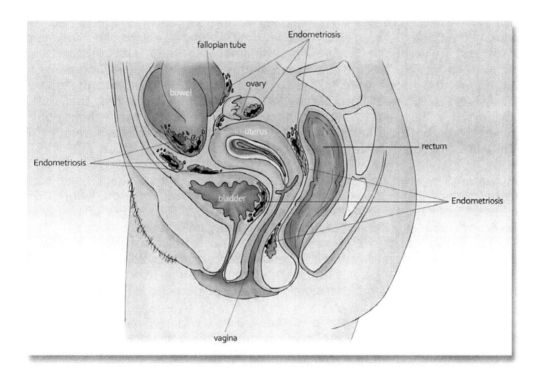

*Illustration of Endometriosis*

## Endometriosis can be categorised into four stages:

**Stage one**: only small patches of endometrial lesions are found on the surface of the peritoneum (the membrane that encases the pelvis), with no resulting scar tissue formation.

**Stage two:** The endometrial lesion can be found in various locations such as the fallopian tubes; ovaries and peritoneum, there may or may not be associated inflammation.

**Stage three**: There is more dispersion of the endometrial lesions throughout the pelvic area. Adhesions and/or scar tissue may also be formed around the reproductive organs and intestines, with chocolate cysts covering the ovaries.

**Stage four:** advanced amounts of lesions are formed over both ovaries, scar tissue is thickened, and spreads to other areas including the all pelvic structures, bladder, and the fallopian tubes may be partially or totally blocked.

### How to treat endometriosis
Many women consult natural therapists for infertility associated with endometriosis. Often they have been treated by gynaecologists and may have

tried IVF without success. This is usually when many of these ladies seek out natural medicines when the conventional medicine approach has been unsuccessful. All of the underlying problems associated with endometriosis really need to be treated to provide the most stable environment for conception to take place. These may include treating: prostaglandin imbalances; luteinised unruptured follicle syndrome – where the follicle develops but the egg is not expelled possible due to lower than normal progesterone causing a luteal phase defect; failed ovarian follicle development; infrequent ovulation; immune dysfunction; and adhesions.

Studies with women with endometriosis wishing to fall pregnant have being treated from 3 to 6 months prior to undergoing IVF procedure with *Gonadotrophin releasing hormone agonists (GnRH)*. The results of this study showed the odds of a clinical pregnancy occurring increased by four fold.

The next generation of treatment for endometriosis is combining *Progestin* with *Aromatase inhibitors (AI);* this method of treatment is directed more at controlling the oestrogen biosynthesis at the endometriotic lesion level.

*Lipiodol Flushing* – flushing the fallopian tubes with an oil-soluble contrast medium Lipiodo in women with mild endometriosis and unexplained infertility has shown to have significant results in increasing pregnancy rates in trials.

Various Natural Therapies have had a long and successful history of helping to alleviate endometriosis problems; some of these therapies may include: Herbal Medicines; Clinical Nutrition; Acupuncture; Massage; Yoga; and Pilates.

Increase aerobic exercise, belly dancing would be very beneficial.

**Natural treatments for Endometriosis:**

***Herbal Medicines:***

- Herbs: Dysmenorrhea – to reduce spasm (pain relief): cramp bark; corydalis; pulsatilla; blue cohosh; wild yam; squaw vine; mother wort; false unicorn root (ovarian pain); dong quai (congestive); black haw; and peonia.

- Decrease blood stasis and clear lymphatics: poke root (use with caution); calendula; dong quai; corydalis; thuja; red clover; and burdock.

- Premenstrual Syndrome (PMS) – hormone balancing (to reduce excessive oestrogen): vitex (chaste tree); sarsaparilla; fenugreek; peony; and tribulus.
- Reduce heavy or prolonged bleeding (Menorrhagia) – shepherd's purse; beth root; lady's mantle; raspberry leaf; cranesbill; golden seal with blue cohosh (combo) may help.

- Anti-allergic – Ephedra (S4 class medication in Australia); albizzia; nettle leaf; and baical skullcap. To assist regulation of prostaglandins: Feverfew in hot conditions and ginger for cold conditions.

- Immune dysregulation – hemidesmus; Echinacea; picorrhiza; astragalus; withania; siberian ginseng; rehmannia; garlic; and noni.

- Anti-inflammatory – ginger; hops (humulus lupulus); turmeric (curcuma longa); liquorice; wild yam; feverfew; rehmannia; white dead nettle; and willow bark.

- Liver herbs – help to detoxify and reduce oestrogens and blood fat levels. St Mary's thistle; dandelion root; greater cheladine; globe artichokes; bupleurum; and schisandra.

- Uterine tonics – True unicorn root; blue cohosh; dong quai.

- Nervines- (support nervous system) valerian; chamomile; verbena; and also spasmolytic herbs.

TCM herbal formulas: Gui Zhi Fu Ling Wan (Cinnamon & Hoelen combination), Dang Gui Shao Yao San (Dang Gui & Peony formula), used with pattern of Qi and blood stagnation.

Jia Wei Xiao Yao San (Bupleurum & Peonia Formula) and Cinnamon Twig and Poria decoction (Gui Zhi Fu Ling Wan) are also beneficial formulas used for treating endometriosis.

Other TCM herbs used for endometriosis may include: Dan shen (Salvia); Chi Shao (Red peony root); Tao Ren (Persica seed); Hong Hua (Safflower); and San Leug (Bur-reed rhizome).

***Homeopathic remedies*** may include: lachesis; graphites; nux vomica; oophorinum; pulsatilla; sepia; and sulphur.

***Nutritional:***

- *Essential fatty acids* (omega 3+6) plus cold-pressed oils such as evening primrose and fish oils can help to reduce the bad series of prostaglandins. Linseed, safflower, sunflower and grape seed prevents platelet aggregation, removes blood stasis, vasodilator improves circulation, anti-inflammatory, reduces abnormal cell proliferation, activates T (immune) cells, reduces cholesterol, enhances insulin and stimulates brown (good) fat metabolism. Dosages of 3000mg or 3 grams daily are recommended.
- Increase dietary intake of fresh fruit and vegetables and reduce animal meats as they contribute to 'bad' prostaglandin production.

- Fish is beneficial. Reduce consumption of dairy food (e.g. cow's milk and cheese) as it is acid and mucus forming and blocks lymph drainage.

### *Other nutrients to consider:*

- Zinc (20-60mg daily)
- Vitamin A (10,000 IU or 6mg Beta-carotene daily)
- Vitamin E (1,000 up to 2,000 IU daily): is one of the most important nutrients used for endometriosis, improving fertility and reducing adhesions.
- Vitamin C (to bowel tolerance 1,000mg-6, 000mg)
- Bioflavonoid (Quercetin, Rutin and Hesperidin)
- Celloids/cell salts: sodium phosphate; sodium sulphate (for liver detoxification); potassium chloride (lymph drainage and endocrine health congestion remover); magnesium phosphate (for nervous system, reduces pain and spasm); iron phosphate (reduces inflammation and replenish iron loss from heavy bleeding).
- Indole-3-carbinol (I 3 C) and/or Diindolylmethane (DIM): to clear excessive oestrogen load
- Iodine
- Increase soy-based foods.
- Reduce saturated fats and incorporate high-soluble fibre intake in the diet.
- Irritable bowel syndrome is also commonly associated with endometriosis. Improving bowel function may also reduce endometriosis symptoms: Include foods such as bitter green vegetables, and additional nutrients such as magnesium, calcium and essential fatty acids.
- Reduce consumption of alcohol and caffeine.
- If tampons are to be used only select ones that are made from guaranteed natural *'pure cotton'*; some bleaching agents still used today contain a known cancer-causing chemical called *'Dioxin'* that is toxic to the reproductive system. When a tampon is removed fibres can remain behind that can cause disruption of the endocrine and immune systems. Dioxin is also linked to lowering male sperm counts and toxic shock syndrome. Another nasty that can be found in some tampons is asbestos; this dangerous substance is also well known to cause many health-threatening problems. It is absorbed through the mucosa in the vagina, and ironically can increase bleeding. Ergo more bleeding = more tampons sold = more $!

### *Medicinal Treatments for Endometriosis:*

### *Danazol (synthetic 3-isoxazole derivative of 17-ethinyl-testosterone):*
Works basically by blocking FSH from the pituitary gland and so preventing a menstrual cycle from occurring. In a sense it is like creating an artificial state of pregnancy. The idea is that after months of FSH suppression the endometriosis should dry up. When Danazol (or gestrinone) is stopped the pituitary rebounds by pouring out abundant FSH, and if treating for infertility a

pregnancy has a better chance of occurring. Danazol has in recent times been the hormone suppressant of choice to use in endometriosis. Danazol has shown to reduce the size and extent of the endometrial lesions with 80-90 per cent symptom relief and 20-35 per cent recurrence rate after treatment cessation.

Danazol is unsafe for the developing foetus; common side effects synonymous with menopause.

The individual response to treatment with Danazol may vary dependent upon dosage. Even though the medication may assist in clearing the endometriosis, conceptual problems still appear to remain for many women. The prescription medical drug Danocrine is often used in conditions such as:

*Endometriosis* and *Menorrhagia*: – abnormally heavy bleeding during menstruation.

*Hereditary Angioedema* – an inherited condition associated with repeated episodes of abdominal pain and swelling of the throat.

*Severe Fibrocystic Breast disease* – lumps in the breast, which are very painful.

The active ingredient of Danocrine is Danazol. Danazol has been associated with a variety of side effects such as:

1    Allergic reactions, including asthma attacks, skin rashes, and hay fever symptoms.
2    Masculinising effect on the female foetus if taken in the early months of pregnancy.
3    Excessive intake can cause nausea, indigestion and fluid retention.
4    Vomiting; constipation; moderate weight gain; acne; oily skin; muscle cramps or tremors; joint pain; mood changes; hot flushes; skin rash; itching; blood in urine; headaches; weakness; irritability; dizziness; depression; and sleep disorders.
5    Menstrual disorders in the form of spotting, alteration of the timing of the cycle and cessation of menstruation.
6    Vaginal dryness and irritation.
7    Changes in breast size.
8    Abnormalities in semen volumes, viscosity, sperm count and motility may occur in males receiving long-term therapy.

Other serious side effects may include excessive facial hair growth; jaundice (yellow skin); visual disturbances; voice deepening or hoarseness; chest pain; pain or redness in any portion of the leg; and difficulty breathing.

Danazol is a medical hormonal treatment, which shrinks the abnormal endometrial tissue by suppressing the hormones that cause the endometrial tissue to grow and thicken each month. Danazol must NOT be taken during pregnancy or breast-feeding and there are also many health conditions and drug medications that Danazol should not be used with.

Consult with your doctor and/or pharmacist to have the safety aspects of using such medications thoroughly explained to you.

### Buserilin/Goserlin
Gonadotrophin-releasing hormone medications (also known as LHRH analogues). These medications are also used to suppress menstruation and help to shrink down fibroids. These drugs are not taken orally as they destroyed within the stomach.

Buserlin is taken via a nasal spray and Goserlin by syringe. These drugs work by 'down regulating' or 'switching off' the pituitary production of LH and FSH. LHRH analogue drugs appear to have fewer side effects in comparison to Danazol but mild hot flushes and vaginal dryness are known symptoms.

### Gestrinone and Medroxyprogesterone
Are capsulated forms of progesterone hormone that is also used in the treatment of endometriosis.

### Endometrial atrophy

Endometrial atrophy or the diminishment of the endometrium can be caused by a lack of oestrogen, such as occurs in Turner syndrome (but not endometrial atrophy caused by tissue destruction). It is usually readily and quickly overcome in the two weeks it takes to administer a course of oestrogen. These conditions can be confirmed via a premenstrual endometrial biopsy (PED). There is no good evidence to suggest that the endometrium needs to be any particular thickness for implantation to occur. Pregnancies have been maintained even with endometrial lining measurements of 4-5mm.


## Polycystic Ovary Syndrome (PCOS)

### The hormone domino effect – 'ovaries with acne'
Polycystic Ovarian Syndrome (PCOS) (Also called *Stein-leventhal Syndrome*) is estimated to affect approximately 6-10 per cent of women of reproductive age, making it one of, if not the most common hormonal (endocrine) disorder among women in this age group. Researchers agree that PCOS is responsible for the majority (perhaps 90 per cent) of adult female acne and is a culprit in excessive facial/body hair (Hirsutism), scalp hair loss and obesity. It may also account for as many as 50 per cent of all female hormone-linked cases of infertility.

Despite these astounding figures, most women who have PCOS are completely unaware they have this condition. Although PCOS was first recognised in 1930, it is only in the past 10 years that there has been research into its cause and only in the past 2 to 3 years that practitioners have started to become aware of this research and so are starting to recognise the syndrome in their patients.

In this condition, there are multiple follicular cysts on the ovaries, which may show as enlarged and have a peripheral 'necklace' pattern of relatively uniformly sized, small follicles when diagnosed via ultrasound or during laparoscopy. Multiple follicles start to grow, and, in the more severe conditions, none ripen sufficiently to release an egg. There is often, therefore, irregularity or an inability to ovulate. This can be confirmed through temperature readings or blood tests to show progesterone levels. Thirty-five per cent of female infertility, and 40 per cent of amenorrhoea (absence of menses), may be due to PCOS.

PCOS is the most common disorder that affects ovulation! The adrenal glands that are situated on top of the kidneys may slightly over-produce the male hormones such as testosterone, which are later converted in the body fat, to oestrogen. This in turn leads to a disturbance in the normal production of FSH and LH. LH may be excessively released in comparison to FSH, this can stimulate the ovaries to become packed full of these many tiny cysts.

The levels of LH to FSH can be greater than 2.5:1 ratio. The pituitary hormone Prolactin may also be over-produced, which may be evident by a milky secretion from around the nipples of the breasts. Very occasionally, PCOD may cause the ovaries to 'run out of viable eggs' much earlier than normal, thus, leading to a state of Ovarian Failure or Premature Menopause.

**Symptoms of PCOS**

About 50 to 75 per cent of women with PCOS do experience symptoms and not all are seen in every woman.
- Excessive, dark, coarse hair growth on the face, chest, abdomen, etc.
- Scalp hair loss (in classic 'male baldness' pattern)
- Acne (may be severe in adolescence and may last into adulthood).
- Skin tags (acrochordons) – teardrop-sized pieces of skin (typically in the armpits or neck area).
- Darkening and thickening of the skin, mainly on the neck, groin, and underarms or in skin folds.
- Obesity - apple shape (often sudden and unexpected weight gain), difficulty losing weight.
- Irregular or infrequent periods (less than eight per year), no periods, or frequent heavy periods.
- Infertility and recurrent miscarriages.
- Chronic fatigue.
- Depression.

*Polycystic Ovaries* - It is important to note that polycystic ovaries are not present in all women diagnosed with PCOS. Also many women with regular menstrual periods and normal testosterone levels may have multiple ovarian cysts. An interesting observation has been made by researchers in Australia; They discovered that most women they examined with PCOS had a shorter 2nd finger on their hand compared with their 4th finger length. This pattern is mostly observed in males; hence the researchers suggest that these women may have been exposed to too much male hormone in the womb.

It is not known what the full cause of PCOS is, but it has been suggested that the problem stems from the ovaries, which are unable to produce the hormones in the correct proportions. It develops when the ovaries overproduce androgens (male hormones e.g. testosterone), upsetting the normal hormone messages to the pituitary gland in the brain.

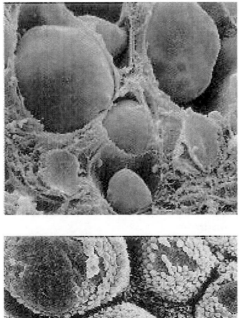
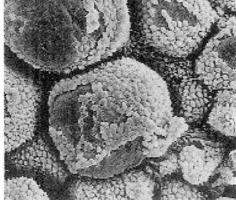

*Figure.18. PCOS – Ultrasound microscopy view*

It is estimated that 1 in 70 women with PCOS have a definite abnormality in the steroid hormone production of the adrenal gland that leaks excessive male sex hormone called adult-onset congenital adrenal hyperplasia (CAH). The hormones that may be excessive are serum testosterone, and the precursor serum 17-hydroxyprogesterone.

In the normal ovary, one dominant follicle matures and releases as an egg (ovum) every month, but in a polycystic ovary, there are only immature follicles that either don't produce eggs at all, or, if they do, may only do so inefficiently. The follicles that fail to completely release an egg then develop into cysts on the ovaries, hence the name.

Many women with PCOS have been found to have a condition known as Insulin Resistance, in which the cells 'resist' the effects of insulin, so the body has to produce more insulin to compensate. It seems that these high levels of insulin then affect the ovaries, stimulating them to produce abnormal proportions of hormones, particularly testosterone, which causes the hair abnormalities and acne. High insulin levels also lead to altered fat and cholesterol usage in the body, which can ultimately cause obesity and high blood cholesterol problems. Elevated insulin levels contribute to or cause the abnormalities seen in the hypothalamic-pituitary-ovarian axis that lead to PCOS. Specifically, hyper-insulinaemia causes a number of endocrinological changes associated with PCOS. These changes may include: Increased GnRH pulse frequency; LH over FSH dominance; decreased follicular maturation; decreased sex human binding globulin (SHBG) binding; and increased ovarian androgen (male hormone) production.

The 'cysts' in polycystic ovaries are not harmful, do not require surgical removal and should not lead to ovarian cancer (?). However, the hormonal imbalance in women with PCOS can make them more susceptible to certain health problems in later life.

These may include:
* *Type - II Diabetes* (particularly from Insulin Resistance),
* *Cardiovascular Disease* - with blood fat abnormalities such as elevated cholesterol and triglyceride levels in the blood.
* *Endometrial Cancer* - the lining of the uterus (endometrium) may thicken with abnormal cells - a precancerous condition, if periods very infrequent (less than every three months at least).

### Microscopic examination of PCOS has shown various pathologies:

1   Enlargement to the whole ovary
2   Thickened capsule
3   Increased number of small cysts under the capsule
4   Absence of follicles that have ovulated or are in the process of maturing
5   Thickening and increased fibrosis of the inner surface of the ovary.
6   Decreased thickness of the lining of each cyst.

There may be situations that may require surgical intervention in abnormal polycystic ovary disorders, these procedures include:

* Ovarian wedge resection;
* Laparoscopic ovarian drilling.

## Possible Signs and Symptoms of PCOS

1   Excess ratio luteinising hormone (LH) to follicle stimulating hormone (FSH)
2   Increased levels of male hormones androstenedione and testosterone.
3   Elevated body mass index (BMI).

Thirty to fifty per cent of women with PCOD are calculated as overweight. The fat is also distributed in a way that more is deposited around the waist (central obesity or apple shape) waist: hip ratio. Studies of women with PCOS and suffer from increased body fat levels (BMI) have shown that even 5-10 per cent loss of body weight can help to restore a regular cycle and lead to ovulation.

### *Body Mass Index (BMI)*
BMI= weight (kg)
Height x height (m2)
Underweight=21, normal=21-26, overweight=27 and greater.

***Insulin Resistant*** – is an abnormality of carbohydrate metabolism which increases the requirement of the secretion of insulin from the pancreas in order to metabolise blood sugars. Glucose tolerance tests (GTT) should be done to measure basal, (fasting) blood sugar, and insulin and glucose levels. Imbalances of inflammatory factors in the body is associated with insulin resistance, some of the mediators include *C-reactive protein (CRP)* and peptide *Adiponectin*. By balancing inflammation reactions in the body will in turn improve insulin utilisation.

It is estimated that 20 to 40 percent of women with PCOS have impaired insulin function; this is approximately seven times higher than women without PCOS.

Medical drugs to counter insulin resistance are Metformin, Glucophage and Glitazones, ACTOSO, Rosiglitazone (AvandiaO), and Rezulin (Troglitazone). Approximately 30 per cent of patients started on Glucophage will experience gastrointestinal nausea, vomiting, abdominal bloating, flatulence, and appetite loss. Generally, these symptoms greatly reduce or decease after several weeks of continued therapy.

The 'Glycemic index' of food is a reflection of how much that food raises your blood sugar. Simple carbohydrates usually have a higher glycemia index than complex carbohydrates. High glycemic foods demand a vigorous insulin response from the pancreas. Choose foods from a low-glycemic index group.
High insulin levels inhibit growth hormone (GH) production from the pituatury gland; this promotes increased fat storage / and affects control of blood cholesterol levels. Elevated insulin also accelerates celluar turnover (speeds up

300

ageing) and stimulates the release of cortisol from the adrenal glands, competing with DHEA. This in turn, affects sex hormone conversion leading to impaired fertility.

**Leptin -** is a hormone secreted by adipocytes that regulate body weight via an effect on metabolism. Leptin may play a possible role in triggering puberty by initiating LH release once body fat levels are adequate to cope with the physiological demands of adolescence.

Leptin has a role in regulation of the follicular development indirectly by control of LH and FSH secretion. This may have an important action of assisting follicular maturation and ovum development therefore affecting fertility and pregnancy. Women with increased weight gain may also show increased leptin levels and leptin resistance (poor utilisation of the hormone) that adversely affects gonadotropin release causing elevated LH levels common with PCOS, therefore contributing possible directly or indirectly to obesity and infertility. Studies have shown that supplementing the trace mineral zinc has been shown to help boost leptin regulation.

**Ghrelin –** is a hormone that is involved with appetite regulation. Studies have found that women with PCOS have 70 per cent increased levels of ghrelin in comparison to women without PCOS. Therefore, appetite regulation may benefit women with PCOS obesity.

**Obesity** – the typical obesity of PCOS is described as 'centripetal', related to fat distribution in the centre of the body, as opposed to the thighs and hips. The, 'apple' opposed to 'pear' type of fat distribution clearly is associated with greater risk of hypertension, diabetes and lipid abnormalities. With increased numbers of fat cells or *adipocytes* also increases the production of inflammatory factors called *cytokines* (including C-reactive protein, tumour necrosis factor, and interleukin as examples).

Medical drugs used to reduce obesity may include: Orlistat (Xenical) reduces fat absorption, and Sibutramine (Reductil) an appetite suppressant. Even a 5 per cent reduction in body fat has shown to greatly improve IVF success and the ability to achieve conception.

**Diabetes -** type II diabetes (non-insulin dependent diabetes mellitus-NIDDM): Women with PCOS have an increased tendency toward this condition.
Medical drugs for this type of diabetes may include: 'Starch blocker agents' - Precose *(acarbose)*; Glyset *(miglitol)*; *Biguanides*; *Thiazolidinediones-Actos (pioglitazone)*, Avandia (rosiglitazone – though, may contribute to weight gain), whereas Metformin is often associated with weight loss.

**Atherosclerosis** - the condition of increased thickening of the arteries is suggested to be of greater risk of developing in PCOS leading to increased cardiovascular diseases. Raised cholesterol and triglycerides may also be elevated in PCOS sufferers (elevated serum, lipids and fats).

**Increased Male Hormones** - raised LH increases recreation of male androstenedione and subsequently increased circulating testosterone. This is worsened by the effect of raised insulin levels, which causes the liver to decrease its secretion of sex hormone-binding globulin (SHBG) that normally binds to and inactivates testosterone.

**Anti-Androgen Medications**: Testosterone receptor blockers may include: Aldactone *(spironolactone)*; Cyproterone acetate; Tagamet *(cimetidine)*. Testosterone metabolism blockers may include: Propecia *(ministered)*, *and* Dutasteride.

**Increased hair growth – (Hirsutism):** the increase in male hormone activity stimulates the hair follicles to increase growth.

Medical drugs such as (oral diuretic) spironolactone have been used; Cyproterone acetate *(progestogenic anti-androgen)*; Diane 35; Brenda; and Flutamide are anti-androgen medications that have also been used to decrease hair growth and acne. Climen is also a progestogenic anti-androgen used to prevent hirsutism. Cosmetic treatments involve bleaching; shaving; plucking; depilatory cream; electrolysis; laser; and thioglycates. Vaniqa Cream *(eflornithine)* is an anti-hair inhibitor agent.

In the majority of **Potential Genetic Links to PCOS**: The possible candidate genes that have been investigated include those involved with the synthesis of steroid hormone, including CYPIIA (cholesterol side-chain cleavage gene) which alters androgen production; CPY19 (the gene encoding P450 aromatase) and CYP17 (17-hydroxylase-17, 20-lysase gene); insulin receptor gene (VMTR); follistatin gene, involved in gonadotropin action.

All have been considered as genetic causes but to date none have been conclusively proven.

**Androgenic Alopecia** - (progressive, non-scarring scalp hair loss) can be diffused over crown with preservation of the frontal hairline.
Medication may include; anti-androgen drugs; weight loss to decrease circulation to male hormones. Camouflage with hair styling (wigs). Drugs - Minoxidil (Rogaine solution) topical lotion.

**Acanthosis Nigricans** - this is an eruption of skin, with increased keratin, papillomatosis (giving the skin a velvety appearance) and pigmentation. Usually occurs in the armpits, nape of neck and under breasts – associated with insulin resistance.

**Hidradenitis suppurtiva** - is other skin condition seen in PCOS that involved inflammation of the specialised sweat gland in the armpit and groin areas.

*Acne* –chronic inflammation of the sweat ducts of the skin. It usually occurs during the early teenage years and in most people it disappears by the age of 21 though PCOS sufferers it may persist.

Acne can be due to the increased male hormone circulation associated with PCOS, the sebaceous glands at the base of the hair follicles increase their secretions of sebum. As the androgens become more active, further enlargement of the sebaceous glands occurs and even more sebum is produced which promotes the growth of a bacterium called *Propioni-bacterium* acne (P-acnes), which thrives in the sebaceous environment.

The bacterium digests the sebum, making it more viscous, as well as producing inflammatory by-products. In response to this inflammation, there is increased formation of the protein *Keratin*, which plugs up the follicles, resulting in the development of small cysts called comedones, which are the initial lesions of acne.

If these cysts are disrupted, they release inflammatory mediators, which result in the formation of a papule, pustule or cyst.

Acne primarily affects the face, and less often the back and chest. It may present in blackheads (these are non-inflamed lesions with a black colour due to the laying down of the pigment melanin). When closed, these are known as white heads.

The various lesions of acne often change from one type to another. They can result in scarring, which becomes significant in only a minority of people.


**Medical treatments for Acne:**

*Mild Acne*: topical creams to break down keratin may include azelaic acid or retinoids, or antibiotics such as benzoyl peroxide, clindamycin lotion or erythromycin gel. Other agents that alter the growth and/or shedding of skin cells may include: Retin-A; Avita; tretinoin; Tazorac/tazarotene; Differin/ adapelene; or Accutane/isotretinoin. Topical agents such as glycolic acid (fruit acid) skin peel are also useful for removing dead skin and to keep the pores open.

*Severe Acne*: oral antibiotics – may include tetracycline (Minnomycin, Mysteclin, Tetrex, Vibra-Tabs), erythromycin or trimethoprim group.
Anti-androgenic medications: spironolactone and cyprotene acetate> progesterone containing, (triphasic pill), and (Diane35, Schering).

Heavy-duty medications such as Isotretinion *(Roaccutane)* have also been used in the most severe cases of acne. This drug belongs to the retinoid class of compounds, which are derivatives of Vitamin A. Studies have stated that sebum excretion was decreased by 80 per cent with this medication.

Consequently, the P-acne also decreased over a 4-8 period of use, as did inflammation and comedogensis production.

Long-term remission of acne symptoms has been observed in 70 per cent of cases. However, **Roaccutane** has been linked to many, potentially dangerous side effects. A pregnancy test must first be carried out before any consideration of use of this drug. Major foetal abnormalities have been associated with this medication among many other complications.

Roaccutane may also interfere with other medications such as tetracycline antibiotics, other acne medications, Vitamin A and progesterone-based contraception preparation. Some of isotertinoin side effects may also include: severely irritated conjunctivitis; nose bleeds; cracked lips; soreness of nasal passages; certain forms of eczema; increased photosensitivity (sunburn); blood lipid abnormalities; muscle and skeletal pains.

### Natural acne treatments:

Topically – comfrey; witch hazel; colloidal silver; tea tree oil; aloe vera and calendula cream/gel. poultice – (carrot, avocado skin, raw potato).
Eucalyptus, thyme and wintergreen essential oils - added to a steam bath.
Avoid over-washing and minimise any use of soaps on affected skin areas.
Aromatherapy essential oils – lavender, bergamot and geranium oils combined in a carrier oil are also good to use in a steam bath.

Medically - dermatological topical creams containing *Hydroquinone and Benzoyl Peroxide 5% w/w* are also used for treating acne externally.

### Herbal medicines
1 Burdock root - counter/decrease sebum production, alterative, anti-bacterial, restores oil and sweat gland function.
2 Calendula – lymphatic, vulnerary, heal skin.
3 Yellow dock and berberis aqua folium (oregan grape) if constipation and sluggish liver function is involved, dandelion root (taraxicum).
4 Vitex Agnus Castus (chaste tree), balance hormonal factors.
5 Iris Versicolor (blue flag), for lymphatics, pustules, comedones – alternative and gland stimulant
6 Poke root, echinacea, gallium (clivers) – also lymphatic tonic herbs.
7 Red clover, clivers, nettles – kidney depurative herbs.
8 Baptisa and myrrh – anti-microbial herbs
9 Sarsaparilla – alterative and diuretic.
10 Barberry, chlorophyll, lecithin, garlic, and bioflavonoids.
11 Kelp – rich in iodine, stimulate thyroid metabolism.

## Nutrients

**Vitamin A** (micellised, emulsified) high dose up to 50,000 IU may be used for several months then cut down. (High doses are only to be recommended for short term use and after a medical check up).

**Vitamin B6** 50-250mg twice daily helps menstrual related acne, decreases oily and greasy facial skin.

**Vitamin C.** 250-1000mg x 3 times daily. It is an effective antibiotic, antioxidant, stress reducer, and it induces cytochrome P450 detoxifying enzyme.

**Vitamin E and Selenium.** Improve erythrocyte glutathione peroxidase to reduce free radical damage to tissue and are antioxidants. Vitamin E 200-1,000 IU daily.

Fifty per cent of acne patients have increased circulating endotoxins, which increases the **copper to zinc ratio**, thus increasing complement and fibrin formation.

**Bromelain** supplements can break up fibrin complexes.

The **enzyme 5-alpha-reductase** has been shown to be greater in acne skin. It converts testosterone to a more potent androgen – dihydrotestosterone. **High protein diets** and Vitamin C can help lower this enzyme.

Acne skin appears to have a defect in metabolism of Vitamin A that cannot be converted to retinol.

**Essential fatty acids** have been shown to be low in sebum and pilosebaceous epithelium in acne skin. Thus may lead to the characteristic follicular hyper-keratosis in acne. Essential fatty acids such as in cod liver oil and Vitamin B5 supplementation can reduce this hyper-keratosis.

Low Vitamin B5 Levels can impair fatty acid metabolism, sex hormone and Co-enzyme A production.

**Chromium** is needed for glucose tolerance factor (GTF) which is required to normalise blood sugar and insulin levels and convert linoleic acid to prostaglandins.

**L-Cysteine** provides sulphur essential for skin maintenance.

**Zinc** supplementation has shown to be as effective as tetracycline in trials.

**Bifidus** supplementation can be beneficial to recolonise bowel bacteria.

**Vitamin B12** supplementation is useful in acne rosacea.

# Diagnosis of PCOS

This is performed by your GP Doctor and/or Specialist.
- An ultrasound scan to check for polycystic ovaries.
- Blood test to detect elevated levels of androgens (e.g. testosterone), Luteinising Hormone (LH), and possible low (FSH) Follicle Stimulating Hormone.
- Other advisable blood tests include - Fasting blood sugar (glucose tolerance test); Prolactin (PRL) (another Pituitary Hormone); Oestradiol (E2); Progesterone (P4); Dehydroepiandrosterone sulphate (DHEAS); Thyroid Function Hormone Profile; Cholesterol and Triglycerides (blood fat) levels; and Full Blood Count (check for Anaemia).

## *Medical treatments for PCOS:*

Medically, there is currently no 'cure' for PCOS. Though, at present they attempt to manage the syndrome with prescription drugs such as:

- The contraceptive pill; anti-androgen medications (Diane 35, Estelle - ED, and Spironolactone, for example); and frequent antibiotics may be used to help 'regulate' the period, and other common symptoms (e.g. facial hair, acne). But neither actually addresses the underlying 'cause' or problems and are associated with potential side effects.

- Biguanides: e.g. Metformin (Diabex) is a drug traditionally used for the treatment of insulin resistance in non-insulin dependent diabetes mellitus (type 2), and is now being used in PCOS. By improving responsiveness to insulin, it may also improve a number of features of PCOS, including lowering the serum LH and serum-free testosterone. Women who are overweight tend to lose more weight with a low-calorie diet if metformin is added. Metformin alone does not appear to enhance weight loss but may help to decrease the risk of hypertension in PCOS sufferers. The suggested dose of Metformin is 850mg twice daily or 500mg three times daily. As a result of Metformin's action, ovulation is improved naturally and if ovulation induction is still needed, there are improvements also in the response of follicles to clomiphene or to FSH. Insulin-related chemicals are involved in the development of ova.

- Approximately 20 per cent of women taking Metformin experience some side effects such as: nausea; diarrhoea; abdominal discomfort or cramping; weakness; more rarely jaundice; extremely low blood sugar; palpitations; blurred vision; fainting; sweating; hunger; bleeding; bruising; and skin rashes.

- Metformin should *not* be used with various medications as they can interact: ACE inhibitors; alcohol; anticoagulants (e.g. warfarin); beta blockers; diclofenac; cimetidine; corticosteroids; diuretics; thyroxine; and numerous herbal medicines. Metformin is not to be used during pregnancy;

breast feeding; by those with type 1 diabetes; individuals with alcoholism; dehydration; blood clots; pancreatitis; advanced heart, kidney, or liver disease. Thiazolindinediones drugs have also been used in PCOS to improve insulin sensitivity by allowing glucose to enter the cells.

- D-chiro-inositol (INS-1) is a nutritional factor that is found in most fresh fruits and vegetables. Preliminary studies conducted using this substance are showing potential promise for the application in PCOS as it has demonstrated insulin- and testosterone-lowering properties. To date no side effects have been reported during trials of the substance. In the future D-chiro-inositol may be isolated and available in concentrated medication form. INS-1 is high in foods like Buckwheat (particularly in the bran).

- Surgical procedures, involving the excision, 'Drilling' or Diathermy (Burning) of part of the ovary, have been shown to provide short-lived benefits and often produce scarring. Studies suggest that laparoscopic ovarian drilling (LOD) gives similar pregnancy rates in women with PCOS when compared to induction of ovulation with FSH. The cost of LOD is approximately 50 per cent less than FSH and the risk of multiple pregnancies is a lot less. LOD requires 3-4 holes per ovary and is best suited to those with low Body Mass Index (BMI). LOD is shown to be superior to Metformin alone in achieving pregnancy.

- Ovarian stimulation drugs such as Clomiphene citrate (Clomid)/Serophene have been medically used to trigger ovulation through FSH release from the pituitary gland. Clomiphene citrate is not a hormone, but a synthetic 'anti-oestrogen'. This drug works by fooling the body's regulatory mechanisms into perceiving that more oestrogen is needed. This stimulates gonadotropin release to provoke follicle growth that will hopefully lead to successful ovulation. Clomiphene's action may help to improve ovulation, but the down side of its anti-oestrogen affect can also target other organs and tissue such as the lining of the uterus and cervix. This action can have negative results by retarding the endometrial development thereby possibility decreasing the embryo's ability to implant to the uterine wall successfully.

- Clomid does not treat the cause of PCOS, and may in fact exacerbate (worsen) the problem, as many follicles are stimulated simultaneously, and normal hormone balance may be further disrupted. An oversensitive response to the ovarian stimulant drugs can actually induce a polycystic condition as well as thicken cervical mucus production. If Clomiphene is to be used the lowest dose is recommended to be commenced on that can result in ovulation.

- Other ovulation inducer medication may include: Gonadotropin - releasing hormone antagonists such as: Clomid; Lupron/Leuprolide; HMG – Pergonal; Humegon and Repronex; FSH - Follistim, and Gonal F; Human chlorionic gonadotropin (HcG) – Profasi; and Pregnyl. Many of these medications work directly on promoting ovulation release. Clomiphene works more indirectly to provoke ovulation.

- Bromocriptine (Parlodel) or the newer and more potent Cabergoline (Dostinex), have been used to treat hyperprolactinemic amenorrhea. These drugs mimic the action of dopamine, the natural inhibiting factor for prolactin in the pituitary.

## Natural Treatment Protocols for PCOS

**The first protocol may require a liver and bowel detoxification program,** to reduce toxic overload on the body that may be contributing to the condition. Natural treatments are very similar to those used in other ovarian cyst conditions with slightly more focus on the balance of the endocrine system.

## Herbal Medicines for PCOS

- **Black Cohosh** can help to lower LH, as can bugleweed and hops. To enhance oestrogen levels herbs like false unicorn root, dong quai and black cohosh again could be considered.
- **Peony** has shown to normalise follicular development because of its effect on the aromatase enzyme and prevent cyst formation. Peony also contains paeoniflorin (a monoterpene glycoside), that acts on the aromatase enzyme on the ovary to promote the synthesis of oestradial from testosterone and therefore reduce the production of androgens. Progesterone levels may also be improved by using peony as it normalises ovarian function.
- **Liquorice** contains an active substance called glycrrhetinic acid that seems to inhibit the enzyme 17B-hydroxysteroid dehydrogenase which converts androstenedione to testosterone in the ovary and hair follicle. Therefore may lower excessive androgen production.
- **Natural Progesterone** creams rubbed into the skin when used in the second half of the menstrual cycle may help balance luteal phase defects.
- **Saw palmetto** has also shown to be very beneficial particularly to reduce excessive androgen levels.
- **False unicorn root** is used for ovulation complaints during the follicular phase of the menstrual cycle (Day 4 to 14). False unicorn root was considered the herb of choice to use for PCOS, though world supplies are diminishing.
- **Tribulus** may be useful as it is a steroidal-saponin containing herb and can substitute for herbs such as False Unicorn Root. Tribulus appears to weakly bind to oestrogen receptors in the hypothalamus, which reduces the feedback from oestradiol and increased hypothalamic FSH secretion. Other herbs that may be considered for PCOS include Wild Yam and Shatavari.
- **Chaste Tree** (Vitex Agnus-Castus) may be used to lower elevated testosterone levels, (but not if luteinising hormone levels are also

elevated); although vitex may help to stimulate ovulation, it has not to date proven reliable in PCOS and may potentially worsen menstrual cycle irregularity in some cases.

- *Homeopathic remedies may include: Calcarea carbonica, sepia and* pulsatilla.

Due to the usual involvement of poor insulin utilisation in PCOS these *clinical nutrients* may be of benefit to regulate blood sugars levels: chromium; co enzyme Q 10; Vitamin E; manganese; vanadium; lipoic acid; magnesium; n-acetyl-cysteine; and zinc. Omega-3 fatty acids and dietary fibre may also be considered.

*Herbal medicines* that may be useful to treat insulin resistance may include: acacia (acacia nilotica); gymnema; goat's rue; hops (humulus lupulus); blue flag; cinnamon; ipomoea batatas (caiapo, white sweet potato); jambul (syzygium jambolana); codonopsis; panax; Siberian ginseng; fenugreek; and sarsaparilla (smilax spp).

*Weight management* may require to be addressed; these fat loss programs may be recommended: Ketogenic (high protein/low carbohydrate) Diet, or Insulin Zone (balances ratios of fats/carbohydrates/proteins) diet.

*Increase exercise or physical activity* - 25 per cent of ovulatory infertility is estimated to be caused from being overweight. A large study conducted by Harvard in 2002 examined physical activity and body fat as risk factors for infertility due to problems with ovulation. The study showed that an increase in exercise of only thirty minutes per week was found to be associated with a 7 per cent reduction in infertility relating to ovulation.

*Other supplements* that may assist with weight loss management are: carnitine; methionine; conjugated linoleic acids (cla); calcium pyruvate; proteins/hummus; phenylalanine; tyrosine; ginger; cayenne; eca stacking; brindleberry; gymnema, green tea; omega-3 oils (fish: salmon, tuna, mackerel); increase dietary fibre; moderate amounts of soya (organic); legumes; flax seed; celery; and Vitamin B complexes.

*Avoid* foods containing saturated animal fats, trans fatty acids (hydrogenated) – fat molecules that have had added hydrogen to slow rancidity – commonly used in hardened stick margarine, commercial baked goods and fried foods. A better alternative is mono-unsaturated fats (MUFAs) derived from vegetable sources including avocados, nuts and olives, or polyunsaturated fats (PUFAs, essential fatty acids) such as Omega-3 fatty acids linolenic acid (EPA/DHA) derived from cold water fish.

*To help reduce insulin resistance* consider increasing low glycemic index foods in your diet; examples of these may include: types of breads – pumpernickel and heavy mixed grains; breakfast cereals – all bran, toasted muesli, psyllium-based cereal, oatmeal; dairy – soy, skim, no fat, low-fat yogurt; fruits and vegetables – grapefruit, peaches, apples, pears, oranges, grapes, kiwis, sweet potatoes; rice, grains, and pastas – fettuccini, whole-wheat spaghetti, spaghetti, long-grain rice, bulgur; legumes – peanuts, soybeans, lentils, chickpeas and baked beans. If you can't live without a sugar fix – substitute commercial refined sugar for Xylitol (all natural sweetner); it has a low-GI of only 7. Normal sucrose / pure table sugar GI value is 100. Xylitol also has other health benefits.

**Consume an adequate diet** of a variety of insoluble and soluble fibres. Clinical studies have shown that up to 50 grams of fibre per day can improve glycemic control as well as reduce lipid levels. When increasing fibre intake, you should also increase your water consumption.

**Herbs** that show anti-cystic activity include: thuja; poke root (use with care); chelidonium; red clover; violet leaves; and blue flag.

**Lymphatic herbs** - clivers and calendula.

**Liver Tonics** – bupleurum; St Mary's thistle; dandelion root; schisandra; and turmeric.

**Anti-Congestive herbs** - garlic, fenugreek, and golden seal.

In TCM, PCOS is regarded as a Dampness pattern. **Chinese herbal formulations** such as: Gui Zhi Fu Ling Wan (Cinnamon & Hoelen combination), Two Cured Decoction (Er Chen Tang), Six Gentlemen Decoction (Liu Jun Zi), and/or Gleditsia (Zao Jiao Ci) may be considered for this condition. Ganshao capsules have been studies with positive results in women with Clomide resistant PCOS.

**Acupuncture** points that can be stimulated to help with PCOS may include: St 40 and Sp 9.


## Hormone Imbalance – Summary
* Need to know timing of ovulation as length of pre- and post-ovulatory phase important as length of cycle.
* Basal temperature reading best guide to ovulation/progesterone levels.
* Ovulation is at the beginning of the rise. Good progesterone levels indicated by immediate, substantial rise sustained with no dip for 12–16 days to allow for implantation (1 week after ovulation).
* Luteal (post-ovulatory phase) < (less than) 12 days inadequate, < (less than) 10 days infertile.
* Progesterone levels rely on adequate corpus luteum, which is determined by size of follicle at ovulation, which in turn depends on length of pre-ovulatory (follicular) phase.
* Ovulation after day 17 less reliable, after day 20 miscarriage extremely likely. Optimum time for ovulation is day 14 or slightly earlier (chances of

successful fertilisation producing healthy offspring > (greater than) 90 per cent), day 15 or later - chances down to 43 per cent, > (greater than) day 16 associated with changes in corpus luteum, and efficiency of progesterone production, > (greater than) 20 (20 - 25) higher incidence of miscarriage and abnormal eggs (ovum). Follicle < (less than) 16 Millimetres (mm) - eggs (ovum) possible won't survive.

- Length of follicular phase dependant on oestrogen levels. Long follicular phase may be result of: * too much oestrogen, * too little oestrogen, * inefficient elimination of oestrogen through the liver.
- Oestrogen prepares endometrium, triggers ovulation and production 'fertile' mucus, which can be used as an indicator of oestrogen levels and a prediction of approaching ovulation, to time conception.
- Oestrogen imbalance leads to: * long follicular phase, * inadequate endometrium, * inadequate mucus.
- Progesterone imbalance leads to: * short luteal phase, * inadequate endometrium.
- Imbalances in both oestrogen and progesterone can therefore, contribute to miscarriage.

### Normal blood serum test ranges during a menstrual cycle

- Oestradiol – day 2 or 3 of menses: 25-75 pg/ml (70-630)pmol/l
- Oestradiol – mid cycle (about day 14): Greater than 150 pg/ml
- An Oestradiol level that is over 50pg/ml may indicate ovarian cysts. Oestrogens can also be measured using urine tests: ug/24 hours
- Menstruating women – Oestrone 5–20 ug/24 hours, Oestradiol 2-5 ug/24 hours, Oestriol 5–30 ug/24 hours.
- Post menopause – Oestrone 0.3 – 2.4 ug/24 hours, Oestradiol 0 – 1.4 ug/24 hours, Oestriol 2.2 – 7.5 ug/24 hours.
- Blood measurements are considered more accurate when testing for a specific type of oestrogen. High levels of oestrogen may be indicative of sex hormone therapy. Low levels may indicate ovarian abnormalities, infertility or menopause.
- Progesterone – day 2 or 3: Less than 1.5 ng/ml
- Progesterone – post ovulation: Greater than 15 ng/ml, reduced progesterone levels can indicate luteal phase defects and/or anovulary cycle.
- LH (Luteinising hormone) – day 2 or 3: Less than 7 mIU/ml (0.8-12.0)IU/l
- LH – mid cycle (around ovulation): Greater than 20 mIU/ml
    Fertility female: 2 – 20IU/L; at ovulation (10 -50 IU/L)
    Adult Male: 2 – 9 IU/L
- LH:FSH ratio – About 1:1
- Low levels of LH may indicate hyperprlactinaemia, infertility or hypogonadism.
- High levels of LH may indicate polycystic ovarian disease (PCOS), or ovarian dysfunction.
- FSH (Follicle stimulation hormone) – day 2 or 3: Less than 13 mIU/ml
    Follicular phase – 3.5 to 16 IU/litre

Mid-Cycle – 8 to 30 IU/litre (10 – 30 IU/L)
Luteal Phase – 1.8 to 12 IU/litre
Post-Menopausal – 25 IU/litre (40 – 200IU/L)
Adult Male – 1 – 5 IU/L
Low levels of FSH may indicate PCOS or hyperprolactinaemia. Elevated FSH levels indicate poor follicle development and consequently, anovulation cycles.
High levels may indicate disease or failure of the testes or ovaries. Ovarian reserves may be diminishing. A blood test on day 3 of your periods for Inhibin B may help to indicate ovary function. Low levels of Inhibin B may identify decreased ovarian function.

- Prolactin – 50 to 600 mU/l (milli-international units per litre) Australia
  Females: 3 – 25 ug/L; Males: less that 450 mU/L (2 – 15 ug/L)
  (Ug/l) micro-grams per litre (Australia), (ng/ml or nanograms/ml) USA
  Elevated prolactin levels may interfere with ovulation and cause infertility.
- Continuously elevated FSH levels may indicate Peri-menopause and that Androstenedione – 2-10 nmol/L
- Dehydroepiandrosterone sulphate (DHEAS) – DHEAS is a mild androgen produced by the adrenal glands. Elevated levels may indicate PCOS. Reproductive female: 0.8-10.2umol/L
- Testosterone – female: 0.4 – 3.6 nmol/L; male: 12-34 nmol/L
- Free Testosterone – female: puberty to 40 years: 3-12 pmol/L. Elevated levels of testosterone in women can lead to infertility. Increased androgen production often leads to lowered SHBG.
- **Note**: American units (ng/ml) are equivalent to Australian readings expressed as Ug/l to convert these readings to mU/l multiple ng/ml or Ug/l by 21.

# Interpretation of pathology results

### Conditions causing female infertility

**Ovarian Failure** – FSH - increased (>25 IU/l), LH - increased (>25 IU/l), LH: FSH ratio - normal, Prolactin - normal, Oestradiol – decreased, Androstenedione – normal; and Testosterone – normal.

**Hypothalamic or Pituitary failure** – FSH – decreased, LH – decreased, LH: FSH ratio – normal, Prolactin – normal, Oestradiol – decreased, Androstenedione – normal, Testosterone – normal.

**Hyperprolactinemia** – FSH – normal, LH – normal, LH: FSH ratio – normal, Prolactin – increased, Oestradiol – decreased; Androstenedione – normal, Testosterone – normal.

**Polycystic ovarian syndrome** – FSH – normal, LH – normal or increased, LH: FSH ratio – often 2.5:1, Prolactin – normal or increased, Oestradiol – normal, Androstenedione – increased, Testosterone – increased, Sex Hormone Binding Globulin (SHBG) – decreased.

## The normal semen test

Volume: 2.5 – 10 mL (average 4 mL);
Colour: Cream
Number of sperm (count): more than 20 million/mL
Motility (activity of sperm): more than 70 per cent activity
Morphology (sperm structure): more than 60 per cent normal formation
Leucocytes (white blood cells): less than 15/HPF;
Erythrocytes (Red cells blood): nil;
Haemoglobin (Blood, Hb): nil
Abnormal sperm: less than 70 per cent.

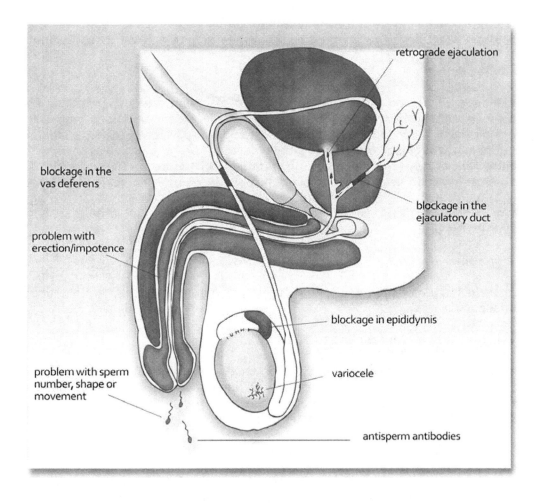

**Figure.19. Unhealthy male reproductive system – causes for infertility**

# Chapter 11

# *Abnormalities of the Anatomy – Males*

There are many congenital and structural abnormalities that can afflict the male reproductive system that may impact on his reproductive capacity. These are some examples of such conditions that may require medical investigation.

### Balanoposthitis

Balanoposthitis is an inflammation of the penis head and the prepuce. This condition may be caused as a result of infections, skin eruptions, or having a tight prepuce. Individuals with diabetes are more predisposed to this condition. The ability to clean under the foreskin may be difficult. *Phimosis* is a contraction or narrowed opening in the foreskin of the penis. Phimosis may be cause by infection in or under the foreskin. It is common for male boys under six to have this; the foreskin should never be forced to retract under this age. Skin conditions or localised swelling will aggravate the problem. Early treatment is best.

### Epispadias

Epispadias is a condition where the opening of the penis opens onto the upper surface.

### Cryptorchidism (undescended testes)

Cryptorchidism is usually detected during childhood where one or both testicles remain in the abdomen. If corrected early enough the testicles may develop normally. The prolonged over heating can damage the delicate seminiferous tubules and testicular tissue can potentially lead to sterility if not reversed.

### Hypospadias

Hypospadias is a condition where the opening of the urethra is on the underside of the penis instead of the end. It has been found that approximately 5 -10 per cent of all infertile males are affected by this condition. It has been estimated that since 1970 hypospedias had doubled.

## Retrograde Ejaculation

Retrograde Ejaculation is estimated to affect approximately 2 per cent of men, due to weakness in the sphincter valve of the bladder. The seminal fluid flows backwards into the bladder but does pass down the ejaculatory duct as normal. Urine may be present in the seminal fluids on ejaculation, which may cause it to appear milky in colour. Oral alkalising agents may be considered. Several causes can be linked to this condition, sphincter valve relaxing drug, which is used to treat asthma, depression and high blood pressure. Spinal injuries, diabetes and prostate problems may also be causal factors.

## Kallmann's Syndrome

Kallmann's Syndrome is a hypothalamus abnormality that affects the production of the release of (GnRH) Gonadotropin Releasing Hormone. Men with Kallmann's Syndrome often lack testosterone and secondary sexual characteristic development.

It is possible that no sperm is manufactured in men with this condition, although hormone therapy may be helpful in treating this problem.

## Vasectomy – 'The big chop'

A Vasectomy is a surgical sterilisation procedure that involves the male vas deferens tubes to be cut to preventing sperm from mixing with the semen on ejaculation. In the USA approximately 50 percent of the population of child-bearing age elect to have surgical sterilisation and about 500,000 vasectomies are performed in the US alone each year.

Reversing the results of this procedure can have mixed results. The reversal procedure is known as a *vasovasostomy*, or *vasoepididymostomy*.

Never say never again, approximately 2 percent of males have vasectomy reversals performed largely due to remarriage, accidental loss of children and S.I.D.S.

Vasectomy reversal operations are also a common culprit for potentially leaving behind scar tissue from microsurgically reconnecting the vas deferens to re-promote the flow of sperm between the testicle and ejaculatory ducts. The success rate of this reversal procedure is fairly low with much of the outcome dependent on the length of time since the initial vasectomy was performed.

Another problem with vasectomy reversal procedures and blocked ducts is the issue of developing anti-sperm antibody reactions found in about 50 per cent of men after the procedure. If the antibody blood levels are high, there is a less likelihood of a reversal procedure being successful.

Sometimes the sperm may be trapped behind an obstruction which can produce the release of a protein into the circulation, therefore initiating a response against what the immune system indicators have recognised as a foreign substance which needs attending to, thus, antibodies are formed, which in reality, is to attack the proteins of the sperm cells and not the foreign invading substance that the body thinks is occurring. This is a classic example of allergic reaction.

A similar response can occur when the female's immune system develops antibodies against the sperm and also the embryo, due to it also assuming that it is under attack from a foreign invader. This inflammatory reaction can affect blood flow through various tissues and can contribute to infertility due to immunological incompatibility or miscarriage of the embryo.

In a large number of cases a sperm aspiration procedure may be recommended instead and the sperm is then used in IFV or ICSI to conceive a baby. If a reversal procedure is performed it may take up to two years before the sperm quality returns.

### Varicocele – 'The silent strangler'

Varicocele is a condition where there are veins in or around the testes. This condition is estimated to affect some 25 per cent of men, of which 40 per cent have fertility problems. A varicocele is the most common correctable abnormality associated with male infertility. Varicoceles form from veins becoming engorged due to weak or defective valves causing the blood to flow away from the testicles/abdomen leading to a blood pooling effect. Blood is supplied to the testis and epididymis by an artery and is drained away by a network of veins known as the *pampiniform plexus* which partially surrounds the testis, the epididymus where sperm are stored, and the vas deferens which conveys sperm away from the testes during ejaculation.

Varicocele may be more common in men who suffer from obesity, pelvic and liver congestion, and elevated scrotum temperature and pancreatic dysfunction. Varicocele can result in elevating the testicular temperature, thus, resulting in sperm defects and lowered testicular volume. Other blockages within the male reproductive system can be extremely tiny and still may cause fertility problems. Over eighty percent of varicoceles are present on one side only, usually on the left. This is thought to occur due to the fact that the left testicular vein is anatomically more likely to suffer back-pressure. Sperm is best produced in the testes at a temperature around ten degrees lower than that of our body's normal temperature which is 37 degrees C.

Some of the tubules within the testes for example, may only be as wide as one and a half times that of a human hair. Damage, scar tissue and trauma to this delicate tissue can quite easily contribute to impairing the passage of sperm through the various mazes of ducts and tubules.

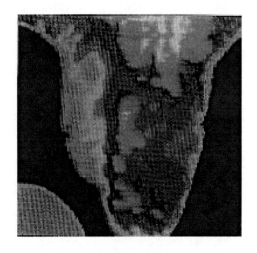

**Varicocoele**
The grey patches in the middle
are a varicocoele (enlarged veins).
This discoloration indicates a
raised temperature, which can
affect normal sperm production.

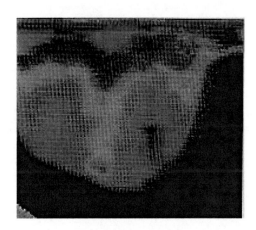

**Healthy testes**
This thermal photograph shows
Heat at the very top whereas the
Bottom portion is on the normal/cool
Side.

*Thermal photos of a varicocele and healthy testes*

If the obstructions are minor various natural therapies can be very helpful, though in more severe cases surgical intervention may be necessary to reverse the blockage. A physical examination by your doctor or urologist is the first step of assessment to determine if a varicocele is present and if it may be causing a problem with fertility. A thermography may then be used to measure the temperature of the testis to examine if over-heating could be affecting the sperm quality.

If surgical corrective measures are recommended, a ligation procedure *(varicocelectomy)* is performed under general anaesthetic on some of the veins to reduce the amount of venous blood pooling around the testis and epididymis. The success rate of improving sperm parameters is around sixty percent (60%) after one year after having the varicocele ligation. The presents of a varicocele has been also shown to be associated with increased levels of damaged DNA in sperm. To further assess if a varicocele has affected sperm DNA and/or quality, a Sperm Chromatin Structure Assay (SCSA) can be performed with advanced laboratory equipment at most fertility specialist clinics.

**Natural treatments that may be used for varicoceles include:**

**Herbal medicines**: bilberry; butcher's broom (ruscus aculeatus); cayenne (capsicum spp); cranesbill root (geranium maculatum); ginger (zingiber officinale); hawthorn berries; horse chestnut (aesculus hippocatanum); ginkgo biloba; gota kola; oak bark (quercus robur); prickly ash; St John's wort (hypericum perforatum); and witch hazel (hamamelis virginiana). Aloe vera gel can be rubbed into the area topically. Arnica and comfrey creams are also beneficial.

**TCM herbal formula**: Cinnamon twig and Poria pill.

**Nutrients**: Co enzyme Q 10; dimethyl glycine (DMG); dimethyl sulfoxide (DMSO); essential fatty acids (EFAs), glutathione; grape seed extract or pycnogenol; Vitamin C with bioflavonoids; quercetin; rutin; Vitamin E; selenium; glucosamine; chondroitin sulphate; proline; lysine; glycine; lecithin; Vitamin A; B complex vitamins (esp. B3, B6, and B12); and zinc.

**Homeopathic**: Ferrum metallium, hamamelis virginiana, and pulsatilla may help.

**Male Hormonal Conditions of the Reproductive System**

**Impotence – 'I've lost my mojo!'**

***Putting the lead back into the pencil – straightening out the situation***
Impotence, or chronic erectile dysfunction, is the constant inability to maintain an erect penis sufficiently for sexual intercourse. The functional processes that are involved to achieve erection are linked to a combination of body activities;

these include correct brain stimuli, hormone secretions, blood vessel and nerve function.

It is estimated that *150 million* men worldwide are affected by erectile dysfunction (ED) as reported by the American Medical Association back in 1999. Approximately 80 per cent of the causes of impotence are due to an organic disease such as *penile arterial insufficiency* and the side-effects from numerous types of drugs.

Diseases such as diabetes, cardiovascular disease, and hypertension can also adversely affect erectile function. The blood vessels that are needed to help form an erect penis can become congested with atherosclerotic (hardening) plaque. This congestion can reduce the blood flow to the penis and result in poor erections. Low levels of the biochemical *nitric oxide* can contribute to erectile dysfunction, also high levels of the hormone *Prolactin* can cause problems as well.

Hormonal imbalances may also cause problems such as having *low thyroid hormonal* levels, having low testosterone levels does not usually affect the direct functional cause behind impotence, but can cause the lack of desire (loss of libido) for intercourse, that may prevent an adequate erection from occurring. Testosterone hormone replacement should not be used until blood pathology is taken to ascertain if the hormone is indeed low as high levels of testosterone can inhibit follicle-stimulating-hormone (FSH) production, which in turn will decrease sperm production.

Diseases or abnormalities of the testes or pituitary gland may be responsible for reduced testosterone production. Without testosterone a male is impotent and cannot produce sperm. The amount of testosterone the testes (Leydig cells) produce is governed by the pituitary gland under the brain. This gland should release FSH and LH in response to low testosterone levels. Correct function of this feedback mechanism (hypothalamic-pituitary-gondal axis) is what keeps testosterone levels in a state of balance. As we age testosterone levels naturally decline; the testes normally produce about 4-7 milligrams of testosterone daily.

Most males over the age of forty will invariably suffer erectile problems at one time or another. The percentage of males affected seems to increase with biological age. Loss of libido may be caused by a depression illness, effects from certain medications or a decline in sexual interest with their partner. It is estimated that 85% of impotence problems have a known physical cause; the remaining 15% may be psychological in nature.

A condition known as *Peyronie's disease* results in a twisting of the penis when it is erect; this prevents the penis from retaining its overall elasticity and may appear contorted. Some of the other possible causes of impotence may include: over consumption of alcohol; extreme stress; strict sexual upbringing; various prescription/recreational drug use; psychiatric disorders; testicular/

erect penis injury; pituitary disease; diabetes mellitus that is poorly controlled; high blood pressure/cholesterol; pelvic surgery; multiple sclerosis; prostate cancer; spine injuries; Parkinson's disease; Alzheimer's; lead poisoning; Klinefelter syndrome; and Frohlich syndrome.

***Medical drugs used for impotence may include***: Viagra (Sildenafil); Tadalafil (Cialis) dosage 10 to 20mg once daily; Vardenafil (Levitra) dosage 10 to 20mg taken 30 to 60 minutes prior to intercourse; Apomorphine (Uprima); injectable Papaverine (Pavabid); Phentolamine (Regitine); Prostaglandin E1 (PGE1); and Alprostadil (Caverject). Penile pump/inflatable implants and penile prostheses are also available if other methods are ineffective.

## Natural treatments for Impotence include:

***Herbal Medicines*** that may benefit include: tribulus; panax ginseng; rhodiola; schizandra; morinda (noni); withania; stinging nettle root; sarsaparilla; damiana; oats; yohimbe; wild yam; maca root; gota kola; hydrangea; pygeum; saw palmetto; bee pollen; and Siberian ginseng.

***TCM Herbs***: Eucommia (Du Zhong), Epimedium (Yin Yang Huo), Morinda Root (Ba Ji Tian), and Deer Antler (Lu Rong).

***Nutrients***: L-arginine; essential fatty acids (dha/epa); kelp; histidine (may improve libido and orgasm when balanced); Vitamin E; quercetin; dhea; Vitamin B1, B5 and choline (to balance the parasympathetic nervous system function); Vitamin C; zinc; Octacosanol (in wheat germ); tyrosine; Dimethylglycine (DMG); and selenium.

*\* Refer to specific herbal medicine and nutrition sections for additional information!*

## Prostatitis / Benign Prostatic Hypertrophy / Hyperplasia

### 'When bigger doesn't mean better'

The prostate is a male sex gland, located beneath the urinary bladder. The function of the prostate gland is to contract muscles within to squeeze fluid into the urethral tract during ejaculation that make up the bulk semen fluid.

Prostatic hypertrophy is characterised by the gradual enlargement of the prostate that is non-tender, non-cancerous and can cause a bladder outlet obstruction. The symptoms that may be present are progressive urinary frequency and urgency, the need to urinary during the night, a hesitancy and intermittency with reduced force to urinate.

For males, dysfunctions of the prostate are the most common cause of genito-urinary problems. Prostatitis is another condition that involves inflammation of the gland; this is usually caused by a bacterial infection (usually E.coli) that can result in fluid retention due to the inflammation. As a consequence the bladder itself may become infected causing distension, tenderness and weakness of the bladder; this in turn can also progress to an ascending infection to the kidneys via the urethra.

There are basically three types of prostatitis: Acute infectious, Chronic infectious, and Non-infectious.

***Benign prostatic Hypertrophy (BPH) / Prostatomegaly*** is estimated to affect more than 50 per cent of males over the age of fifty and is attributed to hormonal changes where the male hormone testosterone is converted to *dihydrotestosterone* (DHT) (a very potent form of testosterone) in the prostate gland. As a general rule of thumb, males over the age of fifty tend to have a decline in testosterone levels. As testosterone seems to fall, other hormones like estradiol, FSH, LH, sex hormone binding ligand, and prolactin all increase. The rise in prolactin increases the uptake of testosterone by the prostate. This will result in an increased production and concentration of DHT within the prostate that also results from its poorly removed.

An enzyme called *5-alpha-reductase* is involved in the conversion process of testosterone to DHT. When DHT increases this will also increase the risk of coronary heart disease, prostatic hyperplasia (overproduction/growth of prostate cells), that can eventually resulting in prostatic cancer. DHT also stimulates protein synthesis, and prostaglandin release in the cells.

A blood test that measures for PSA (prostate-specific antigens) is a marker for identifying prostate cancer. A PSA level below *4 micrograms* per litre is considered normal, elevated levels over 10 may be an indicator of possible prostate cancer. High levels of leucocytes in a semen analysis may indicate prostatitis or an infection of the urinary-genito system. A physical prostate examination may also be recommended by your doctor to manually feel for roughness, size and hardness to the prostate gland, this requires putting a gloved finger into the rectum through the anus opening.

**Natural treatments For Prostate Disorders:**

***Herbal Medicines***: saw palmetto; sabal serrulata; pygeum (pyguem africanum); stinging nettle root (urtica dioica); buchu (barosma betulina); willow herb (epilobium spp); parsley; horsetail; marshmallow leaf; turmeric; golden rod (solidago virgaurea); cough grass (agropyron repens); hydrangea; gravel root; corn silk; African potato (hypoxis rocallidea); pine (pinus spp); spruce (picea spp); red clover; olive leaf; and panax ginseng.

***Nutrients***: essential fatty acids (EFAs); soluble fibre (psyllium seed husks, guar gum, rice bran, oat bran, slippery elm); beta-sitosterol; boron; Vitamin C; Vitamin E; quercetin; selenium; Vitamin B Complex (esp. Vitamin B6); zinc; isoflavones; lignans; genistin; glycine; alanine; beta carotene; Vitamin D3; conjugated linoleic acid (cla); indole-3-carbinol (i3c)/(dim); and melatonin.

**Food to Increase in diet**: tomatoes (for the lycopene they contain), soy products; garlic; onions; cabbage; raw pumpkin seeds (pepitas) (high in zinc and essential fatty acids); bee/flower pollen (contains flavinols); brewer's yeast; plant-based foods; grapeseed extract; and oily fish (for DHA/EPA).

**Avoid**: High cholesterol foods; saturated fats; acid-forming foods; cigarette smoking; pesticide exposure; toxic heavy metals such as cadmium; PCBs; beer; wine; caffeine; stress; and excess tryptophan.

Alternate hot and cold sitz baths reduce congestion and increase circulation.

## Medical procedures and drugs used for prostate disorders may include:

A procedure called Transurethral vaporisation of the prostate (TVP) involving an electric current to vaporise excess tissue may be used.

**Medical drugs** such as: Finasteride (Proscar); Prazosin (Minipress); Terazosin (Hytrin); and Doxazosin (Cardura) are available to help shrink enlarged prostates. Alpha-blocking drugs such as Alfuzosin or Indoramin may be used to help relax the smooth muscle around the urethra to improve the flow of urine and help reduce BPH symptoms. Other medications used may include anti-androgen drugs such as Finasteride, which prevents the activation of testosterone in the prostate gland with the aim of shrinking the swollen tissue; this may have the effect of improving the symptoms and reducing complications. Injectable drugs like Aleuprolide (Lupron) may also be considered to decrease prostate enlargement.

**For Prostate cancer** – A surgical procedure called a *radical prostatectomy* involves removal of the gland. Side-effect of this procedure may cause impotence in 75 per cent of men and urinary incontinence in 25 per cent of men undergoing the surgery.

Medications such as Nilutamide. an anti-androgen drug, may be used to slow the progression of advanced stages of the disease. Other methods used to contain the cancer are *Radiotherapy* – directing an external beam of radiation at the target prostate to destroy the cancer cells and *Brachytherapy* – injecting radioactive particles into the prostate. Irritable bowel and increased bladder frequency can be potential complications of these procedures.

# Chapter 12

# *Prescription – Fertility Medications*

**'When Science steps in to help with fertility'**

There is a wide variety of prescribed medications available today that can be used to improve the odds of conception. Some of these medications may be used to increase ovulation chances and can be utilised in conjunction with timed intercourse or IUI. Other types of medications are used with medical assisted reproductive technology (ART) such as egg retrieval, IVF and ICSI to enhance either the number of eggs available to create embryos for implantation such as FSH, and others are used to help reduce the odds of miscarriage in hope of maintaining a viable pregnancy such as supplemental progesterone and HCG.

As with all medically prescribed drugs, the types also used in fertility come with both positive and potentially negative effects. Throughout this chapter I have discussed both the upside and downsides to the major prescription medications that may be medically recommended. The information in this section may help to assist with your understanding of how these chemical drugs work and what possible side-effects can occur. Advancements in providing more pure chemical drugs and better administering methods such as pen injections are constantly on the improvement! The majority of problems that arise from prescription fertility drugs are usually based upon dosages used and the frequency of back-to-back courses.

## Clomiphene Citrate/USP (Traded as Clomid, Clomhexal or Serophene)

Clomiphene has been commonly used since the 1970s as the primary medical treatment to stimulate ovulation. Clopmiphene is an anti-oestrogen drug that tricks the brain into thinking there is little to no oestrogen in the blood. The pituitary gland responds by increasing FSH supply to stimulate the ovaries and egg production. The dosage of clomiphene is taken orally in tablet form once daily for a period of five days, most commonly from days 2 to 7 of the menstrual cycle. Clomiphene should only be taken over a maximum of six consecutive months. Three by three monthly with breaks in between would be more preferred as Clomiphene residues can accumulate and absorb into the body's adipose fat tissue.

The ovulatory response to cyclic Clomiphene therapy appears to be mediated through increased output of pituitary gonadotrophins, which in turn stimulates the maturation and endocrine activity of the ovarian follicle and the subsequent development and function of the corpus luteum. The role of the pituitary is indicated by increased urinary excretion of gonadotrophins and the response of the ovary, as manifested by increased urinary oestrogen excretion.

Clomiphene citrate is indicated for the treatment of anovulation in carefully selected infertile women who wish to become pregnant. In such patients, approximately 70 per cent will ovulate and (provided that there is no other cause of infertility in them or in their partners) about 30 per cent will become pregnant. It is worthwhile to note those patients who were single and some who either did not desire pregnancy at the time of treatment or had impediments to achievement of the pregnancy other than ovulatory dysfunction.

Ovulation most often occurs from 6 to 12 days after a course of Clomiphene. With this in mind, coitus (intercourse) should be timed to coincide with the expected time of ovulation. Spontaneous ovulatory menses have been noted after Clomiphene therapy has been used in some patients. Individuals that are usually considered for Clomiphene treatment may include infertile patients with polycystic ovarian syndrome (PCOS) who have not responded to wedge resection of the ovary but may respond to Clomiphene (short term)!

Clomiphene is ineffective in patients whose primary pituitary or ovarian failure precludes the possibility of stimulating normal function. Clomiphene and injections of Human Chorionic Gonadotropin (HCG) may be considered as medical options administered at about the expected time of ovulation where anovulation still occurs after sole use of Clomiphene has not achieved ovulation, and/or whose luteal phases are so short that the opportunity to conceive is limited.

Clomiphene is probably not a safe drug in pregnancy; at least once the embryo's genital tract is developing, around eight to ten weeks from the start of the conception cycle (from the last menstrual period). Clomiphene as an oestrogen-blocking medication happens to be very similar in structure to the estrogenic drug *diethylstilbestrol* (DES), which was widely prescribed in the 1950s for miscarriages, and which is now notorious for having caused deformities of the upper vaginal and uterus in female foetuses and of the epididymis and vas deferens in male foetuses.

Experiments show that Clomiphene and DES do similar harm in pregnant mice. What they have in common, in disturbing these oestrogen-sensitive events in the embryo, is prolonged attachment to the oestrogen receptors, distorting the normal sequence of events in the development of the relevant organs and tissue. Clomiphene has also been used in males to stimulate the testicles to produce more sperm and testosterone.

The use of Clomiphene citrate (Clomid) has also been linked to many undesirable side effects. The drug is used to stimulate follicle stimulating hormone (FSH) release from the pituitary gland. Excessive usage of this medication is involved in an increased incidence of ovarian cancer (one study has suggested a potential increase of 400 per cent incidence of ovarian cancer was observed after (1) year of continual monthly administering, though other studies have not reported incidences of this extent!). It has been recommended that all women considering using this (or similar) medication/s should have a 'base-line' ultrasound to assess the tendency to benign or malignant tumour development. Other side effects may include: 'explosive ovaries', ovarian hyper-stimulation syndrome (OHSS) and subsequent polycystic ovarian syndrome (PCOS). (Ironically, Clomiphene is one of the drugs used to also treat PCOS.)

Stimulation of the ovaries to 'harvest' multiple eggs for fertilisation, though, can use up viable ovum supplies if the process is unsuccessful and may shorten the female's potential reproductive life-span, and may exacerbate pre-existing pelvic or cervical infection.

A host of hormone-related side effects such as hot flushes; nausea; gastrointestinal problems; ovarian enlargement; blurred vision; increased nervous tension; depression; fatigue; dizziness; light-headedness; insomnia; breast soreness; heavier menstrual bleeding; intermenstrual bleeding; urticaria (hives); increased urinary frequency; moderate reversible hair loss; bloating; weight gain; increased incidence of thrush (Candida); jaundice (skin yellowing); and headaches. Clomid also can cause thickening of cervical mucus, which may actually lower one's fertility, in some instances.

There is very little research or information available on the connection between IVF, fertility drugs and deformity, but we do know that spina bifida is five (5) times more frequent in IVF births, and when mice are given Clomid (Clomiphene citrate), their babies are smaller and have an increased incidence of birth defects. Interestingly, the Clomid product information states quite clearly that there is a chance Clomiphene may cause birth defects if it is taken after you become pregnant. Drugs of this nature may have potentially a longer-than-desired life span in the body tissues; therefore, it may interfere with the natural regulation of your body's hormones after stopping the medication! Women with ovarian cysts and fibroids must be cautious when taking Clomid, which ironically is most often the underlying condition that the Clomid is being prescribed for in the first instance. Women with abnormal uterine bleeding, hormone tumours or liver disease should not take Clomiphene medication. The reported birth defect rate of Clomiphene use is one in two hundred (1:200) births.

A study in 1989 showed an increased response to Clomid when combined with a TCM herbal formula called *Wen Jing Tang* (warm the menses decoction). During this study woman that didn't ovulate after three cycles of Clomid, were given Wen Jing Tang formula, which then made them ovulate. Also other

325

studies comparing Clomid use when taken with Vitamin C had improved ovulation results. Recommended dosage of Clomiphene usually starts from 50mg (one tablet); most successful pregnancy results usually occur with doses of 150mg or just over. Higher doses of Clomiphene can have the opposite effect. The right dose is the key!

## Recombinant Human Follicle Stimulating Hormone (FSH) or Follitropin

Beta (Active composition), (marketed under trade names for example 'Puregon'). The active ingredient of products such as Puregon, (Human FSH), is produced by Chinese hamster ovary cell line transfected with the human FSH sub-unit genes (i.e. by recombinant DNA technology). Other FSH prescriptions include: Gonal-F (Active ingredient is Follitropin-Alfa) (genetically synthesis FSH), and Merodin HP, Bravelle (Highly purified Urofollitropin - HFSH).

FSH is indispensable in normal female and male gamete growth and maturation, and in gonadal steroid production. FSH is secreted by the pituitary gland in response to stimulation by gonadotropin. In females, FSH is essential for the normal cyclic growth of ovarian follicles and then prepares the follicles for the action of luteinising hormone (LH). The most important effect resulting from parental administration of FSH to females is the development of mature Graafian follicles. In males, FSH stimulates spermatogenesis without significant effect on the androgen-secreting interstitial cells of the testes. In the female, the amount of FSH is critical for the onset and duration of follicular development and consequently for the timing and number of follicles reaching maturity. Recombinant human FSH can thus be used to stimulate follicular development and steroid production in selected cases of disturbed gonadal function.

Furthermore, Follitropin-Beta/Alfa can be used to promote multiple follicular development in medically assisted reproduction programs (e.g. in vitro fertilisation/embryo transfer (IVF/ET) and gamete or zygote intrafallopian transfer (GIFT/ZIFT). In the absence of an endogenous luteinising hormone (LH) surge, treatment with human FSH is generally followed by administration of Human Chorionic Gonadotropin (HCG) to induce the final phase of follicle maturation, leading to ovulation.

In the male, in deficient spermatogenesis due to hypo-gonadotropic hypogonadism, Recombinant Human FSH is given to substitute FSH for the stimulation of the Sertoli cells. The high LH activity needed to stimulate the Leydig cells is provided by an HCG preparation given in addition the human FSH. The FSH is administered via either intra muscular/subcutaneous injection. Conditions that human FSH is indicated for may include: anovulation; defective follicle ripening; and/or corpus luteum insufficiency.

The potential list of side-effects or adverse reactions are similar to those seen of the use of Clomiphene citrate (Clomid) such as: ovarian hyper stimulation syndrome (ohss); ovarian enlargement; nausea; abdominal pain; increased ectopic pregnancies; vaginal haemorrhage; miscarriage; pain over body; flu-like symptoms; swollen abdomen; pain at injection site; pulmonary and vascular complications such as atelectasis, acute respiratory distress syndrome, and possible venous thrombo-emboli events.

Since follicles of over 15 millimetres (mm) may produce pregnancies, a maximum of two additional follicles exceeding 15mm is accepted. If this limit is exceeded, HCG may be withheld and pregnancy should be avoided (under consent) in order to prevent large multiple gestations/births (if carried to term)!

## Human Chorionic Gonadotropin (HCG)
## (Traded as 'APL Injections', 'Pregnyl', and 'Profasi', recombinant-HCG 'Ovidrel')

The action of HCG is virtually identical to that of Pituitary Luteinising Hormone (LH), although HCG appears to have a small degree of FSH activity as well. It stimulates production of gonadal steroid hormones by stimulating the interstitial cells (Leydig cells) of the testis to produce androgens (testosterone) and the corpus luteum of the ovaries in women to produce primarily progesterone, though it also assists with mild oestrogen production.

Androgen stimulation in the male leads to the development of secondary sex characteristics and may stimulate testicular descent when no anatomical impediment to descent is present. This descent is usually reversible when HCG is discontinued. During the normal menstrual cycle, LH participates with FSH in the development and maturation of the normal ovarian follicle and the mid cycle LH surge triggers ovulation; HCG can substitute for LH in this function. During the normal pregnancy, HCG secreted by the placenta maintains the corpus luteum after LH secretion decreases, supporting continued secretion of oestrogen and progesterone and preventing menstruation.

The gonadotropins stimulate the synthesis of oestradiol, progesterone, and testosterone by the gonads after in vivo administration or after addition to ovarian or testicular slices. Luteinising hormone causes a rapid accumulation of cyclic AMP in slices of bovine corpus luteum. Since cyclic AMP mimics the effects of luteinising hormone on steroid genesis, it has been suggested that the cyclic nucleotide is a mediator of the action of the gonadotropin. In certain cases, this preparation is used in combination with Human Menopausal Gonadotropin (HMG).

Conditions that HCG and HMG may be used for include: Hypo gonadotrophic hypogonadism; delayed puberty (associated with the above); cryptorchism (undescended testis), sterility; selective spermatogenesis; corpus luteum inadequacy; and sterility in females due to absence of follicle ripening or ovulation.

Profasi and Pregnyl are manufactured for utilising the hormone produced by the placenta of pregnant women and is extracted and purified from the urine of the pregnant woman. Ovidrel (by Serono) has be produced using the latest in recombinant technology and is injected subcutaneously under the skin in pre filled syringes and is much easier to administer than older versions (of Profasi and Pregnyl) that required intra-muscular injections.

## Human Menopausal Gonadotropin (HMG)
## (Traded as Humegon, Repronex and Pergonal)

One of the key ingredients used in female fertility drugs is a chemical derived from post-menopause urine. In the early days of medical fertility drugs one cycle of fertility treatment could require as much as 30 litres of the stuff. Serono, one of the world's largest infertility drug manufacturing companies, reported in 1995 receiving 40,000 gallons of urine per day, collected by road tanker; most but not exclusively was supplied largely from Italian nuns' urine (Yes, 'nuns', you did read it right, what a mind-blowing thought – maybe the urine was divinely blessed! Isn't it ironic that post-menopausal women are able to help young childbearing age women to conceive is this way; how bizarre!)

The problem with urine-derived preparations is that they contain unwanted impurities and proteins which can cause allergic reactions. Furthermore, administering these drugs can be quite painful as they have to be injected directly into the buttock in large quantities, and necessitate daily visits to a clinic. Advances in extraction technology are improving with the newer generation of medication.

After menopause has occurred the ovaries stop producing oestrogen and in response to this the levels of FSH and LH are very high. These raised levels of hormones are excreted into the urine. The FSH and LH are extracted from the urine and purified.

If you are given HMG your ovaries should respond to the FSH in the preparation and egg maturation will take place. As a result oestrogen levels will rise and this provides a very handy method of assessing your response to treatments.

The oestrogen can be easily measured by 24-hour urine collection testing. The aim is to produce adequate levels of oestrogen. If the final oestrogen amount measures below 180nmol, pregnancy is unlikely to occur using this line of treatment. If levels are above 514nmol there is an increased risk of multiple pregnancies potentially occurring. (This is the medication that has usually been used when a large number of babies are born in a single pregnancy).

Having ultra-sound scanning after using HMG can assist in monitoring the number of follicles that are growing that can assist in assessing the effectiveness of the treatment. Dosage of HMG may be increased until desirable oestrogen is reached. Sometimes Clomiphene may be given with

HMG to enhance results. HMG only produces follicle growth; to bring on ovulation HCG is given. Intercourse should also take place about the time of the treatment cycle. If a pregnancy has not taken during that cycle and your oestrogen levels have risen very high, then HCG may be withdrawn to avoid complications such as hyper ovarian stimulation syndrome and potential multiple pregnancy.

HMG is used in patients with amenorrhoea due to pituitary failure or when ovulation was not satisfactory using Clomiphene though results are not as successful. A possible benefit of combined HMG/HCG therapy around ovulation time is an increase in cervical mucus production; this may be useful for women whose mucous production is not quite so good.

## Gonadotrophin Releasing Hormone (GnRH)

The hypothalamus in the brain directly controls the pituitary gland. GnRH is released by the hypothalamus normally in a pulsating manner. This signals the pituitary to release its stores of FSH and LH.

At times the hypothalamus may fail to function correctly and the GnRH may not be released in this pulsating pattern. The domino effect to this is that the pituitary will poorly produce FSH and LH and amenorrhoea will occur. Medically, a possible solution is to administer GnRH, though this will only be effective if it is delivered in the rhythmic pulsating manner to artificially mimic the action of a normally hypothalamus. Administering the GnRH is via a pump delivering system that is pre-set to pump GnRH into the body at a metered and measured time (every 60 to 90 minutes for about two weeks the normal length of a follicular phase) and dosage.

An advantage that GnRH has over other treatments is that hyper stimulation of the ovaries does not occur and multiple pregnancies are much rarer and fairly in line with the general population averages. Pulsatile GnRH may work effectively for hypothalamic anovulation and hyperprolactinemia, but not so good in PCOS.

Miscarriage rates and birth defects have been shown to be no different to normal percentages.

## Ovarian Hyper Stimulation Syndrome (OHSS)

This condition can occur in women who have had follicle stimulating hormone (FSH) injected for egg growth. Some ladies respond excessively to the drug and/or the dose given. If large numbers of eggs grow and are subsequently released, the high hormone levels coming out of these hyper stimulated ovaries combined with the increased size of the ovaries may cause a series of unpleasant side effects (to say the least) over the next several weeks. This combination of symptoms and signs is called *Ovarian Hyper stimulation Syndrome (OHSS)*.

OHSS can occur in women who have had ovulation induction where the ovaries are stimulated, the eggs released and then the woman has artificial insemination or intercourse. It most commonly occurs, however, in the IVF program when the ovaries are deliberately overstimulated to grow as many eggs as possible.

The incidence of significant OHSS occurring in woman during IVF programs is approximately 1 to 5 per cent. This level of OHSS means that the lady would be quite ill and may require hospitalisation. Almost all women who go through IVF have some of the minor symptoms of OHSS but these are usually managed at home with only minimal disruption to normal lifestyle.

### Signs and symptoms associated with OHSS
- Lower abdominal pain due to swollen ovaries.
- Increased abdominal distension caused by collection of fluid in the abdomen.
- Nausea, vomiting and diarrhoea.
- Fluid collected in the base of the lungs in severe cases causing shortness of breath.
- Increased coagulation of the blood potentially causing clots in the veins in severe cases.
- Significant fluid and electrolyte imbalance in the body.
- Dehydration on severe cases.

### How does hyper stimulation occur?
The cause of OHSS is still poorly understood. Some women seem to have a particular susceptibility towards OHSS and even with small numbers of eggs may have quite severe symptoms.

The majority of women usually need quite intensive ovarian hyper stimulation before the symptoms occur. It is rare to see OHSS in women who have less than 10 eggs collected in the IVF programs. The more eggs that are grown and collected, the higher the risk of OHSS!

A variety of hormones and chemicals that are released by the ovary and other organs in the body seem to change the permeability of small blood vessels in the body. This causes a shift of fluids within the body to places where they should not be, e.g. in the abdominal cavity instead of in the arteries and veins and in the tissues beneath the skin. This causes a lot of swelling and discomfort. As there is less water flowing to the kidneys there is less urine output and the balance of compounds like sodium and potassium in the body become quite disturbed.

You should contact your doctor if you are worried about OHSS and have any of the following symptoms:

- Severe continuing lower abdominal pain which is causing sleep disturbance and needing recurrent analgesia.
- Persisting nausea, vomiting and/or diarrhoea.

- Abdominal distension (swelling) which is causing discomfort and/or shortness of breath.
- Swelling of one leg, calf tenderness or chest pain.

### Mild Hyper stimulation
Mild OHSS is characterised by some abdominal distension and lower abdominal pain and can generally be managed by bed rest and mild pain relieving medication such as Panadol. Hydration should be maintained by good oral intake of fluids, approximately 2-3 litres of fluid per day

Mild fluid retention and lymph oedema may be benefited by drinking several cups of dandelion leaf tea per day and additional Vitamin C with bioflavonoids.

Eat small amounts of food, especially high protein foods, at frequent intervals. High protein foods include meat, fish, eggs, chicken, lentils and raw nuts.

Protein supplement powder drinks such as Sustagen are recommended prior and following egg pick-up procedures.

Hospitalisation is rarely required in mild OHSS.

### Moderate to Severe Hyper stimulation:
This level of OHSS requires hospital admission for observation and bed rest.

Medical treatments may include:
- An intravenous line to maintain fluids and to provide extra protein for the body.
- Anti-nausea/vomiting agents usually given by injection.
- Heparin injections given under the skin to stop the blood from clotting excessively.
- Daily blood tests to measure electrolytes and fluid balances.
- Paracentesis: This is a process which involves draining the large pool of fluid in the abdominal cavity with a Teflon catheter and is probably the most helpful treatment for moderate to severe OHSS.
- It is a relatively painless procedure performed under ultrasound control. Most women usually show marked improvement within several days after having the procedure.

Women with underlying conditions such as Poly Cystic Ovarian Syndrome (PCOS) are particularly at risk and should discuss the risks of this condition with their doctor if they choose to proceed with IVF programs. The OHSS does not decrease your chances of getting pregnant but is often associated with a positive result.

# Chapter 13

# *Miscarriage*

### *'The Silent Epidemic'*

To firstly become pregnant and then to lose a child can be a soul-crushing ordeal to experience during a person's life. For those who have sadly lost a child due to miscarriage, you will know the experience is a very unpleasant one and we all grieve and cope one way or another very differently depending on our beliefs and circumstances. The following information will hopefully shed some light about the reasoning behind why miscarriages may occur and what active measures that can be taken to minimise and potentially prevent miscarriages occurring in future conceptions.

A miscarriage by definition is the delivery of or the process of delivering a *conceptus* before there is a viable *foetus*. There are many different types of miscarriage that can occur, due to many different known and unknown causes. Here are some examples of the names used to describe the various types of miscarriages: threatened miscarriage; inevitable miscarriage; incomplete miscarriage; complete miscarriage; menstrual miscarriage; subclinical miscarriage; missed abortion; and recurrent (habitual) miscarriage

- *1 in 5* pregnancies now ends in miscarriage

- *1 in 10* pregnancies now end in premature birth or 'small for dates' babies.

- *1 in 30* infants are born with congenital defects (despite apparent improvements in diagnostic techniques). The Miscarriage Association in the UK estimates the miscarriage rate may be as high as 1 in 3 or even 2 in 5.

- *1 in every 250* pregnancies is ectopic.

- The harsh reality is that **5 out of 6 embryos** will not have survived out of 8 weeks gestation in the womb.

Each individual conception is uniquely a one-off prototype (in a sense), designed from a genetic blueprint that has never been tried before, therefore the struggle for life is fraught with many potential problems and complications that can go wrong within the microcosm of the human body.

## Chances of miscarriage

Week 1-2        75 per cent pre-implantation, 30 per cent post- implantation

Week 3-6        10 per cent at 14 day post ovulation when hCG reaches 50-80

Week 6-12       5 per cent (or less if heartbeat heard)

2nd Trimester   3 per cent (considered stillbirth after 20 weeks)

3rd Trimester   1 per cent (after 24 weeks)

***Miscarriage affects 12 to 22% of clinical pregnancies.***
IVF and medical assisted fertility procedures has an increased miscarriage rate in comparison to natural occurring pregnancies.

The majority of miscarriages (75-90 per cent) usually occur during the first trimester of pregnancy before 13 weeks.

***Causes of miscarriage*** are - chromosomal 10-50 per cent, anatomical defects 5-12 per cent, endocrine dysfunction (e.g. diabetes, thyroid imbalance) 10 per cent, immune coagulation 30-50 percent, and unknown 15-50 per cent.

***Causes of recurrent miscarriage*** (from medscape review) - anatomic 10 per cent; chromosomal 10 per cent; endocrine (e.g. luteal defect; elevated LH, FSH, Prolactin) 20 per cent; and immune/coagulation 60 percent. Elevated levels of uterine natural killer cells (UNKC) white blood cells has show to be a major contributing factor to a large percentage of recurrent miscarriages.

**Causes of miscarriage can be found in 50%/50% in men and women.**

***Genetic/Chromosomal*** - more common in older women and men; Environmental toxin link including: radiation; free radical/ROS link in both eggs; and sperm. Down 's syndrome and Turner Syndrome are examples of chromosomal abnormalities. Wilson's disease, a genetic condition affecting the liver, may also contribute to problems. Between 30 to 40 per cent of birth defects are caused by medical, environmental, genetic and psycho-social factors that could, to some degree, be prevented.

Certain individuals that come from various cultural backgrounds are more prone to different types of inheritable diseases. People from ethnic or Eastern Jewish ancestry backgrounds have a higher likelihood to Tay-Sachs. In Latino and African-American (or Negro descent), Sickle-cell anaemia. Caucasian white people to cystic fibrosis and people from Mediterranean, African, and Southern Asian tend to get thalassemia.

Apart from ethnic backgrounds that are linked to inheritable diseases, you may simply have a higher incidence of conditions such as autism or forms of mental retardation in your family, a specific gene that has been identified to contribute to these problems is the fragile X gene. Other forms of inheritable health conditions may include certain types of cancers, lung diseases, and neurological or neuromuscular diseases such as muscular dystrophy.

Our genetic code (put simply) is made up of a sequences of a 4-lettered alphabetic code (A, G, C, T) (A is always paired with T, and G with C) A – adenine, T – thymine, G – guanine, and C – cytosine; that are randomly alternated along the genetic chain. When there is a glitch in the coding sequence (e.g. one or more of this letters are out of place) then this will result in a specific genetic defect determined by the position this code break is located. The human genome has been identified to have over 30,000 genes on DNA chromosomes.

Scientists have recently discovered that the male Y-chromosome where many genetic defects are to found is not as weak and fragile as once believed. Studies have shown that this chromosome is actually able to self-repair by over laying or looping upon itself to regenerate. This is big news to geneticists and offers great hope, because Y-chromosome defects were previously thought to be incurable, but now there will be future research into decoding the genetic sequence and stem cell research.

These conditions may one day be a thing of the past with further investigations into this new era of medicine. Even though many of these aforementioned genetic problems may not be a direct cause of miscarriage or infertility as such, they are important factors that are well worth knowing about.

**Anatomical -** septate uterus (a wall dividing the cavity of the uterus into two or more compartments); fibroids; endometriosis; cervical incompetence; (the most common structural failure of the uterus in containing the pregnancy is a prematurely opening, dilating, cervix, called cervical incompetence). Hydro salpinx (also increases ectopic pregnancy risk); CVS and amniocentesis (esp. after 13>40 week) procedure.  Risk is higher in IVF patients and those with a history of abortion.

**Endometriosis -** increased risk associated with exposure to chemicals such as Xenoestrogens, and DDT. Reduced implantation due to macrophage defect, 50 per cent reduction in fecundity.

**Endocrine -** Luteal phase defect (LPDs) - low progesterone after day 11 of cycle high prolactin. High FSH and morning LH on day 2 of cycle. (Progesterone pessaries and human chorionic gonadotropin injections may be considered during the first trimester). Thyroid disease (over active thyroid gland –

thyrotoxicosis) can also be subclinical condition. Metabolic diseases such as: Diabetes; chronic kidney disease; liver condition – Wilson's disease; and Coeliac disease.

***Poly Cystic Ovarian Disease*** - associated with high LH androgens and poor body mass index (BHI). Low basal metabolic index (slow metabolism) and immature eggs. Dysregulation of leptin metabolism and/or function in the placenta may be implicated in recurrent miscarriages, gestational diabetes, intrauterine growth retardation and pre-eclampsia.

***Elevated BMI - very obese*** (over 35 per cent body fat) risk of miscarriage is extremely high, (over 80 per cent). Women with recurrent miscarriages have significantly increased prevalence of insulin resistance when compared with matched fertile controls. (Craig LB. KA.RW.Kuttab, WH Fertile Steril 2002; 78(3); 487-90).

***Poor egg quality*** - immature eggs due to early ovulation before day 11; polycystic ovarian disease; age over 40 years ovulation later than day 18 on cycle. An egg that receives poor blood supply is more prone to chromosomal breakages.

***Infection*** - fever due to systemic infection (bacterial, viral); food poisoning e.g. Listeria that can transfer to foetus; gastro intestinal infections; chlamydia; urealyticum primary genital herpes; hepatitis A,B,C; HIV/AIDS; rubella (German measles); cervical infections such as ureaplasma, urealyticum and mycoplasma hominis; toxoplasmosis; glandular fever; B streptococci; treponema pallidum; coxsackie virus; listeria; campylobacter (causes gastroenteritis); and cytomegalovirus (CMV). Medically, many of these micro-organisms are treated with antibiotics such as: metronidazole (Flagyl), tetracycline and erythromycin.

***Toxicity*** – cigarette smoking triples infertility rates and the risk of ectopic pregnancies and miscarriages is up to 50 per cent. Exposure to pesticides, heavy metals, solvents including cleaning products, alcohol, caffeine and decaffeinated drinks are also implicated. Elevated concentrations of chlorinated hydrocarbons (with long half-lives) were observed, especially in women with uterine fibroids, endometriosis, miscarriage, persistent infertility and hormonal disturbances. (Gerhard Environ Res. 1999:80 (4): 299-310. Increased risk of miscarriage associated with maternal serum DDE. (DDT metabolite) levels. Mercury exposure from seafood linked to infertility and miscarriage.

***Stress and related emotional states*** - Hypothalamus-pituitary-adrenal/ ovary axis link. Reduced/stagnated blood supply to/in pelvis. Spasm to fallopian tubes and uterus (impatient). Depleted kidney energy and adrenal function. 1st and 2nd Chakra issues – related to fear.

***Coagulation (thrombophilia) and Immune Factors*** – Antiphospholipid Syndrome – anticardiolipin antibodies, Factor v Leiden (the G1691A allele) and Prothrombin G20210A (gene) mutations, MTHFR C677T allele (which stand for methyl tetrahydrofolate reductase – is responsible for turning folic acid into metabolites that have several critical roles in the developing foetus and in the mother. This is a major reason why folic acid supplements are so important prior and during pregnancy. In males, this molecule can predispose him to increased risk of heart disease and oligospermia.

**Elevated serum Homocysteine** - Auto-immune thyroid, joint, CT disease, lack of blocking antibodies. T-Helper Immune Cell (TH1 /TH2) imbalance, (in both directions). Leucocyte population skew (CD 4, 8). Natural Killer (NK) cells and Macrophage dysfunction.

**Blocking antibodies** such as DQ Alpha may not be adequately produced that are required the stop the women's immune system from attacking or rejecting the foetus. Blocking antibody imbalances is particularly problematic when the mother and father share the same antibodies or the DNA is too similar. Lymphocyte immune therapy may be recommended as a treatment option.

**Natural Killer Cells (NK cells)** make up approximately 50 per cent of all white blood cells and are needed to regulate rapidly dividing cells such as cancer cells. Women who produce excessive amounts of NK cells may be at increased risk of miscarriage. NK cells give the body protection from cancer cells formation, but NK cells can also attack other cells that divide and grow rapidly, the fast developing cells of an embryo can easily be mistaken by the aggressive NK cell activity and turn on the embryo.

Treatment options to balance excessive NK cells may include: steroids; rheumatoid arthritis drugs (e.g. Prednisone); lymphocyte immune therapy; intravenous immunoglobulins; and natural alternatives like fish oils high in EPA, and Vitamin E.

**T-Helper 1/T-Helper 2** (Th1/Th2) cytokine ratio – are essential for maintaining correct immune system balance. If Th1 (autoimmune response) becomes to dominate in ratio to Th2 (suppressive response) this can greatly increase the risk of failed embryo implantation and is a major factor in recurrent miscarriage and infertility. T-Helper 1 is involved with responding to microbial infections: virus, bacteria, fungus and cancer. Treatment options may include: anti-TNF drugs, IVIg and natural alternatives such as fish oils high in EPA and Vitamin D. Fish oil supplementation has shown to inhibit TNF alpha and decrease cytokine production. Vitamin D is known as an immune modulator and regulates the T-helper cells and decreases the auto-immune response that is driven by excessive Th1. Vitamin D has also shown to increase the balance of Th2 cells that help to maintain pregnancy. Polypodium leucotomos is a fern found in Central America and is an effective remedy for Th 1 dominant tissue specific auto-immune conditions such as protecting pregnancies.

**Note**: Anti-phospholipid syndrome (or anticardiolipin syndrome) is a Th 2 mediated auto-immune condition associated with a higher incidence of foetal loss. In cases or recurrent spontaneous miscarriage, this should be eliminated as a potential cause before using Polypodium.

*Thyroid antibodies* – thyroid-related disorders are becoming an ever-increasing problem in society today. Women may produce antibodies that attack the thyroid gland and cause an abnormal reaction to immune T-cells. More and more evidence is showing that these thyroid antibody reactions may be responsible for contributing to causes of infertility, embryo implantation failure and recurrent miscarriages; even when thyroid hormone production levels are medically investigated as being normal. Raised blood levels of thyroid-stimulating hormone (TSH) are a marker for hypothyroidism, as are low levels of TSH being indicative of hyperthyroidism.

Faulty proteins that can be corrected with administrated replacement proteins are errors in the blood coagulation proteins *Fibrinogen* and factor XIII (factor thirteen), which are needed to provide the scaffolding for the newly invading trophoblast and therefore for construction of the placenta.

Blood levels of **anti-nuclear antibody** (ANA) are often increased in women with failed embryo implantation, recurrent miscarriages and in patients with Lupus (SLE). Anti-nuclear antibodies can affect structures within the cell's nucleus and attack cells within the womb and fertilised eggs. Treatments for anti-nuclear antibodies may include anti-inflammatory medications such as steroids like Prednisone. Break-throughs in gene/immune medicine is ever changing; these are some of the current areas being investigated: Leukaemia inhibitory factor (LIF); interleukin 10 (IL-10); regeneration and tolerance factor (RTF); vascular endothelial growth factor (VEGF); complement; and sticky adhesion molecules called integrins. LVF (www.riala.com - Reproductive Immunology Associates).

1. **Placenta praevia** – if the embryo attaches to the lining of the uterus, the endometrium, in the lower part of the uterus, the placenta will get into the way of the foetus during labour. This is known to have complications; a caesarean section can be needed for the baby to be delivered safely.

2. **Blighted ovum** – is a variation of chromosomal errors. Blighted ovum occurs when the placenta and amniotic sac develop and put out pregnancy hormones but the foetus itself doesn't develop. So you may test positive as being pregnant, but there is no foetus forming. Usually a blighted ovum will not progress past 11 weeks, and spotting may occur.

3. **Molar pregnancy** – or '*Hydatidiform mole*' may occur in one in every thousand conceptions. This type of chromosomal anomaly results in the egg being abnormal, as no chromosomal content are passed on and therefore is no foetus, only the placenta. The placenta usually grows very quickly; signs of pregnancy may be evident very early and have unusually high beta levels. To stop the abnormal cell division, a chemotherapy drug known as Methotrexate may be used. Molar cells can spread very rapidly to

other areas, not unlike how cancer cell proliferate. This condition can cause serious complications and future pregnancy attempts should be withheld for 6 or more months to make sure no abnormal cells remain in the body.

4. **Ectopic Pregnancy** – In an ectopic pregnancy, the embryo may be developing normally, but it is growing in the wrong place and the embryo has implanted somewhere other than in the uterus, usually the fallopian tubes. Ectopic pregnancies are not a rare occurrence – 3 to 4 out of 100 pregnancies are ectopic and the percentage has been rising over the last several decades.

When a pregnancy is ectopic, the normal pregnancy hormones are still produced and the HCG test is positive. Women who have a pre-existing tubal disease may be at greater risk. Further investigations to rule out an ectopic pregnancy may include having an ultrasound to find evidence if a pregnancy has occurred in the fallopian tubes or elsewhere other than in the uterus.

An ectopic pregnancy may show symptoms such as lower abdominal pain and discomfort, particularly on one side. Bleeding is common and may last for several days. Because the embryo is still forming, this can cause a potentially very dangerous situation as the fallopian tube can rupture and cause internal bleeding, which if untreated can be life threatening.

The embryo needs to be removed; this procedure may require undergoing laparoscopy with general anaesthetic. The fallopian tube will also be lost with this method. If the ectopic has been picked up very early in the pregnancy then drug therapies such as Methotrexate (commonly used in chemotherapy) may be trialled first. Even if a fallopian tube may need to be removed the chances of successfully conceiving again is believed to be approximately 75 per cent of the capacity if you were to have both tubes functioning.

5. **Placentae abruptio** – This is a term that refers to the detachment or coming away of the placenta from the uterine wall prior to birth. This condition is still not fully understood why it occurs but the condition appears to affect more women who are smokers, use recreational drugs, have had physical trauma, polyhydramine (too much fluid around the baby), severe pre-eclampsia, high blood pressure or are heavy alcohol drinkers. Signs and symptoms to be aware of may include: Vaginal bleeding; severe abdominal pain; tight and/or hard stomach area that is sore to touch. These symptoms may be an indication of blood pooling and clots behind the placenta. Seek immediate medical assistance in this situation. Ultrasound observation, medical oxygen, pain relief medication, IV drip and a possible blood transfusion may be required if the abruption is severe.

6. **Rh (rhesus) factor** – If both mother and baby are Rh-negative then there is usually no concern, but if mother is Rh-negative and the baby is

Rh-positive there can possibly be problems as the baby grows, particularly if some of the baby's red blood cells pass through the placenta into the mother's blood. Her body can then produce antibodies to the Rh-factor. These antibodies then can re-cross the placenta and attack the baby's red blood cells. This can increase the risk of the baby having abnormal blood cells, risk of blood transfer is usually more likely to occur being birth. Conditions such as Erythroblastosis may develop which can lead to anaemia, jaundice and even stillbirth. Medical treatments are available if risk has been assessed: an injection of a blood product called *anti-D* immunoglobulin is usually given within 72 hours of giving birth.

## Miscarriage tests for men

***Sperm chromatin structure assay*** – simply put, measures DNA breakage in sperm. If the proportion of the sperm cells in the sperm count showing DNA damage is more than 15 per cent, then sub-fertility or miscarriage is more likely. More than 30 per cent of sperm cells damaged are likely to cause sterility or recurrent miscarriage. This is a useful addition to just having a careful sperm count done.

The second structural feature the fertilising sperm endows to the embryo is the centriole, a minute rod-shaped structure at the head-end of the sperm's tail filament, or flagellum. After fertilisation the centriole replicates, forming the two poles that the chromosomes are oriented towards in the cell divisions of mitosis. Faults in the centriole mean faults in cell division, and faults in cell division mean faults in the embryo's constitution.

A study in Karolinska hospital, Stockholm, showed that males with 14 per cent abnormal sperm count contributed to 14 per cent miscarriage rate. But, males with 43 per cent abnormal sperm counts contributed to a miscarriage rate of 83/84 per cent (a compounding problem). These findings quite simply show that *the less viable quality the sperm is the much higher ratio of miscarriage* caused potential occur; this is why the male contribution to good conception should never be overlooked.

Even good sperm counts could possibly be improved to excellent sperm quality, thus enhancing the overall percentage of success to carry a healthy pregnancy to full term!

A major advance in sperm biology has been the advent of powerful *proteomic* tools, which basically enable us to know how cells work. Using this technique (Proteomic profiles) a strong relationship has been indentified between *reactive oxygen species (ROS)* attacking the sperm's DNA leading to oxidative DNA damage, which in turn impairs fertilisation, and results in poor pre-implantation development, increased rates of miscarriage and morbidity in the offspring.

This new technique can help with identifying better sperm being selected prior to ICSI procedures. Males taking in adequate anti-oxidant nutrients have shown great reductions in sperm DNA oxidative damage.

## Recurrent miscarriages

The term *recurrent miscarriage* is medically defined when a woman has had at least three miscarriages in a row, with no successful pregnancy in between. Recurrent miscarriage is believed to be fairly rare and only affects less than 2 percent of woman.

In 50 per cent of these cases an isolated cause may be detected. If a woman's LH levels are high prior to ovulation there is an increased the risk of a miscarriage.

The most common type of miscarriage results from random chromosomal faults known as *aneuploidy*. Aneuploidy is where there is an abnormality in the correct number of chromosomes; one or more of the resulting pair may have an additional chromosome known as *trisomy,* such as trisomy 21 or more commonly referred to as Down's syndrome.

Chromosomal errors that may have only one chromosome are known as *monosomy.*

A less common chromosomal abnormality is a condition known as *translocation;* this is where part of one chromosome is knocked off and ends up attached to another one. Generally, the cells where this occurs can still contain the correct total amounts of genetic material and the individual in which this occurs normally will not be aware of this condition known as *balanced translocation.*

In some cases, however, when the pair of chromosomes divides some may end up with either too little or too much genetic information; this condition is known as *unbalanced translocation* which may affect 2-4 percent of people with recurrent miscarriage and IVF implantation failure.

***In acupuncture*** the UB 42 (Door of the corporeal soul) point located three inches on both sides of the third thoracic vertebra is often used after miscarriage to help resolve grief and may help to resolve future conception difficulties.

**One of the most important tests may include**:

***Premenstrual endometrial biopsy*** – this test assists in establishing that there is a normal decidual reaction. Unless the lining of the uterus is hospitable to the penetrating blastocyst, the pregnancy has no hope of becoming established properly.

The procedure is performed during the month the woman is not trying to fall pregnant, with local anaesthetic and sedation I.V. The test assists to reveal the following information:

1.  That progesterone production in the women's luteal phase has been adequate,
2.  That there is no disease of the endometrium such as endometritis that is limiting it or which might indicate a infection that could cause miscarriage unless treated with antibiotics,
3.  That there is not an abnormal population of Natural Killer (NK) immune cells poised to mount an immune reaction against the implanted embryo, and
4.  That the material genes of the decidual reaction are intact. Some of the areas looked into may include – leukaemia inhibitory factor (LIF); interleukin 11; prolactin and the receptors; growth-promoting factors for blood vessels; and structural cells called fibroblasts.

*Nuchal translucency (NT)* – This is another test to access for chromosomal abnormalities. This involves using ultrasound technology to measure the fluid under the skin at the back of the baby's neck. The nuchal cord is primitive nervous tissue the runs along the length of the foetus spinal cord. If the level of measurement is above a certain level then there is a risk of chromosomal abnormalities such as Down's syndrome, spina bifida (spinal cord defect), Edward's syndrome and Patau syndrome. This procedure is usually performed between weeks 11 to 14 of pregnancy. If a high level of risk is ascertained then a Chorionic villus sampling (CVS) may be recommended to verify preliminary findings.

*AFP Blood Test* (Alpha-fetoprotein - AFP) – This test assesses the likelihood that an unborn baby will have a neural tubal defect, but cannot definitely tell if a defect exists. Blood is taken between weeks 16 to 18 of the pregnancy; after week 18 accuracy is less reliable. Alpha-fetoprotein slowly decreases during a normal pregnancy and present in the amniotic fluid surrounding the foetus in the uterus. A rise in AFP may indicate foetal distress, spinal defects, kidney damage or multiple foetuses e.g. twins. Very high levels of AFP detected in the mothers blood can possible indentify Down syndrome (trisomy 21); liver disease; cancers of the liver, bowel, stomach, ovaries or testes.

*Triple test (Maternal test or Bart's test):* This blood test measures alpha-fetoprotein for neural tubal defects and two other hormones to assess the risk of the baby having Down's syndrome. Abnormally high AFP may indicate neural tubal defect, whereas an abnormally low result may indicate Down's syndrome.

This test is usually taken at about week 16 of the pregnancy. An ultrasound may be recommended to support any pathology findings.

A new and easy Pap test has been developed by Gribbles Molecular Science that in initial trials has shown almost one hundred per cent accurate results in detecting a variety of serious chromosome defects such as Down's syndrome and cystic fibrosis to name a few. The benefits of this Pap test appear to have many advantages over older testing methods. One of the new test's major advantages is that it can be performed as early as six weeks into a pregnancy to yield accurate results. The nuchal translucency ultrasound scan and blood test are only of benefit from twelve weeks of pregnancy and only has 85 to 90 percentage rating of accuracy. Amniocentesis is performed around 20 weeks of pregnancy and chorionic villus sampling (CVS) from 10 to 12 weeks. This test should be widely available very soon and will be a breakthrough in early diagnosis for expecting mothers.

*Antiphospholipid Antibodies – (APAs)* – Antiphospholipid antibodies are the most common abnormal immune problem causing recurrent miscarriages. Phospholipids are glue-like substances needed in the early stages of pregnancy. Excessive blood-clotting APAs can affect the cells necessary that build the placenta and prevent embryo implantation. Antiphospolipid syndrome is a T-helper 2 (Th2) immune Dominate condition.

APAs in the setting of auto-immune diseases (e.g. SLE, primary APS, drug induced APAs), a variety of plasma <u>protein</u> antigenic targets have been identified.

APS definition – the person must have at least one of the major clinical findings.

1.     Venous thrombosis
2.     Arterial thrombosis
3.     Recurrent foetal loss
4.     Thrombocytopenia

A positive (+) lab test result for either ACAs or LA. Retest in 6-10 weeks following initial lab results to rule out transient APAs as a result of intercurrent infection or medications.

## Medical Treatments for APS: examples of protocols study:

In women with APS, the early loss miscarriage rate in the untreated group was 50 per cent; the treated group had significantly better results of 17.5 per cent using **Clexane/Aspirin medications.**

**Anticoagulants (blood-thinners) are one of the first lines of treatment options.**

*Baby Aspirin* (86-100mg) (e.g. *Cartia*) - may be used from ovulation on confirmation of viable pregnancy. Aspirin is part of the non-steroidal anti-inflammatory family of drugs. Studies that have investigated the effect aspirin has on preventing miscarriage and fertility, have yielded mixed results, particularly relating to dosages used. Non-steroidal anti-inflammatory drugs (NAIDS) normally used to relieve pain, can also possible cause a condition call *'luteinising unruptured follicle syndrome'* (LUFS). This condition prevents the follicle from bursting to allow the egg to be released from the ovary. Without egg release natural conception cannot take place, therefore can be a cause of infertility.

Medication-induced LUFS appears to be linked to higher-dose non-steroidal anti-inflammatory use. Conversely, low-dose aspirin use (100mg daily) has been shown to actually improve ovarian response as well as increasing blood flow to the ovaries and uterus. Pregnancy rates to women taking low-dose aspirin almost *doubled* and risk of miscarriage rate significantly reduced.

Like with all medications the correct balance of dosage can make all the difference between helping to fix the problem or it can contribute to actually causing the problem. *More does not more always mean better!*

**Heparin** (a carbohydrate-rich anticoagulant, 'blood thinning' medication) – Heparin is given as an injection under the skin. Its side effects, in addition to accidental or spontaneous bleeding, especially at the injection site, include a loss of some calcium from the bones. Rarely, but a potentially serious depletion of blood platelets and kidney and liver failure are also known. – (Supplementation with Calcium, Vitamin D, and other bone connective tissue nutrients can help to decrease Osteoporosis risks).

**Heparin/Clexane -** may then be considered. Combined with aspirin studies have shown double the improved outcome rate – BMJ 1997. Preliminary trials are taking place to investigate the effectiveness of an immunisation with *beta2 glycoprotein* (beta2GPI) in combating antiphosphlipid antibodies to increase the success of live birth rates.

**Herbal medicines** may include: to reduce blood viscosity – turmeric; hingko biloba; ginger; garlic; dan shen; dong quai; white willow bark; and gota kola; etc.

**Nutrients** such as: Essential Fatty Acids (EFA'S); fish oil; Vitamin C; bioflavonoids; zinc; and Vitamin E are also of benefit.

**Herbs for immune/allergy modulation prior to conception**: astragalus; rehmannia; reishi; shiitake mushroom; feverfew; hemidesmus; Siberian ginseng; withania; albizzia; baical skullcap; and liquorice. Chinese herb perilla frutescence (perilla seed) and mandarin peel (citrus reticulate) extracts are high in the flavonoid luteolin, which has shown to be effective in reducing T helper 2 (Th2) immune dominance.

**Cough Syrup** – This method is a little on the controversial side. Around the time of ovulation the cervical mucus should be thin and stretchy; though in some women, the mucus does not thin enough to allow sperm to get through the cervical bottle neck.

The rationale behind this theory is that using **pure cough syrup or guaifenesin (Robitussin, Benylin)** thins not just the mucus in the nose and chest but throughout the whole body. This may help the sperm to have a running chance at getting through to the egg and achieving fertilisation.

Imagine trying to crawl across a dry desert with no water, you won't last very long. A similar scenario to what the sperm would be going through if the reproductive environment is too hostile.

**Natural Medicines that may also be useful in thinning mucus:**
Herbs – white horehound; garlic; golden seal; golden rod; eyebright; ribwort; fenugreek; and horse radish.

**Nutrients**: Bromelain, Vitamin C, and bioflavonoids.

**Corticosteroid Drugs – Cortisone-like drugs, including Prednisone or Prednisolone**, are commonly used in medicine to suppress the immune system. These powerful medicines are potentially a double-edged sword. Studies to date have not been very endorsing of Corticosteroid use in preventing miscarriages. Though having perceivable benefits, these medications appear to actually do more harm than good in major trials. Premature labour, gestational diabetes and elevated blood pressures are among some of the complications observed. In situations of recurrent miscarriage due to elevated uterine natural killer cells (UNKC) steroid therapy may have warranted application.

**Progesterone** – No pregnancy can survive without it. In human pregnancy, it is made not in the ovaries but next to where it is doing its work, between the foetal trophoblast and the maternal decidua. Progesterone has beneficial effects not just in keeping the uterus quiet; it also directly and potently suppresses the immune cells responsible for rejection, while at the same time promoting the friendly Natural Killer (NK) cells, promoting the travelling extra villous trophoblast cells responsible for conversion of the material arteries feeding the placenta, and inhibiting the sequence of inflammatory events that precede the muscle contractions in the uterus that push out the pregnancy.

Therefore, having an optimal balance of this hormone indeed appears to have its crucial place in miscarriage prevention. Natural progesterone is available for use vaginally (needed to get high doses directly into the uterus) as pessaries or vaginal gels such as Crinone. Studies comparing the success of implantation and pregnancy rate after IFV procedures (during the luteal phase post embryo transfer) using progesterone only compared to vaginal micronised progesterone combined with 100 micrograms per day of transdermal estradiol. The results of these studies show significantly better outcome by combining both progesterone and low dose estradiol than using progesterone alone.

**Immune Gamma Globulin Infusions** - are collected and pooled from the natural antibodies from healthy individuals and are being investigated for their role in stopping hostile molecules such as immune T cells and unfriendly Natural Killer (NK) cells that may be involved in miscarriages. Normally, these immune cells are very important for protecting the body for cancers, but when they are overworking they can mistakenly attack the sperm or embryo and can affect fertility and contribute to miscarriage. Treatment with highly purified intravenous immunoglobulin (IVID) can assist in the body forming blocking antibodies to bring about a state of balance to reduce excessive immune cells some they can't affect the baby.

*Viagra* (Sildenifil) - is more commonly known as a drug used for impotence disorders. It has been reported that the drug has also been applied to assist with the thickening of the endometrial lining in conditions where it was considered to be too thin to maintain a viable embryo implantation. Conditions may include endometritis or endometrial atrophy. Research to date has been very sketchy in regards to its real benefits.

Viagra is believed to improve blood flow to the uterus, which may assist the endometrial lining to thicken. The endometrium can be examined via ultrasound or by having a premenstrual endometrial biopsy performed which may help to shown the action of oestrogen and progesterone on the endometrial tissue.

Individuals with a history of heart, liver, kidney disease; angina (especially if taking nitrate medications); and/or stroke may be excluded as a candidate to use Viagra or similar medications. Side effects may include headaches, flushing, blue haze in vision and indigestion. Many types of erection enhancer medications may also interact with other cardio-vascular, blood-thinning and antibiotic medications.

*Viagra suppositories* are a new innovation that are showing great promise as a better method of delivering Sildenifil directly to the uterine lining, bypassing many of the potential side effects the oral version may cause.

*Labour inhibitors* – Medications classified as Tocolytics such as: *Ritodrine hydrochloride, Terbutaline and Magnesium sulphate* are used under medical/ hospital supervision to prevent premature labour. These drugs work by relaxing the smooth muscles of the uterine lining to stop contractions occurring.

*Condoms* – The female body can develop an inappropriate immune reaction against the sperm, which can prevent it from even fertilising the egg. This immune response is basically the same as any allergy reaction, say, to certain foods or environments factors such as flower pollen.

The use of condoms during intercourse for a period of time can help to reduce the female's immune system's response to the sperm. This method can help to desensitise the allergy reaction, so at such time when conception is to be attempted, there is less likelihood of the immune system turning on the sperm or the embryo if conception is successful.

## Natural Treatments that may benefit in preventing miscarriage

- **Endometriosis** – Essential fatty acids; bupleurum; rehmannia; calendula; castor oil pack; and red clover.

- **Luteal Phase Defect** – vitex; paeonia; lady's mantle; Siberian ginseng; Vitamin B6; flaxseed; and progesterone cream.

- **Improve Egg Quality**: shatavari; ginkgo biloba; helonias; paeonia; cauliphyllum; folate; EFAs; Vitamin E; selenium; and CO Q 10 (increased folate levels may be required in older women).

- **Uterine Health:** wild yam; cramp bark; black haw; blue and black cohosh.

- **Stress:** withania; liquorice; Siberian ginseng; schizandra; motherwort; verbena; passiflora; zizyphus; valerian; pulsatilla; magnesium; and Vitamin B6.

- **Recurrent miscarriages** – homeopathic remedies may include sepia, and kalium carbonium.

# Threatened Miscarriages

## Natural supportive treatments
- False unicorn root (helonias); true unicorn root (aletrus); wild yam (dioscerea); paeonia; lady's mantle; black haw; cramp bark (viburnum opulus); and vitex – separately in morning. These herbs can help to balance the hormones, reduce spasms and cramping, tonify the uterus and reduce uterine bleeding.
- Herbs to help stop excessive bleeding: cranesbill; beth root; and shepherd's purse.
- Extra amounts of calcium/magnesium (balanced 2:1 ratio) can help to reduce cramping and spasm.
- Vitamin C and bioflavonoids can help to strengthening vascular integrity.
- Mild immuno-suppressant or anti-allergy herbs such as hemidesmus and albizia can be used if allergy reactions may be a factor in threatened miscarriage.
- Get plenty of bed rest (sleep on your *left side* to increase blood flow to the baby) if suspecting a threatened miscarriage.
- Avoid strenuous exercise and heavy lifting.

- TCM herbal formulas: Shou Tai Wan (Foetus Longevity Formula) – made from equal amounts of Tu Si Zi (Cuscuta), Sang Ji Sheng (Loranthus), Xu Duan (Dipsacus), E Jiao (Gelatin). Dang Gui Shao Yao San (Danggui & Peonia formula). Tong Jing Wan (Danqqui & Notogingeng formula), and Morinda combination.
- There are numerous individual herbs that may also have relevant application to help prevent threatened miscarriage: Atractylodes (Bai Zhu), Gelatin (E Jiao), Dipsacus (Xu Duan), Sangjisheng (Sang Ji Sheng), Scutellaria (Huang Qin), Eucommia (Du Zhong), Perilla fruit (Zi Su Ye), Amomum (Sha Ren), Cuscuta (Tu Si Zi), Artemisia (Ai Ye), and Astragalus (Huang Qi).

***APCA*** – *anti-paternal cytotoxic antibody test*: To determine whether or not you are making antibodies to your partner's white blood cells, that could be leading to rejection or recurrent miscarriage. Immunisation treatments are available to reduce these reactions.

***Diminished Ovarian Reserves*** (DOR) 'Fertility Potential'– Premature ovarian failure (POF) affects 1 in 100 women; it is recognised that genetics is the basis for this condition. A study of 1,034 patients with DOR with FSH level equal to or less than 14.2 IU/L only 28 (2.7%) conceived.

Four out of the 28 pregnancies (71.4%) were lost in the first trimester. Pregnancy loss rates in women with DOR were 57.1 per cent in women under 35 years of age. 63.5 per cent in women 35-40 years old and 90 per cent in women over 40 years. Significantly higher compared to age matched patients with normal ovarian reserve. Levi.AJ.fertile sterile 2001 1:76 (4): 666-9. The *anti-mullerian hormone (AMH)* testing is of significant help for assessing the degree of ovarian reserve.

### Self-help – things to do to reduce miscarriage risk

- Reduce or avoid: smoking; caffeine drinks; alcohol; excessive weight loss; exposure to toxic chemicals; excessively vigorous intercourse; and laxative intake. If an infection is suspected seek immediate medical attention to be on the safe side.

- The warning signs of miscarriage may include: spot bleeding or bleeding of any type; abdominal cramping; dizziness; burning headache; swelling joints; excessive nausea or vomiting; fever; extreme sudden fatigue; fainting; severe or sudden backache; pelvic pain; and sudden loss of pregnancy symptoms.

# Premature Births

One in 10 births are premature (under 37 weeks gestation). The cause of why premature births occur is still not fully understood. Research conducted during the last 10 years has largely linked *inflammation* as one of the major probable causes to premature labour occurring. The main origin of this inflammation is believed to originate from the oral cavity due to periodontal/gum disease (gingivitis/pyorrheal). The mouth harbours some of the nastiest micro-organisms in the body.

These micro-organisms release endo-toxins (xenobiotics) into the body that can affect many bodily functions such as uterine activity. These endo-toxins interfere with immune mediators and prostaglandins, which can induce labour and affect foetus white/grey brain matter development. Therefore correcting and maintaining good oral hygiene may be an important factor to consider as a preventative measure to avoiding premature births.

**Remedies for oral health may include**: Herbal medicines – thyme; sage; golden seal; Echinacea; myrrh; and neem (though has contraceptive properties).

**Nutrients for Oral Health:** zinc gluconate; Vitamin C; bioflavoniods; Co enzyme Q 10; lactobacilli/bifidus; Vitamins A, E and D.

**Nutrients for controlling inflammation:** quercetin (bioflavonoid); EPA/DHA (Omega 3 – fish oil); Vitamins C, E; beta-carotene; zinc; and selenium.

**Herbs for controlling inflammation** may include: turmeric; ginger; and rosemary.

**Other methods** may include: brush teeth using bicarbonate soda and salt, gum massaging, daily teeth flossing, and mouth washing with Listerine (contains benzoic acid), Closys11 (contains chlorine dioxide) and Colloidal Silver.

Other studies have shown that when women were given supplements containing folate, zinc and iron from the start of the first trimester it led to a 4-fold reduction in the risk of a very preterm delivery and a 2 to 7-fold reduction in risk of low birth weight. Similar supplementation that was started during the second trimester reduced the risk by half of that of the first trimester results.

Infant cardiac defects have also shown to reduce by 25 per cent when women started taking a preconception multivitamin during the first trimester.

After conception, embryonic growth is so rapid that unless all building blocks are present and toxins absent, vital stages of development can be compromised. There is growing evidence that suggests that the very first few days, even hours, of the embryo's life are of critical importance. During the first trimester, foetal mass increases over *2.5 million* times; during the following trimesters the foetal growth slows to increase in mass by *230 times*. This phenomenal rate of growth has exceptional nutritional requirements and there is mounting evidence to support the addition of extra nutrient supplementation to reduce the risk of birth defects and premature delivery.

Advances in neonatal care have come a long way in recent years; very premature babies are now able to survive from as young as 23 weeks gestation, which is an incredible 3 months prior to their true due birth date. In the future premature babies may also be saved from even a much earlier age.

## Causes for premature birth

- Premature ruptures of membranes (waters break early)
- Severe urinary/kidney infections
- Multiple pregnancies
- IVF and ART - have approximately 15 per cent chance of premature births compared to 6 per cent for natural conceptions
- Incompetent cervix (Cervix opening unexpectedly)
- Heavy vaginal bleeding
- Trauma (e.g. Car accident, or fall)
- Excessive over lifting
- Domestic violence
- Extremely stressful events (e.g. death of someone close, job loss)
- Excessive abuse of alcohol, smoking and drugs
- Many of the causes to why premature births occur are still scientifically unknown.

**I'm stuck on you baby**

Researchers have discovered how an embryo initially attaches to the wall of the uterus – what appears to be one of the earliest steps needed to establish a successful pregnancy. About six days after fertilisation, the embryo is shaped like a sphere. The surface of the sphere is made up of a layer of specialised cells called the trophoblast. At this phase of development, the embryo is called the blastocyst. The trophoblast later gives rise to the cells that will form the foetus' part of the placenta. The placenta is made up of both maternal and foetal tissues.

The trophoblast is coated with a protein known as **L-selectin**. The wall of the uterus is coated with carbohydrate molecules. The researchers believe that as the blastocyst travels along the uterine wall, L-selectin on its surface binds to the carbohydrates on the uterine wall, until the blastocyst gradually slows to a complete stop. After this happens, the cells that later become the foetus contribute to the placenta develop.

The placental tissue from the foetus then invades the uterine wall by sending finger-like extensions into it. These projections make contact with the maternal blood supply, becoming the pipeline through which the foetus derives nutrients and oxygen, and rids itself of carbon dioxide and waste.

The embryo's journey is arrested by the sticky interaction with the uterine wall. Some cases of unexplained infertility and early pregnancy loss are thought to derive from a failure of the trophoblast to properly attach to the uterine wall.

Findings from the study may also offer insight into pre-eclampsia. In this condition, pregnant women develop dangerously high blood pressure that may lead to convulsions and even death. Pre-eclampsia appears to result from a failure of placental cells to convert to blood vessel-like cells that perform their secondary function of conveying carbon dioxide, oxygen, nutrients and wastes between the uterus and the foetus. If trophoblast cells fail to securely attach to the uterine wall, then it's possible they may not successfully convert to this secondary function.

Tissue samples were taken during the women's monthly cycle both before the uterus is receptive to the blastocyst's implantation and at the time when the uterus is most receptive to implantation. The researchers found that the amount of carbohydrate on the uterine wall was greatest at the time when uterine receptivity to the blastocyst was greatest.

At the time of implantation, the blastocyst expresses much larger amounts of **L-selectin** than it does before implantation. Researchers then exposed isolated trophoblasts to carbohydrate-covered beads under conditions resembling those found inside the uterus. They found that the trophoblasts bonded to the carbohydrates on the beads. They also found that isolated trophoblasts bond more firmly to sections of uterine lining collected when the uterus is most receptive to implantation than to those collected when the uterine lining is least receptive. The researchers determined that the isolated trophoblasts were able to bond with the uterine carbohydrates for up to the 16th week of pregnancy.

Infection-fighting white blood cells known as leukocytes use the L-selectin on their surface to roll to a stop on the lining of blood vessels, which are coated with carbohydrate molecules. The discovery of L-selectin's role in embryo implantation means that the wealth of knowledge scientists have amassed on this sticky molecule can now be applied to questions related to early pregnancy.

There are now available several adhesive agents – **embryo glues** – used with some medically assisted reproductive procedures that are designed to mimic this attachment process that occurs when the embryo and uterus are connected with one another. Future advancements in the development and refining of these special types of adhesive agents will hopefully greatly increase the embryo's chances of sustainability and improve the success rates to couples that may benefit from the application of this substance.

## Amniocentesis/Chorionic Villus Sampling (CVS)

The amniocentesis test involved removing a small quantity of amniotic fluid (liquor amnii) the substance that is formed from foetal urine, faeces and the placenta. Amniotic fluid is necessary to help cushion and protect the developing foetus. The amount of this substance slowly increased throughout the pregnancy. The amniotic fluid is syringed out of the mother's abdomen using a long needle to be analysed for different genetic defects such as Down's syndrome. This test can also identify the baby's sex and is performed after week 14 of the pregnancy.

Performing these medical procedures may contribute to a significant miscarriage rate, which is higher in those previously infertile and/or with a history of abortion (conservative findings state 1 in 250 pregnancies). Many apparently resulting miscarriages seem to be ignored/unreported, so ratios may be higher than published. The blood tests, which now precede amniocentesis and CVS, have a high rate of false positives (and false negatives) results and can lead to unnecessary and risky procedures.

Other blood pathology has also come under some scrutiny in recent times, such as early blood tests in pregnancy that may be taking away some vital blood and nutrient supply that could be potentially robbing the uterine lining and/or placenta (when forming) from sustaining the viability of the embryo. Procedures also like excessive abdominal or uterine ultrasounds during the early stages of pregnancy have been under investigation for many years now. Individuals who have or were having previous difficulties conceiving should bear in mind that over intervention unless critically necessary many not always be the best course of action!

## Summary of common drugs that may be used in IVF procedures

**Clomiphene** – increases the natural production of follicle stimulating hormone (FSH) and luteinising hormone (LH), which stimulates the ovaries to produce follicles. It is taken in tablet form and the most common brands are Clomid and Serophene.

**Follicle Stimulating Hormone (FSH)** – stimulates the ovaries to produce more follicles and therefore eggs. Used in the stimulation phase of down regulated and flare cycle. Administered by subcutaneous injection and, increasingly, by an injection 'pen' version. Common brands are Puregon (in solution form) and Gonal F (in powder form and in multidose vial form).

There are four kinds of FSH available:

1.  Human menopausal gonadotropin which comprises a high content of LH, such as Humegon and Pergonal. These preparations contain contaminating urinary proteins that some people develop allergies to (they need to be given by muscular injection), and they can contain variable amounts of

Human chorionic gonadotropin (hCG) to make up the required amount of LH activity.

2. Purified human menopausal gonadotropin with low LH content, such as Metrodin and Menopur.

3. Highly purified human menopausal gonadotropin with absent LH activity, such as Metrodin HP or known as Fertinex (in the USA) and Menogon also known as Repromex. These are the newer preparations of FSH, free of the contaminants of early types of FSH products and are easier to administer.

4. Recombinant FSH with absent LH activity, that is, follitropin alpha (Gonal-F) and follitropin beta (Puregon, or Follistim).

**GnRH agonists** – these preparations first stimulate the pituitary gland to produce FSH and LH, thereby stimulating ovulation and then gradually suppress the natural FSH and LH hormones and therefore inhibit the pituitary from competing with the FSH injections. This group of drugs is closely related to the natural hormone gonadotropin-releasing hormone (GnRH), which is released by the hypothalamus in the brain every hour or so to keep the activity of the pituitary gland functioning. Their purpose is to prevent an unwanted LH surge but maintains hormone synthesis within the follicle. Used in the suppression phase of a down regulated or flared (initial increase in FSH and LH) protocol. GnRH-agonists are stopped when ovulation has been stimulated and triggered with hCG.

Common brands are: Synarel (Nafarelin acetate) is given by nasal spray usually twice daily and Lucrin (Leuprolide / Leuprorelin acetate) by daily subcutaneous injection. Other versions may include: Buserilin (Suprefact) by nasal spray usually requiring to be taken four time daily, Goserelin (Zoladex) and triptorelin (Decapeptyl), both given as monthly depot injections.

Skin rashes are an occasional side effect of these medications due to histamine release.

**GnRH antagonists** – immediately suppress the natural hormones and inhibit ovulation. These preparations antagonise the FSH and LH output without the initial flared phase as occurs with the GnRH- agonists. There are several types of protocols that may be used to assist conception in different ways: (1) Short, (2) Long, & (3) Ultra short protocols.

Common brands used are: *Cetrotide (Cetrorelix) and Orgalutran (Ganirelix).*

**Human chorionic gonadotropin (hCG)** - triggers ovulation and provides luteal support. Used in down regulated, flared, antagonist, and clomiphene cycles. HCG is the hormone of pregnancy and in early pregnancy acts like LH in stimulating the corpus luteum to make progesterone. HCG injection/s can replace and mimic the body's natural surge of LH, setting in motion the body's processes of egg follicle maturation to ovulation (to egg retrieval). HCG is administered by subcutaneous or intramuscular injection. Most common used brands are *Profasi* (by Serono), *Pregnyl* (by Organon) and *Choragon* (by Ferring), recombinant, synthetic LH (*Lutropin, Luveris),* some countries may provide recombinant hCG – *Ovidrel* (by Serono).

***Oestrogen (oestradiol)*** – enhances the development of the endometrium. Used in artificial thaw cycles and is taken orally as a tablet. Most common brands used: *Progynova.*

***Oral contraceptive pill (OPC)*** – helps to program the cycle and begin the process of suppressing the natural hormones. It is taken orally as a tablet. Most common brands used in conjunction with IVF are Microgynon *20 or 30 ED.*

***Progestogen*** – regulates menstrual bleeding. It is used to bring on a menstrual period and is taken orally in tablet form. Most common brand used is Primolut.

***Progesterone*** – supplements the natural production of progesterone and provides luteal phase support. Used in some stimulated cycles and within artificial thaw cycles. Taken either as a vaginal pessary, gel or administered by intramuscular injection. Most common brand used of injectable progesterone is Proluton and Crinone as a vaginal gel.

***Crinone -*** may be recommended for women who have low progesterone or luteal phase defects that may be contributing to infertility or miscarriage problems. Crinone does have some side effects including: cramps; abdominal pain; perineal pain (around the genital and back passage); headaches; breast enlargement or breast pain; feelings of severe sadness and unworthiness; decreased sexual desire; sleepiness; feeling emotional; constipation; nausea; passing urine at night; bloating; dizziness; vaginal discharge; itching of the vaginal area; vaginal thrush; diarrhoea; vomiting; painful sexual intercourse; and painful joints.

***Glyceryl Trinitrate – (Nitro-Dur 5)*** – Is a vasodilator medication that is more commonly used for the prevention of angina attacks.  In recent times these types of drugs are now being use in fertility and IVF preparation.  The vasodilation action helps to supply blood flow to the reproductive system.  By improving nutrient and oxygen to the inner layers of the uterus, the embryo when attached to the wall of the womb may have increased chances to develop due to enhanced uptake of nutrients and oxygen.  The Glyceryl trinitrate is applied to the foot area using a patch (transdermal delivery system - usually dosed at 5 mg).  The patch is put on the foot in the morning and removed before bedtime to reduce headaches as a side effect.

# Chapter 14

# *Plan C: Medically Assisted Reproductive Techniques (ART)*

### *'More than one way to make a baby'!*

*Down to serious business, life under the microscope. The high-tech approach to boosting your chances of success.*

Medically assisted reproductive techniques (ART) may be tried if all other methods have been attempted. Medically assisted conception may increase the chances of pregnancy as it can directly increase the number of sperm getting to the egg and/or increase the number of eggs available for fertilisation. ART requires an increased level of invasive intervention in comparison to other conventional lower-level intervention methods, though depending on the cause behind the infertility it may be a considered (sometimes only) treatment option for achieving the appropriate result.

Like all other forms of increased intervention procedures also comes the possibility of increased risks. So it is advisable to be well aware of the 'fors and againsts' of the various medically assisted reproductive techniques available and the types of medications used when venturing down the road of this line of treatment.

There are many different levels of assisted intervention that may be considered. Depending upon your particular circumstances you should consider beginning gently with the lower-tech treatment options first before jumping straight into the more high-tech options unless they are absolutely necessary. Thorough preliminary assessment will help to gauge which assisted method is right for you.

There has been much advancement in ART in recent years; some of these include the refinement of fertility medication to reduce undesired side effects and the development of better culture mediums to protect and maintain the viability of embryos (early embryos nutrients, Ph level, and oxygen requirements differ from older embryos), and the list goes on. Between 1.5

and 2 per cent of all conceptions are now achieved through ART. *(this does not indicate take-home-baby percentage).

IVF was first pioneered in Australia; since then Australia has also achieved many of the world firsts in ART. More than 65,000 IVF babies have been born in Australia, and 35,000 of these babies have been born in the last five years (2001-2006) (due to the pregnancy rate increasing 10-fold over the last 25 years from 4 per cent to 40 per cent). One in every 35 births in Australia is a result of IVF. During the last 12 years the utilisation of ART has increased by 77 per cent. There are now more than one million babies that have been born though IVF since *Louise Brown* was the first 'test tube' baby to be born on 25th July in 1978; British IVF pioneers Dr Patrick Steptoe and Dr Robert Edwards were the ones to successfully achieve this breakthrough technique. Louise is now a mother herself with her first baby born in January 2007 from natural conception.

Reports by the American National Center for Disease Control and Prevention (CDC) stated that in the USA alone in 2003, 48,756 babies were born from 122,872 ART procedures, which was an increase from 2002 figures of 45,751 ART births from 115,392 reported procedures.

Statistics correlated in 2001 by the National Perinatal Statistics Unit has stated that the average conception success rate per IVF cycle was 20.6 per cent; women aged 25-29 achieved more success with embryo transfer cycles resulting in live births with 34.7 per cent. Women between the ages of 40 – 44 years the percentage rate was 7.8, 45 years and over 1 per cent. Women using their own thawed eggs (about a third) achieved a pregnancy in only 16 per cent of cycles.

In 1991 a study conducted at Charles University in Pilsen, Czech Republic, showed an increase in Zona pellucida antibodies after failed IVF, as a reaction to egg (oocyte) collection. 20 per cent after 1 IVF attempt (same as non-IVF group), but 64 per cent after 2 procedures, 91 per cent after 3. This auto-immune response may compromise potentially compromise future conception, natural or ART. Most successes are on the first two attempts.

In 2004, the average age of women using ART in Australia was 35.4 years (up from 34.4 years in 2002); the average age of all mothers during the same years was 29.4 years. Of all births in Australia during 2002, 2.3 per cent were from ART. The average age of males involved in ART was 38 years.

During 2004 in Australia and New Zealand, there was 41,904 reported ART (IVF or similar technique) cycles started resulting in 6792 healthy babies born. This figure is greater than 20 percent up for the 2002 report. Just over half of women using ART used their own fresh eggs, with about 22 per cent of cycles resulting in a baby.

ART processors, simply put, are essentially a transport delivery system and ovulation induction method.

Recent studies in the UK by Foresight have showed that conception rates *doubled* for IVF procedures when the couples were incorporating natural pre-conceptual health care programs as opposed to couples that were not.

**Some of these techniques may include:**

### Ovulation Induction

When the primary cause of infertility is diagnosed as *ovulation dysfunction* and both the male and female are absent of any other obvious problems that may be contributing to infertility, then ovulation induction drug therapy may be recommended to help promote ovulation.

The woman will be given a course of *clomiphene* to increase the natural production of FSH which is responsible for maturing the follicles in the ovary. In some cases where the clomiphene has not produced the desirable result, the doctor may suggest a lose dose injection of FSH to complete the maturation of the follicle/s. The FSH injections work in most cases except in women that are menopausal.

The dose of FSH will depend upon how sensitive you are to it; generally the dose is quite low – aiming to stimulate 2-3 follicles at most. The doctor will request for the patient to undergo ultrasounds to monitor the response in the ovary and may even require blood tests, to check hormone levels especially oestrogen.

When ovulation is close there is a surge of LH which indicates you will ovulate in approximately 24-48 hours. This is the time you will be asked to have regularly timed intercourse to attempt conception. Some women may need to be given an injection of HCG to initiate the release of the egg from the ovary.

Once one of the follicles reaches approximately 18mm the injection is administered and ovulation will mostly occur within 48 hours. Some specialists may also recommend using progesterone pessaries or cream after the ovulation phase (luteal support) if the body's natural progesterone levels are low to help maintain the pregnancy when conception occurs.

As HCG is the hormone which is secreted by the implanted embryo, women who have had the injection to trigger ovulation may get a false positive pregnancy test result if a test is taken before 10 days of the injection. Therefore to avoid the disappointment it is best to wait until at least 14 days before conducting either a urine or blood test to confirm a possible pregnancy.

Polycystic ovarian disease (PCOS) and hypothalamic anovulation are some of the common conditions for which ovulation induction may be recommended.

### Artificial insemination (by the husband or partner's sperm)

*Artificial insemination (AIH)* is a procedure where sperm is injected directly into uterus during the fertile phase of the woman's cycle.

Medically advised for males with low or weak sperm count, this procedure may place stress on the male to produce viable sperm; the female must undergo insemination treatment timed to coincide with ovulation.

AIH may be considered when there are physical difficulties with intercourse such as impotence, paraplegia, or were the sperm cannot penetrate past the cervix to the uterus for one reason or another such as excessive scar tissue. Sometimes a uterus catheter may be required. Artificial insemination is considered when the woman is ovulating and there is no obstruction or damage to the fallopian tubes. AIH has shown to be not as effective as IVF if the sperm counts are low.

### Main points why AIH may be recommended
- The sperm motility is poor
- Cervical abnormality or sperm-mucus problems
- Anti-sperm antibody problems
- Unknown cause of the infertility

### Artificial insemination by a donor sperm, or (AID)
AID is typically used when the husband or sexual partner has a very low or zero viable sperm counts and fertilisation is not thought possible (the same as the above procedure but using donor sperm). The woman receives the donated sperm at the precise time in her fertility cycle. The 'father' responsible for the care of the future child is not the genetic father. Donated sperm may carry genetic faults/infection (despite careful screening).

### Blastoplast
This is a procedure where the fertilised egg is left to grow and cells to develop in a controlled laboratory environment until the embryo is five (5) days old, at which time the embryo is transferred for implantation using IVF technique.

### Embryo Transfer (ET)
This procedure involves having the embryo or embryos transferred into the woman's uterus after the egg/s and sperm have been retrieved and fertilised in the lab. The transfer of the embryo usually takes place two to five days after fertilisation. Depending upon the circumstances; the number and quality of embryos that are transferred will vary. Normally, less than two or three embryos are transfer at any given attempt.

If the procedure proves to be too successful then there may be a very high probability of carrying multiple pregnancies. This is an important issue that needs to be anticipated when discussing this treatment option with your partner and specialist.

### Frozen embryo transfer (FET)
FET is basically the same procedure as transferring a fresh embryo; the difference is that the embryo had been cryopreserved (stored in a cryoprotective solution to prevent cellular damage and frozen at minus 30

degrees C in a tank of liquid nitrogen) and then thawed before implantation into the uterine cavity.

### Fertility Drugs
Typically used for men with low hormone levels. A supplement of GnRH, a hormone that promotes growth and function of the gonads, is given. The success rate is not very high with this line of treatment.

### Sub-zonal Insemination (SUZI)
SUZI is a procedure used for men with low sperm count, no motile sperm, or immature sperm. Sperm is placed under the zona pellucida (protective coat around the egg (ovum) using a micropipette.

### Zona Drilling (ZD)
Zona drilling involves having a chemical applied to the outer ovum shell that dissolves the zona pellucida to create a small hole. Sperm is then placed next to the egg (ovum) so it can be penetrated for fertilisation to occur.

### Gamete Intrafallopian Tube Transfer (GIFT)
In this procedure, after ovarian stimulation and egg retrieval, the ovum and sperm (gametes) are mixed and transferred into the fallopian tube immediately, without waiting to see if fertilisation has taken place, usually via laparoscopy.

This method requires at least 100,000 sperm to proceed, therefore a reasonably normal motile sperm count is needed. Usually, it is needed to transfer 3 or 4 eggs to achieve results with this technique. Because of this reason, there is a higher chance of multiple pregnancies to occur.

GIFT is a procedure that is quickly falling out of vogue, as IVF and ICSI have been showing better results, though GIFT has had slightly better results than IUI.


### Mitochondrial injection technique (MIT) or Cytoplasmic 'mitochondrial' transfer – 'getting super-charged'
This is a new procedure that involves the extraction of a relatively small quantity of cytoplasm material from a healthy egg and injected into the recipients egg by ICSI procedure at the time of fertilisation.

This technique has shown warrant when the egg used for insemination appears aged and/ or resistant to fertilise.

The transfer of cytoplasm contains the energy-producing mitochondria (where there can be over 400,000 in a typical fertilised human egg), enzymes, and RNA/DNA molecules. Either of these may be potentially inefficiently functioning in the aging egg.

During egg retrieval (or pick up) the eggs are surrounded with cumulus and granulosa cells, which assist the development of the eggs. These cells are normally discarded but with MIT they are retained to be specifically treated to extract the mitochondria.

The granulosa cells are washed free of red blood cells after egg retrieval and then homogenised to free the mitochondria; the new mitochondria is injected into the egg to replace to damaged mitochondria.

This technique does have some criticism regarding what future effects or defects may possibly arise from the introduction of this small amount of foreign DNA from the donor egg cytoplasm (enucleated cytoplasm transfer). Many of the embryos that have received this super-charging appear to thrive much better and the increased percentage of pregnancy has significantly improved. Some clinical reports have indicated preliminary results have increased success of conception by 30 per cent.

MIT can utilise either the cytoplasm collected from other eggs from the prospective mother or if mitochondrial function is accessed as been compromised, then donor egg cytoplasm can be transferred. This procedure is very similar to that used in ICSI.

### *Intracytoplasmic sperm insertion or sperm microinjection (ICSI) – throwing everything at it plus the kitchen sink – 'a tough nut to crack'*

In this technique, which may be used if the male has a low sperm count, motility or there are too many abnormal sperm, the woman is injected with healthy sperm extracted from the testes while the egg is held in place with a suction pipette in a dish.

The sperm is microinjected via a thin glass pipette through the outer layers of the egg (mucous-*cumulus* that has a diameter about 10 times that of the egg itself and *zona pellucida* membrane) into the *cytoplasm* of the inner area of the egg for fertilisation to occur. The insemination phase of ICSI is very similar to that of an IVF procedure (that will be discussed soon). Micromanipulation of the sperm and egg has been a major advancement in reproductive technology.

ICSI may also be recommended if conventional IVF appears less viable due to the sperms inability to penetrate the outer layers of the egg and other factors such as sperm antibodies that may prevent natural fertilisation from occurring. ICSI is one of the newer techniques, and is said to be to probably the most successful and becoming one of the most popular medical procedures to date!

ICSI requires only 10 or fewer sperm to proceed.

### Main points why ICSI may be recommended
- The sperm numbers are very low
- Sperm motility is poor
- Antibodies to the sperm are present
- Sperm formation (morphology) is very abnormal
- Fertilisation has not taken place by other means or unknown cause

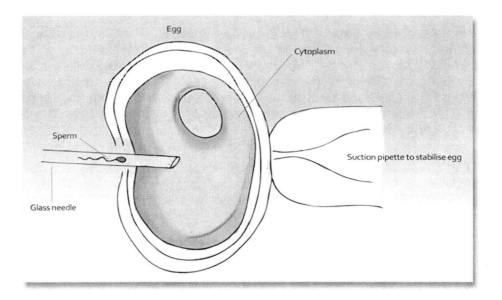

*Figure.20. Illustration of ICSI*

## Intrauterine insemination (IUI) or Intracervical insemination (ICI):

### Getting the 'turkey baster' treatment

This method is one of the first line medically assisted conception procedures used as it is relatively simple and less complicated than procedures such as IVF. A sperm sample is collected and taken to the lab where the sperm is removed from the other seminal fluid to purify the sample of excess cells and chemical substances such as antibodies. This sperm sample can be used fresh for an immediate IUI/ICI attempt or frozen for future application.

The sperm is then concentrated and 'washed' so that the best sperm are used for insemination. In this procedure the sperm is delivered into the cervical mucus, through the cervix into the uterus with the aid of a fine catheter and speculum at the time of ovulation. This procedure may also be performed with ovulation induction drug therapy if it is required.

The level of discomfort that the woman experiences is said to be very similar to that of having a Pap smear examination. IUI usually required about 1 million sperm to perform this technique. Research into treating sperm with platelet activating factor (PAF) for IUI appears to significantly improve pregnancy rates. The expense of an IUI procedure is approximately *10 times* less than that of more advanced procedures such as IVF and ICSI.

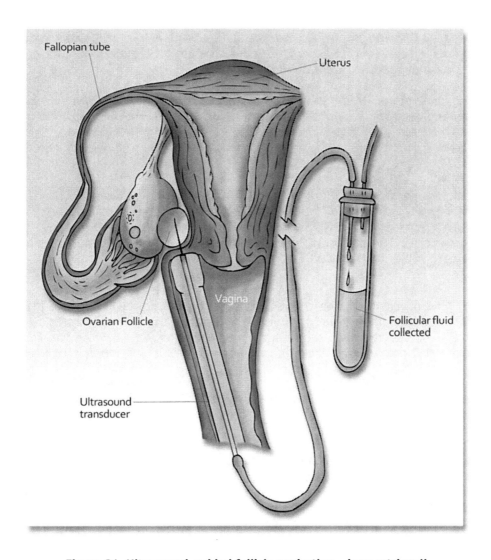

*Figure.21. Ultrasound-guided follicle aspiration – 'egg retrieval'*

# In Vitro Fertilisation (IVF) – 'A storm in a tea cup'

Here a women's ovum (egg) is fertilised outside the womb in a laboratory and inserted into the uterus. This may be done if the fallopian tubes are blocked. IVF require fewer sperm than IUI procedures. In regular IVF, between 50,000 and 100,000 motile sperm are placed with the retrieved egg or eggs (via a 'pick-up' procedure) in a plastic dish.

The sperm swarm around the egg and break down the *cumulus* layer. After 15 hours or so the egg is checked to see if fertilisation has occurred usually by observing the presence of *pronuclei*. If fertilisation has taken place the embryo should have divided twice containing four cells.

By day three stage, there should be eight cells (at this stage one or two cells may be removed to be examine for various genetic disorders). On day four, the forming embryo may have developed to 16 or cells. At this phase, the cells may have fused called 'compaction' and the dense ball of cells is now called 'morula'.

This morula on day five then develops a hollow fluid filled centre, the morula has now transformed to a '*blastocyst*', and this process is called blastulation. The blastocyst may comprise 64 or more cells at this phase and are now known as *blastomeres*. The blastocyst cells are now beginning to differentiate swelling and stretch the zona pellucida membrane to become thinner.

Some of the blastocyst cells stay in the inner mass that will later become the *foetus*. The others form the outer *trophectoderm*, which will become the first trophoblast, the placenta and later the afterbirth. For blastocysts to form to this stage of development requires a special culture medium, as the forming embryo nutrition requires changes. A glucose solution is needed to maintain and facilitate these metabolic changes.

Sometimes before an embryo transfer occurs, the blastocyst cells may start to expand and break through the shell of the zona pellucida membrane. This is referred to as a '*hatching blastocyst*'.

A blastocyst needs to hatch before it is able to attach to the uterine lining. In some instances the zona may be too hard for the embryo to break through normally (this may occur more commonly in women over 37 and embryos created in the laboratory compared to natural embryos) and the intervention with a micro laser or acid-tipped needle may be used to open the zona to help this process. Studies into gender outcome with blastocyst stage transfers appear to increase the likelihood of a *male* child birth.

This procedure is known as '*assisted hatching*' and is still not conclusively proven of its true effectiveness and there is some discussion that it may actually increase the incidence of identical, or monozygotic twins.

Blastocysts have shown to have a higher incidence of split because they are already hatching through the outer shell.

This may also lead to other problematic issues, as identical twins share the same placenta and sac, known as twin-twin transfusion syndrome. One of the twins may be deprived of vital nutrient supply and are at greater risk of being tangled in the umbilical cords. After embryo transfer have taken place, the implantation rate is quite respectable at approximately 50 per cent in some IVF clinic. Due to this reason, some clinics only choose to perform a single embryo transfer as there may be a much higher rate of multiple pregnancies occurring.

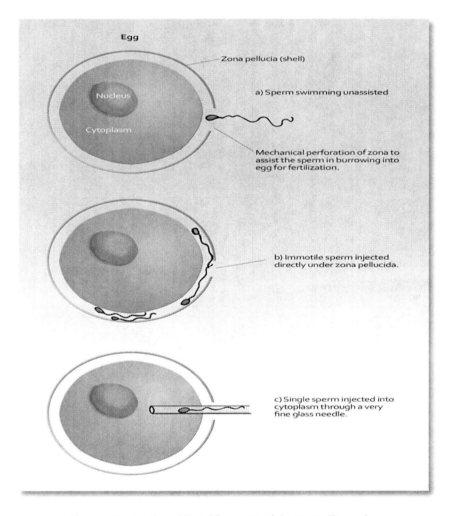

*Figure.22. Assisted hatching – particle zone dissection*

Some clinics may advise attempting to transfer a number of embryos, depending upon various factors such as the lady's age (usually the older you are the more embryos may be attempted to be transferred), the number of

363

stimulated viable eggs collected, the progression of the embryo growth, and reproductive history.

This is a serious topic to ponder over and you usually have little time when it comes to the crunch to make a conclusive decision. 'Be careful what you wish for', because if you go for the full shebang, you many end up with a few extra mouths to feed than you originally plan on all at once. Some may choose to roll that dice and play the odds to see what comes up.
The way sperm is selected for such procedures various between IVF clinics. Though, sperm that are more likely to appear normal in shape contain normal genes, as opposed to the sperms motility. This is not a fool proof method, some specialities state that even very abnormal-looking sperm can be genetically normal and have gone on to develop into healthy off-spring.

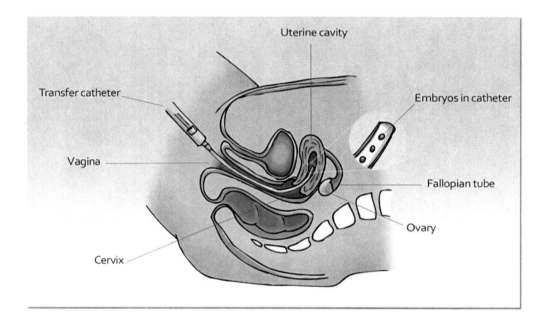

*Illustration of In Vitro Fertilisation (IVF)*

## Main points as to why IVF may be recommended:

- Anatomical or tubal problems that cannot be corrected
- Ovulation difficulties and significant rise of over stimulation due to medications
- Adhesions or inflammation problems that may interfere with fertility
- The sperm is being blocked by an obstruction
- The sperm number are low or sperm quality is poor

- The male may have had a previous vasectomy or a vasectomy surgical reversal has failed
- Unexplained fertility

### The main stages involved during an IVF treatment cycle may include:

- Suppression of hormones
- Stimulation of follicles and control of ovulation
- Surgical egg pick-up and supply of sperm
- Fertilisation of the egg/s
- Transfer of the embryo
- Luteal support for implantation

### Zygote Intrafallopian Tube Transfer (ZIFT)

In ZIFT the ovum and sperm are combined, and if the egg is fertilised, it is inserted into the fallopian tube.

### What to expect during a typical IVF/ICSI cycle

### 'The full shebang – warts and all'

A typical IVF cycle can be basically categorised into several different sections.

### 1. Down Regulation – 'Let's get ready to rumble'

Normally, IVF treatment may commence at the start of a menstrual cycle or alternatively in the 4th week of a predicted cycle. This will be determined when consulting with your IVF specialist. The first stage of the IVF treatment may be what is known as down regulation which there is 3 main types that may be used 1) *Short protocol*, 2) *Long protocol* or 3) *Ultra short protocol*.

Depending upon the clinic or specialist, many women who are under 35 tend to be recommended the 'long' protocol? Woman over 35 are usually put on a modified 'short' protocol. This is done to decrease the suppressing effect of the drug/s, as women over 35 may have fewer viable eggs and the aggressive natural of the drugs may have detrimental effects.

During the **short** protocol, treatment starts on about day 1 or 2 of the menstrual cycle with *GnRH-agonist drugs and FSH injections* within a day or two.

This helps to make use of the *'flare'* of FSH activity that follows the first day or two course of GnRH-agonist drugs to stimulate the ovaries. The short protocol may be recommended to ladies who have experienced over-suppression after trying the long protocol.
A down side to this procedure is that sometimes with this flare of FSH (that is normal at this stage in the cycle) can also stimulate LH to surge also. If there

is still some activity left in the corpus luteum that may be still remaining from the previous cycle many respond to this stimulation and start to produce fresh progesterone.

This could possibly last for a week and detrimentally effect the development of new follicles, their eggs and also the endometrium lining. The Ultra Short protocol involves stopping the GnRH-agonist after about 4 to 5 days. This helps to prevent losing control over the pituitary function and prevent the LH surge for at least a week after the drugs is stopped. This type of method may even further suppress the pituitary activity better than taking the GnRh-agonist continually up until ovulation time.

With ultra-short protocols, the trouble spots can be that the follicles may develop prematurely before the GnRH-agonist is stopped and LH may require to be introduced. Another hitch is that if a further dose of GnRH-agonist given after several days without it, a second flare in the pituitary activity may occur and can also increase the LH output that we need to actually stop.

A 'micro dose' of the GnRH-agonist may be given in a diluted saline form daily. This may be recommended for women who have not stimulated well from the previous cycles or have above-normal FSH levels, though micro-dose protocols appear to have a relatively poor response for women over the 35 age group.

The **long** protocol (as its name suggests) involves starting to take the GnRH-agonist many days, if not weeks, before the FSH injections are started.

This will allow a wider window of opportunity to suppress or wind down the pituitary activity and allows more flexibility with times of the day in which to retrieve the egg. Egg retrieval usually will take place two weeks after the start of the FSH injection. This method can be started at the commencement of menstruation or even a week or so earlier (mid-luteal phases). This can allow the serum oestrogen and progesterone to be monitored, and the FSH injections are not begun until they are both suppressed.

A potential problem when starting a long protocol is that the flare at the start of the cycle can produce transient ovarian cysts with the development of the follicles. There are various GnRH-agonist products that are available, and depending on what country you're in or what your specialist may prefer to use, these drugs go by different names.

Some of these may include: Leuprorelin (Luctin, Leuprolide, Lupron), given as injections under the skin; Nafarelin (Synarel) by nasal spray; Buserilin (Suprefact) by nasal spray; Goserelin (Zoladex), Triptorelin (Decapeptyl) by monthly depot injections; and Signarel.
GnRH-agonists basically are used to block LH surge so that ovulation is temporarily stopped by stimulating the pituitary gland and then de-sensitises it so that the FSH and LH from the pituitary levels decrease.

Your IVF specialist may prefer to choose an alternative type of drugs called a GnRH-antagonist. Some of these drugs include: Cetrorelix (cetrotide); and Ganirlix (orgalutran). This drug is used to prevent premature ovulation by decreasing levels of FSH and LH, but without first causing a flare. This type of drug only needs to be taken for a short time, several days, and may be started on about day 9 of cycle closure to egg retrieval.

Women who can't tolerate large dosages of medications, or due to certain previous illnesses such as breast cancer, may also attempt what is referred to as the *'natural'* protocol; this involves taking little to no drugs prior to egg retrieval.

During the early stages of the IVF treatment protocols, the male at this stage may be required to supply a sperm sample to be tested and examined for the sperm 'swim up' method to assess viability. Research using a developed carbohydrate-antioxidant hybrid polymer has shown to deliver Vitamin E to sperm and is prolonging the sperm's viability; future studies into this polymer may prove very beneficial to enhancing sperm longevity.

## 2. Stimulating Ovulation – 'there she blows . . .!'

The next stage in the treatment protocol is the introduction of ovary-stimulating drugs to 'trigger' the pituitary hormones to stimulate ovulation. During this stage drugs such as *gonadotrophins*, or *follicle-stimulating hormone (FSH)*, are usually prescribed (taken twice daily if oral or once daily by injection). There are recombinant drugs such as Follistim and Gonal-F that are completely made by non-human protein in the lab. These drugs are able to injected subcutaneously and less invasive than older types of gonadotropins such as Humegon, Menogran, Menopure and Purgonal.

The newer recombinant drugs are more expensive, but contain nearly pure FSH, without the LH as in the older varieties that are made from purified urine from post-menopausal women. There are now newer versions of this type of drug made from highly purified human urine such as Bravelle, which is nearly as pure as recombinant drugs.

Other types of ovarian stimulating drugs include: Anti-oestrogen drugs - Clomid, Serophene, and Tamoxifen (Novadex); FSH – Metrodrin highly purified, Puragon; Luteinising Hormone Releasing Hormone (LHRH) - Fertiral and Bromocriptine (Parodel)

Human chorionic gonadotropin (hCG) is known as the 'hormone for pregnancy' and can be given by injection to replace the natural LH surge. The introduction of the drug will cause the egg in the mature follicle to be fertilisable, and trigger the ovulation process. This makes egg retrieval easier as the egg should come away with the aspirated follicular fluid. HCG is used to mimic the LH surge and lasts longer than the natural LH surge so less dosage needs to be given.

The types of hCG preparations that are available include: Pregnyl, Profasi, and Choragon, and Ovidrel (Recombinant hCG). The dosages used for these drugs are best to be discussed with your specialist as differing centres may recommend different dosages. As a guide you may need to be on hCG for approximately 10 days.

Ovulation usually occurs approximately 38 hours or so after the hCG injection (at the appropriate dose). After about 34 hours the eggs are mature and should be floating freely in the follicle. The egg retrieval procedure would then be booked in to be performed around 36 hours after the injection. One of the major downsides to using hCG is that it can cause ovarian hyper stimulation syndrome (OHSS) that is potentially very dangerous (especially in women who are very young or have polycystic ovaries).

Sometimes getting exactly the right dose to suit the individual is more art than an exact science (it's not perfect), but occasionally things may not necessarily go to plan and you may get too much of a good thing and overshoot the mark *(what should work in theory does not always work in reality)*.

If your estradiol rises too quickly, or if you make too many follicles (e.g. 20 or more) OHSS can develop after egg retrieval causing fluid to build up in the pelvis and around the lungs, potentially unbalancing your body's fluid volume and causing increased blood viscosity and clotting. On occasions when higher dosages of FSH are required, the incorporation of low amounts of LH may be recommended to reduce the incidence of OHSS from occurring and to protect the integrity of the developing egg. When a woman's ovarian response to rFSH was suboptimal, adding rLH may result in more eggs retrieved than increasing the dose of rFSH. Starting dosages of FSH usually range between *150 – 250 IU* per day.

### 3. *Monitoring Egg Development – 'tracking events'*

There are several methods that may be used to monitor how the ovary is responding to the drug treatments by measuring and remeasuring the amount of oestrogen in the blood and using a transvaginal ultrasound to visually see the number and size of the ovarian follicles. Monitoring is a handy tool to help troubleshooting any foreseeable problems such as OHSS and can assist in diagnosing when the best times are to administer drugs such as hCG to achieve correct follicle maturation at the right time to retrieve healthy eggs. The monitoring process may begin from the start of your menstrual cycle.

Blood tests to examine your estradiol, progesterone, and LH are done as well as a possible pregnancy test to rule out that the actual bleeding is from a true menstrual bleed and not caused by something else such as a miscarriage or ectopic pregnancy; all these hormones should be low at this stage.

Monitoring the ovaries after the embryo transfer has taken place is used to assess that there is adequate production of progesterone to maintain the pregnancy. This is done also via another blood test to evaluate the serum progesterone levels.

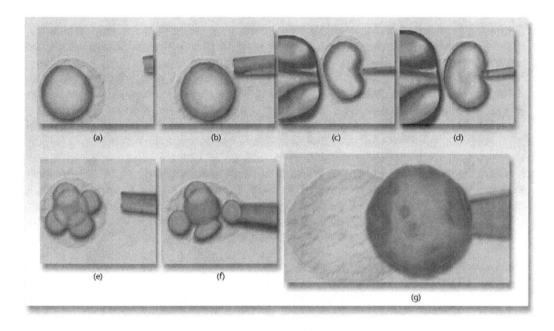

**Figure.23. Micromanipulation of egg to embryo**

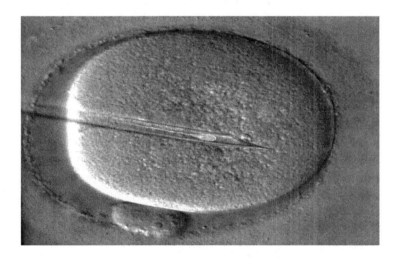

If progesterone levels begin to fall that can indicate a luteal phase defect, then extra progesterone may be needed to boost or substituted lagging progesterone to maintain correct levels. Examples may include: progesterone pessaries; Prometrium capsules; creams such as Crinone, Cycologest; or an additional small dose of hCG may also be considered.

**Grading an Embryo**

*'Finding the diamond in the rough'*

Some IVF centres have a grading system to evaluate the potential quality of a forming embryo; this grading process assists in the selection criteria of picking a well-developing embryo if insemination is required.

***Graduated Embryo Scoring (GES)*** – is a microscopic method for assessing embryo quality. With the GES technique, each embryo is separately examined through a series of microscopic assessments throughout a period of 72 hours following egg insemination. A GES grading score is determined that is scaled to a maximum of 100. The embryos of a women under the age of 40 with a 70 plus GES score have better than 35 per cent likelihood of implantation being successful. In comparison when the GES score is under 70 the percent of implantation is less than 20 per cent. Embryos that have a higher likelihood of implanting successfully appear to have the presence of sHLA-G (soluble human leukocyte antigen-G) in the media surrounding each embryo.

***Embryo Marker Expression Test (EMET)*** – this test measures the genetic marker sHLA-G concentration that is released for from the early developing embryos into the culture media. The EMET is performed 48 hours after the egg retrieval to identify 'competent' or EMET-positive embryos. Studies have reported that single transfers of EMET-positive embryos resulted in 60 per cent pregnancy rate in women under 39 years of age. In women aged between 39 to 43 years the success rate was above 40 per cent.


**Looking for the best embryos to transfer**

*'Survival of the fittest'*

The best-looking embryos are graded as a 1A, with 1 through 3 being the size of the cells and A through D being the degree of fragmentation. (Different levels may be used by different clinics). Some embryologists may choose to do a three-day transfer; if the embryo has reached the 10 to 30 cell division stage then it is classed as a *morula*. Morulas usually have a very high rate of implantation, similar to blastocysts; in fact they are the embryo stage right before blastocyst.

Only a very few number of embryos are usually graded 1A; most embryos that are at least 4 cells are graded 2B or C. These embryos also have a decent chance of implanting as well. The following types are usually not considered for implantation: *Multinucleated embryos* – contains 3 or more 'bundles' of genetic material: at least 75 per cent are abnormal. Embryos with *uneven pronuclei*: abnormality is about 85 per cent. *Embryos that develop too rapidly:* There may be a large number of chromosomes that are abnormal.

When implantation is attempted using procedures such as IVF the uterus lining is usually observed via an ultrasound to assess if the lining appears ready to attempt an implant. Embryos have been shown to implant on lines as thin as 3 to 4 millimetres, though as a rule of thumb a thickness of a least 7 millimetres is usually preferred. The lining may be described as triple lined or *tri-laminar (TL)* that is most often seen to have the best results; the next is *isoechogenics (IE)* pattern, and then *homogenous hyper echoic (HH) pattern*, which has the poorest response.

Choosing to transfer on day 3 versus day 5 – there have been many advances in culture mediums that have allowed embryo development to be more successful than in previous years of sustaining the developing blastocyst. One of the downsides to day 5 blastocyst transfers is that even with these culture advancements, they do not provide all the growth factors that can ideally mimic that of the natural environment of the fallopian tubes. Development of embryos (in vitro) to day 3 in most IVF clinics is estimated to be in the vicinity of 90 per cent.

Blastocyst development to day 5 has been reported to be around the 50% range. Therefore from day 3 to 5 there is a dramatic embryo loss percentage prior to transfer. The upside to blastocysts that survive to day 5 giving the sub-optimal development environment and are of high quality grading may be predestined to develop further when transferred into a more ideal natural environment!

Day 5 transfers are a relatively newer procedure' you should discuss the 'pros and cons' with your fertility specialist and/or geneticist to further understand which method is right for you. Prior to transfer an *endometrial function test* may be recommended by your specialist to assess the endometrium's potential to support implantation and its ability to contribute to the nutrition of the developing embryo.

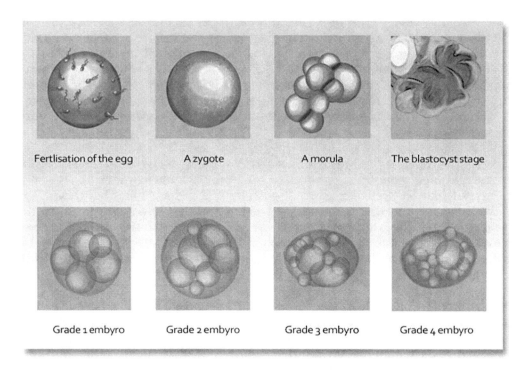

| | | | |
|---|---|---|---|
| Fertlisation of the egg | A zygote | A morula | The blastocyst stage |
| Grade 1 embyro | Grade 2 embyro | Grade 3 embyro | Grade 4 embyro |

*Grading stages of embryo cell division*

## Pre-implantation Genetic Diagnosis (PGD)

Normally in IFV, the embryologist chooses which embryo/s will be transferred to the uterus based on visual observation of the embryo as it develops. PDG allows the scientist to base their choice of embryo selection on the results of these genetic tests.

### Types of genetic disease
1) Chromosome errors e.g. Down syndrome, translocation
2) Errors with in gene e.g. Cystic fibrosis, myotoud dystrophy
3) Errors with in mitochondria
4) Errors in more than one gene

PDG requires the biopsy of cells from the embryos that have been produced from IVF procedures for analysis. Only one to four cells are required depending on the embryo's development stage e.g. 3 days (6 to 8 cells) to 5 days (100 cells). At this stage of embryo development the individual cells have not differentiated into specific tissues, therefore are representative of all other embryo cells at the stage. If one cell's genetic material is analysed as abnormal, then the embryo is classed as abnormal 'Mosaicism'. PGD does not measure the sHLA-G produced by the embryos in culture media, therefore this

372

analysis does not identify if the embryo is competent to adhere to the uterine lining upon transfer.

**The Most Common Tests Used:**

### Fluorescent in sit hybridisation (FISH)
This test involves counting the number of chromosomes and observing their arrangement. The FISH probes adhere to a particular chromosome; each probe has a particular colour. When viewed under a UV light, the probes appear as coloured dots on the cell nucleus. The geneticist counts these dots to tell how many chromosomes are present.

The removal of these cells from the embryo does not affect the embryo's normal development. An example of this can be used for Down's syndrome that has an extra copy of the chromosome 21. The FISH analysis can show an affected embryo's cells with 3 glowing dots in the colour corresponding with chromosome 21.

### Polymerase Chain Reaction (PCR)
This analysis is to detect if problems are at a genetic level rather than at a chromosomal level. PCR makes millions of copies of a part of the DNA code, enabling the geneticist to see whether this part of the DNA in the sample is normal or not! E.g. Cystic fibrosis is caused by gene mutation.

These procedures may be of benefit particularly if either one of the couple has, or is a carrier of, a diagnosed genetic mutation that has been identified, or if recurrent miscarriages have occurred from IVF procedures, to rule out suspected genetic causal factors. At present only a limited number of genetic problems can be identified using current PGD technology. Advancements in these procedures are constantly emerging and in the future many more genetic diseases will be able to be detected and PGD will be used more routinely to improve IFV success rates.

Types of genetic abnormalities that can be currently tested by using PGD: a-l-antitrypsin deficiency; Chatcot-Marie-Tooth disease; Cystic fibrosis; Down's syndrome; Duchene muscular dystrophy; Fragile X syndrome; haemophilia A; Lesch Nyham syndrome; retinitis pigmentosa; sickle-cell anaemia; Tay-Sachs disease; and Turner's syndrome. Many other genetic abnormalities will also be able to be detected in the near future with constant advancement in testing technology.

Oocyte karyotyping by **Comparative Genomic Hydrydization (CGH)** provides a highly reliable method for selecting 'competent' embryos; this breakthrough technique is headed by Geoffrey Sher M.D of the Sher Institute of Reproductive Medicine, Las Vegas, Department of Obstetrics and Gynaecology, University of Nevada School of Medicine, Reno. The results thus far are showing that by transferring euploid embryos has markedly improved

IVF outcome, these findings, if corroborated, could initiate a paradigm shift in assisted reproductive technology (ART).

## When going through with the embryo transfer

*'A Date with Destiny'*

For the actual embryo transfer you arrive at the IVF clinic and the staff will help you get prepped for the procedure. Your doctor or embryologist will discuss with you what will go on throughout the transfer stage and may advise you on how the embryos are looking and the number of embryos you agree upon to proceed with in the transfer.

Many centres prefer to do the transfer with the assistance of ultrasound guidance; this may mean that you have to fill up with lots of water prior to the procedure so that the bladder is full. This helps the doctor to see with more accuracy, and the full bladder may assist in pushing the uterus up giving a straighter path for insertion into the uterus. When you lie down for the procedure, having a full bladder may feel uncomfortable.

Many ladies when going in to attempt a transfer are usually feeling undoubtedly stressed and anxious, not only about the procedure itself but also the anticipation of the success of the final outcome after the procedure.

There are several acupuncture techniques that may be beneficial to try in your preparation before IVF embryo transfer. LI 4, Lv 3, Pc 6, Sp 6, Sp 8, Sp 10, St 36, St 29, and points on the upper and lower segments of the ear are most commonly used. These points may help to regulate the endocrine system, improve the uterus's ability to accept an embryo, and to calm the state of stress.

Some centres may recommend muscle relaxant medication such as Valium (or similar) prior to the transfer as it may help to decrease undesirable muscle cramping, spasming and assist in taking the edge off the anxiety.

The ultrasound probe is place upon your abdomen and the cervix area may be washed to remove mucus from around the opening. A speculum is left in place and a catheter containing the embryos is inserted through the cervix opening and guided into the uterus (via the ultrasound) to find a suitable location to slowly inject the embryos into the uterus. Some cramping sensations are usually experienced during this stage of the procedure, so that Valium you may have taken earlier should have kicked in nicely and is earning its keep by smoothing some of the discomfort.

The catheter is slowly removed and checked to reassure that all embryos have in fact been transferred correctly. After the transfer has been done, some clinics may require you to stay lying on the table for a time. When it's time to leave the clinic you may be advised to restrict strenuous activity for a period of time and should get some reasonable bed rest on your arrival home.

Also when you get home you will more than likely need to empty the bladder and/or bowels. This will not affect the implantation of the embryos and in fact can minimise the negative effects of uterine cramping which can be a potential problem.

By this stage of the whole process you may feel a bit sick and tired of being a human pin cushion, and having to be drugged up to the eyeballs with these chemical cocktails. It is now time for you to take some personal 'me' time to rest, recover, and let nature take its course. Studies into the amount of immediate rest after an IFV embryo transfer compared a 1-hour rest period to a 24-hour rest period. The results for this study were indeed surprising with the shorter rest period group having much more success than the longer rest group in carrying the pregnancy. A rationale for this may be the importance of adequate blood and oxygen supply to endometrial lining post transfer, possibly being sedentary after the procedure may potentially hinder this adequate blood flow during these early stages.

Sexual activity, heavy lifting, and excessive exercise should all be put on hold until you get a bit further down the track. So no bungy jumping, sky diving or kick boxing for a while. You may find that your partner, family and friends may want to sometimes over-involve themselves in this 'event'. It may be best in the early stages to back off from major social situations to allow yourself time to recharge both emotionally and physically. Find simple things to do to keep yourself occupied and entertained to pass the time such as catching up on some reading or so on.

If there is anything that going through IVF or ICSI will teach you is 'time management skills' and to become 'very patient', as the waiting game is mind numbing. Many ladies that are going through medically assisted reproductive procedures may be working or have other commitments to attend to. Your reproductive system time schedule and your personal life time schedule will not necessarily go hand in hand with one another and you may find yourself running around like a chook with its head cut off if you don't anticipate and plan your time well!

Try to maintain a positive outlook and keep things as stress free as possible!

## The pregnancy result

### And the winner is ...?
If you haven't had a nervous breakdown and have survived all the fun and games before today, it now comes down to reading the results.
If you haven't started to bleed heavily within the few weeks after the embryo transfer, your IVF clinic will call you back in to perform a urine test. Many ladies will probably do this at home, as the home tests nowadays are very

accurate, or a blood test to detect the pregnancy hormone *Beta hCG* (that is secreted by the blastocyct into the mother's bloodstream after implantation that signals a successful conception).

If it is present then:

# 'Congratulations, you are Pregnant'

*Or in other less technical words you're 'up the duff' or if you prefer you're 'knocked up' or 'have a bun in the oven'!*

*Possibly some of the sweetest words you'll ever hear!*

The level of hCG begins at 5 IU/litre and roughly doubles ever two to three days. When the level of hCG has reached between 50 to 80 IU/L, this can then be verified as a positive result from a urinary pregnancy test.

This level is normally reached about the time the next menstrual cycle was due, approximately 10 to 14 days after conception. Blood tests can detect positive pregnancy results from as early as eight days after conception with levels of 25 IULml or more. If the hCG levels are higher than expected for the dates than this may indicate that the pregnancy is further advanced, or perhaps a multiple pregnancy (e.g. twins) has occurred!

Your specialist may ask you to come back in several weeks if everything is going well to perform an ultrasound scan to visually observe how it's going. Antenatal care may be recommended in the following weeks thereafter.

**Note**: *If the hCG levels decline or only increase very slightly on follow-up pregnancy tests, this can be a sign of impending miscarriage. If miscarriage has occurred hCG can remain in the woman's blood for 4 to 6 weeks thereafter.*

## The first trimester

**From conception to 12 weeks gestation, the miracle of life begins**
After the fertilised egg, or blastocyst, has completed its journey along the fallopian tube and implanted into the uterine wall, it undergoes a rapid series of cell divisions. These will see it transform into the embryo and the organs that will nurture it throughout the pregnancy. The embedded blastocyst forms two layers. The inner layer of the cells, the endoderm, develops into the baby's digestive and respiratory systems. The outer layer also divides into two parts. The ectoderm, or outer layer, develops into the nervous system and skin. The middle layer, or mesoderm, becomes bone, muscles, circulatory, and reproductive systems. At the same time, the outer layer of the cell mass is

developing into the life-support systems that will nurture the baby – the umbilical cord, the chorion and, later, the placenta.

The outer layer of these membranes forms the chorion, which surrounds the embryo, while another inner layer of membranes becomes the amnion. These membrane layers develop 10 to 12 days after conception. The amnion layer forms the amniotic sac, which fills with amniotic fluid to provide the embryo with a shockproof, temperature-controlled inner environment. By nine weeks, the unborn baby, now referred to as a foetus, is very active and swims about within the amniotic sac in the womb. By the end of the first trimester (12 weeks), the foetus is approximately 7.6 cm long and weighs 14 grams. It can swallow, absorb and discharge fluids. Hands form and fingernails are in progress. Within the next week the vocal cords form. These are the first miraculous stages of how life begins.

## Metabolic changes during pregnancy

During the course of pregnancy maternal weight increases by an average 25 per cent. This is due to foetal growth, enlargement of maternal organs, increased storage of fat and protein, and increased blood volume and interstitial fluid. Metabolic processes significantly increase during pregnancy. Oxygen consumption is raised by 20 per cent; the abterior pituitary gland secretes greater amounts of thyroid-stimulating hormone (TSH); the thyroid gland enlarges in approximately 70 per cent of pregnant woman – increasing iodine uptake and returning it in circulating T3 and T4.

Energy needs are greatly raised during pregnancy; this is achieved by increased fat storage for maternal needs and raised post-prandial serum glucose for placental transfer to supply the foetus. The mechanisms are due to the insulin-antagonist effects of human placental lactogen (hPL) and possibly also to progesterone. There is a rise in serum glucose and decreased glycogen storage in the liver. Reduced motility of the gastric tract (mainly due to increased progesterone) enhances absorption. This combined with reduced de-animation under the influence of human chorionic gonadotrophin (hCG) and hPL, result in an increase in the levels of plasma proteins and a correspondingly increased supply of amino acids for foetal growth. Consequently there is decreased urea in the blood, and decreased urinary output (Dysuria).

Progesterone output from women's ovaries before pregnancy is around 15-20mg. The placental progesterone during pregnancy reaches an output of 250mg per day. Oestradiol and oestrone are increased one hundredfold and oestriol is increased one thousandfold, with total oestrogen output reaching 30-40 mg per day. Cortisol and aldosterone (Adrenal gland hormones) are also produced in increased amounts, promoting serum glucose levels and the retention of sodium respectively.

Maternal levels of FSH and LH (pituitary gland hormones) are suppressed, prolactin levels rise and relaxin is also produced (which softens and relaxes the ligaments and cervix to facilitate birth). The cardiac-circulatory and kidney systems are also put under increased workload during pregnancy. Plasma volume of the blood can rise significantly (particularly by the 3rd trimester) to 40-57 per cent increase. This increased demand on the heart also increases its rate and stroke volume. Red blood cells and clotting factors also rise in the blood, increasing coagulability. Due to this increase, cardiac load causes the peripheral blood vessels to dilate to counter for the extra work demand. During weeks 8-16 due to reduced vascular resistance blood pressure can initially drop, which may cause some woman to experience dizziness; the blood pressure then gradually rises.

The kidneys retain more sodium under the influence of increased aldosterone, resulting in retention of fluid/oedema. During pregnancy, total body water increases by 6-8 litres. Urinary output reduces during pregnancy (dysuria) despite some 100 extra litres of fluid pass through the kidneys tubules each day. This can potentially increase the risk of urinary tract infection.

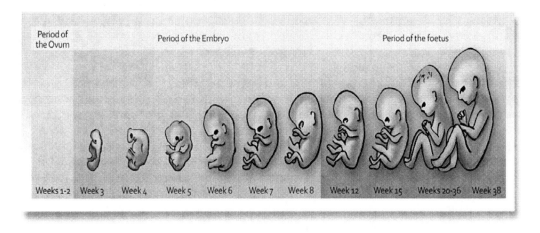

*Figure.24. A developing foetus*

# Chapter 15

# *Symptoms of Suspected Pregnancy*

***Sore Breasts*** - a universal sign of suspected pregnancy is breast soreness, with or without feelings of heaviness or tingling in the nipples. Unfortunately, sore breasts can be caused by increased progesterone and oestrogen, so if suppositories are being used the symptoms could be a side effect on the body rather than the growing embryo. If the woman has recently been on fertility drug medication or commonly experiences breast soreness premenstrually, breast soreness can be mistaken as a sign of pregnancy if hCG levels have not yet been confirmed. The breast areola pigment may darken and the lubrication ducts around the nipples because raised.

***Fatigue*** – Can be a symptom of elevating progesterone and hCG (Human chorionic gonadotropin), both of which are produced from a growing embryo. Progesterone also raises the temperature, which may make you feel more sluggish than normal.

***Nausea*** – Can be due to higher-than-normal levels of oestrogen, progesterone and hCG levels. If a multiple pregnancy has occurred then the hCG levels may be higher therefore contributing to potentially more severe bouts of nausea. Note: Morning sickness most commonly occurs between week 6 to 14 of pregnancy.

***Cramping*** – Discomfort is not untypical, particularly in the first couple of weeks into a pregnancy. If the conception occurred after using fertility drugs (ovarian stimulation), there could be a case of enlarged ovaries. Lowered progesterone levels are also observed with increased incidences of cramping.

***Spot Bleeding*** – This is very common in the very early stages of pregnancy. Spotting may be caused by the embryo burrowing into the uterus and causing leakage of blood from small blood vessels. Irritation from using progesterone suppositories can also cause mild spotting.

***Smell*** – Pregnancy often heightens your sense of smell, and you may find that common odours such as cooking smells may make you nauseous. Due to the changes in your body's chemistry even perfumes may have an altered odour when applied to your skin.

**Cravings and odd tastes** – Again due to the alterations of body chemistry and rising hormones, the saliva often changes and reflects the chemical content of the blood giving a metallic taste in the mouth. Certain food may taste different to normal. It is not uncommon to notice that during the pregnancy that the woman may develop odd cravings for foods that may not usually be eaten in certain combinations, e.g. pickles with ice cream.

**Increased urinary frequency** – when the embryo starts the secrete hCG, and your progesterone rises. The blood supply to the pelvic also increases, which may cause pelvic congestion. This may lead to bladder irritation that can increase the desire to expel urine even if only in small amounts but more frequently. This is called in medical terms *micturation*. This can even occur as early as the first week of pregnancy.

## Troubleshooting Problems during Pregnancy

### 'I've got you under my skin' – The stork is on its way

Pregnancy lasts for approximately forty weeks. This time is commonly divided into three periods called trimesters: The first trimester is calculated from the first day of you last period to week 12; the second trimester is from week 12 to week 28; and the third trimester is from week 28 until the delivery date.

During the first trimester of the pregnancy the mass of the foetus increases by an incredible two and a half million times (2,500,000); in the second and third trimesters the rate of mass growth is approximately 230 times. During the very early stages of foetal development, correct nutrient balance is of vital importance as nutrient demands necessary for proper cellular formation is extremely high. During the first two months of gestation a baby's weight increases twenty-two thousand (22,000) times starting from a single cell.

During the pregnancy you may feel discomforts that occur mostly as a result of hormonal changes within the body, nutritional deficiencies, and anatomical changes that will happen continuously throughout your pregnancy.

### Nutritional requirements

Calorie intake should not be increased in the first trimester of pregnancy; however, for the remainder of the pregnancy the calorie intake can be increased by approximately *10 per cent or 160 to 200 calories extra daily.*

These extra calories should come from **protein** foods such as beans; cheese; fish; meat; milk; and yogurt; preferably getting it from plant sources rather than animal. This is equivalent to approximately 2 serves.

### Other extra important nutrients that may be needed include:

- **Calcium** from dairy products; broccoli; almonds; figs; legumes; peas; and beans.
- **Folic Acid** from broccoli; green vegetables; potatoes; and liver.
- **Iron** from apricots; liver; sardines; tuna; and prune juice.

### Particular nutrients that are important for the health of the growing baby are:

- Essential fatty acids (EPA/DHA), iodine and taurine – are all important of the child's brain cognition and development.
- Make sure that you are obtaining adequate soluble fibre in your diet as constipation and flatulence (gas, wind) are common conditions. Example may be: bran, cereals, and psyllium seed husks.
- Avoid powerful laxative medications where possible, because they may over-stimulate the peristaltic action of bowel that can potentially cause premature stimulation of the uterus and affect the carrying of the pregnancy.
- The raised progesterone hormone levels during pregnancy have a relaxing effect on all ligaments and smooth muscles that may often contribute to the development of varicose veins, piles (varicose vein on anus) and heartburn. The application of witch hazel cream is useful to soothing piles and meadowsweet tea is good for settling down heartburn.
- Eat plenty of a wide variety of fresh fruit and vegetables, such as figs, prunes and raisins. Rotating your type of food intake may also help to minimise developing potential food allergies or sensitivities.
- Drink plenty of clear water; try to maintain approximately two litres of fluid intake daily.
- A high quality multi-vitamin/mineral supplement (designed for pregnancy) may be recommended to cover any nutrient shortfalls throughout the pregnancy.
- Colloidal mineral supplementation yield (over 70) well absorbed and assimilated microscopic minerals and trace element nutrients, which can help to prevent cellular deficiencies in mother and baby.
- Tonic herbs that may be useful in the last 6 weeks of pregnancy and may benefit in preparing for labour (minimise complications e.g. haemorrhaging), improving lactation (breast-feeding) and enhancing recovery include: withania; Siberian ginseng; raspberry leaf (Rubus idaeus) (raspberry leaf tea can also be consumed after the end of the first trimester and slowly increased until labour); vervain; oats; stinging nettles (leaf and root) (Urtica dioica); alfalfa (medicago sativa); cinnamon; horsetail; ginger; blessed thistle (one of the best to improve lactation);

goat's rue; holy thistle; fennel (foeniculum vulgare); codonopsis; and aniseed.

In the last two week before the baby's due birth date herbs such as: blue cohosh; dong quai; false unicorn root; and squaw vine may be also included to aid contractions and prepare the body for a easier birth.
* *Note* - (Not to be taken early in the pregnancy)!

*Homeopathic remedies to help during labour*: caulophyllum 3x; pulsatilla 6x; belladonna 6x; cimicufuga racemosa 6x; chamomilla 3x; and arnica montana 6x. Other remedies that may be considered for use during birth include: aconite; gelsemium; chamomilla; magnesia phosporicum; and kali phos.

*Homeopathic remedies to help lactation*: lac defloratum 3x; bryonis 3x; belladonna 6x; gelsemium 3x; graphites 6x; lac caninum 3x; nux vomica 6x; phytolacca 6x; pulsatilla 12x; and calcium carbonate 3x.

*Acupuncture points used to improve lactation*: SI 1; SI 11; GB 21; and St 12.

*Flower essences*: Rescue Remedy (Bach), and Emergency Essence (Australian Bush Flower Essences).

## Anaemia

During pregnancy, blood volume (the amount of blood in the body) increases by about 40 per cent particularly in the 2nd and 3rd trimesters. This increase in volume is largely due to the increase in blood plasma.

The red blood cells do not increase proportionately and the protein haemoglobin is part of the red blood cells that is needed to carry oxygen to the cells of the body.

Symptoms may include fatigue; a rapid heartbeat (palpitations); paleness of the skin, gums, and around the inside of the eyes.

Another condition called *Pica* can also develop with anaemia, and can also be a sign of other nutrient and tract element deficiencies. Pica can cause the person to crave unusual substances: Clay – iron may be deficient; sugar – chromium; salt – calcium, magnesium, and Vitamin K; ice – iron; and cigarette ash – potassium and possible parasites.

*Natural treatments for Iron anaemia may include:*
*Herbal medicines*: nettle root/leaf (urtica dioica); dong quai (only at the very end of the pregnancy); alfalfa; bilberry; blackstrap molasses; and withania.

**Nutrients**: Iron (best supplemental sources are ferrous sulphate, gluconate, amino acid chelate and phosphate. Some forms of iron are known to cause constipation and are poorly absorbed. There are many other nutrients that also play essential roles in preventing anaemia: folic acid; Vitamin B6; Vitamin B12; Vitamin B2; copper; molybdenum; selenium; histidine; lysine; and Vitamin C. Foods to increase may include: green leafy vegetables; bananas; broccoli; rice bran; apples; asparagus; cherries; egg yolk; plums; parsley; prunes; raisins; raspberries; dark grapes; sunflower kernels; cottage cheese; English spinach; organically raised red meats; and liver. Excessive fibre intake and poor stomach acid production can affect iron absorption.

# Depression

During pregnancy feels of depression are a relatively common condition experienced by many women. Moods may fluctuate during various times throughout the pregnancy. If the symptoms persist, or are worsening, it is advisable to seek professional help. Just having someone else to talk to outside your immediate circle of family or friends may be all that is required to help allay these feelings to get things off your chest.

Moderate exercise can help with depression as it can elevate the body's endorphins to promote feelings of wellbeing. Chemical imbalances such as adrenal hormones and neurotransmitters (dopamine, cortisol, GABBA, serotonin, norepinephrine, noradrenaline, and melatonin) are one of the major causes of depression and through the various stages of the pregnancy your hormones will certainly be changing to accommodate the growing baby's needs. For example when oestrogen levels rise during pregnancy, this can increase the output of a substances called *interleukin 1* for macrophages (a type of immune modulating cell) that can contribute to depression, this can also be an issue with depression with PMS.

*Typical signs of depression may include:*
Low self-esteem; emotional instability; loss of energy or fatigue; loss of interest or pleasure; crying; memory and concentration is poor; difficulty in performing tasks; appetite and/or weight decreasing; binge eating on comfort foods; sleep difficulties; thoughts of suicide and hopelessness.

If you have been experiencing four or more of the above symptoms for over a two-week period, with associated moodiness, then this can be classed as a type of depression.

*Natural treatments for mild depression may include:*
**Nutrient** deficiencies such as: biotin; folate; essential fatty acids (GLA/DHA); omega 3; Vitamins B12, B6, P5P, B3, B2; Vitamin C; calcium; magnesium; potassium; zinc; copper; iron; tyrosine; tryptophan; and DL phenylalanine can be linked to causing depression.

**Other nutrients** that can benefit include: 5-hydroxy tryptophan (5HT); S-adenosylmethionine (SAMe); taurine; choline; inositol; chromium; gamma-amino-butyric acid (GABBA); and nicotinamide adenine dinucleotide (NADH).

**Herbal Medicines** that may also be considered: St John's wort (Hypericum perforatum) *(not to be used with other prescription anti-depressant medications; it may also prematurely increase uterine contractions), lemon balm; oat seed (avena sativa); liquorice (glycyrrhiza glabra); Siberian ginseng (eleuthrococcus senticosus); ginger; damiana (turnera diffusa); panax ginseng; vervain (verbena officinalis);and withania (withania somnifera).

**Aromatherapy oils** that may be considered: Bergamot, chamomile, geranium, or rose.

**Homeopathic remedies**: bamboo (bambusa arundinacea); ignatia; arsenicum album; cimicifuga; calcarea carbonica; aurum metallicum; natrum muriaticum; sepia; and pulsatilla.

**If memory and concentration are poor natural remedies to consider include**:
**Herbs** – bacopa (bacopa monnieri); ginkgo biloba; gota kola (centella asiatica); and schisandra (shisandra chinensis).

**Nutrients**: acetylcholine; acetyl-L-carnitine; Co enzyme Q 10; dimethyl glycine (DMG); DMAE; huperzine A; lecithin (phosphatidyl choline, phoshatidyl serine); pregnenolone; and L-glutamine.

There are many drugs and chemicals that can cross over the placenta barrier and possible affect the developing foetus. These chemicals can potentially filter into the foetus's blood supply and cross the blood-brain barrier that protects the brain tissue. Many prescription anti-depressant drugs also can fall into the category, so if you are currently taking any such medication it is important that you consult with your doctor regarding advice to minimise any undesirable side effects.

## Oedema/Fluid retention (swelling)

Oedema affects more that 50 per cent of pregnant women and is more likely to occur in the third trimester but can arise at any time. It usually affects the feet, legs and hands, and is generally worse at the end of the day. Oedema during pregnancy can be caused by a rise in the body's oestrogen levels. Oestrogen draws fluid to it contributing to a tendency to fluid retention. This is a relatively normal condition that is experienced during pregnancy but if it gets out of control it can lead to a more serious condition called pre-eclampsia.

Oedema can also be caused by protein deficiency so be sure to have adequate amounts in the diet. Avoid commercial table salt, processed food products and strong diuretic medications. Avoid being on your feet for long periods of time; particularly avoid standing in one place without moving about. DO NOT reduce water or fluid intake.

**Natural remedies for oedema** may include: dandelion leaves (tea or extract form); bioflavonoids – quercetin, rutin, and Vitamin C.

**Foods of benefit**: celery; leeks; pawpaw; carrots; oats; avocado; broccoli; lentils; sunflower kernels; bananas; sprouted chick peas; kale; and spinach. Make sure you have adequate potassium foods in your diet such as: legumes, bananas, and spinach.

Walking can also help to relieve fluid retention as the contraction of the large muscle groups move the lymph and circulation.


# Pre-Eclampsia

Pre-eclampsia can be a complication of pregnancy that is characterised by high blood pressure, toxaemia (poison or toxic bloodstream), oedema, and an excess of protein in the urine; it usually occurs in the last trimester of pregnancy. A very small percentage of women who develop pre-eclampsia go on to have seizures and/or comas. Pre-eclampsia affects approximately 7 per cent of all pregnancies and is a major contributor to maternal mortality, premature birth, intrauterine growth retardation, and perinatal mortality.

Pre-eclampsia is more common with women who previously experienced cardio-vascular problems prior to falling pregnant. The raised blood pressure can potentially affect nutrient supply to the developing baby. Pre-eclampsia is associated with a T helper 1 (Th1) immune dominate state. Avoid excess salt in your diet, drink plenty of water, and reduce stress as much as possible.

***Natural treatments to support pre-eclampsia may include:***
***Nutrients***: Increase Vitamin C; L-arginine; bromelain; quercetin; calcium; chromium; selenium; magnesium; (moderate) Vitamin E and Essential Fatty Acids (EFA).

***For Toxaemia***: Scutellaria baicelensis (Chinese skullcap) and ginger.

***Liver support herbs:*** St Mary's thistle. Natural Diuretic: dandelion leaf.

***Anti-clotting foods***: Garlic, coleus forskolli, and capsicum.

***Hypertension:*** Hawthorn berry/leaf.

***Medically:*** Aspirin (only with doctor advice).

*Acupuncture points:* GB 20; GB 34; St 36; Sp 9; P 6; Liver 2; Liver 3; and LI 11.

### Foods to increase in diet to prevent pre-eclampsia:
Broccoli; citrus fruits; guavas; parsley; pineapple; coleslaw; strawberries; rosehip tea; sunflower kernels; corn; green leafy vegies; asparagus; apples; and grape fruit.

## Morning Sickness

### 'Let's go to … Yurp!'

It is estimated that 50 per cent of all pregnant women experience some degree of nausea and/or vomiting during pregnancy, particularly during the 6th and 12th weeks. This is a normal reaction and may occur any time of day, not just in the morning like its name suggests.

A serious version of abnormal vomiting is a condition called *Hyperemesis gravidarum.* This condition affects approximately 1 woman in every 300 pregnancies. It involves severe, continual nausea and vomiting after the 12th week and it can result in dehydration, acidosis, malnutrition, and substantial weight loss. If this condition persists, it can potentially put the developing foetus in danger.

The reasons why this abnormal nausea is caused is still not fully understood, but it may be associated with very high elevated levels of hormones such as oestrogen and chorionic gonadotropin (hCG). HCG is produced by the placenta during the first trimester to increase the placenta's quality.

Another train of thought on why morning sickness occurs is likened to a body self-protective mechanism; many of the types of foods that women develop an aversion to are usually ones that contain a high micro-organism content such as meats. This nausea is believed to occur to protect the developing embryo in the early stages of the pregnancy from foreign organisms being introduced into the body's system that may compromise the pregnancy.

Other possible causes may include: bile duct diseases (e.g., gallstones and cholecystitis); drug toxicity; inflammatory bowel disorders; low blood sugar (hypoglycaemia); molar pregnancy; thyroid imbalances; and poor nutritional status prior to conception.

### Natural treatments for morning sickness may include:
**Herbal medicines**: black horehound (ballota nigra); ginger (zingiber officinale); meadowsweet (filipendula ulmaria); catnip; chamomile (matricaria recutita); chen pi; cinnamon quills (cinnamomum zeylanicum); dandelion root (tarraxacum officinale); fennel; fenugreek (trigonella foenumgraecum); holy

thistle (cnicus benedictus); lemon balm; marshmallow (althea officinalis); peppermint (mentha piperita); peach leaf; spearmint; raspberry leaf; slippery elm powder;and St Mary's thistle (silybum).

**TCM Formulas**: saussurea and cardamom combination (Xiang sha Liu Jun Zi Tang), and bupleurum and peony formula (Jai Wei Xiao Yao San).

**Nutrients**: Vitamin B6 (with Vitamin B complex); magnesium; essential fatty acids (EFAs); and L-methionine. Liquid colloidal mineral supplementation may also be effective at relieving symptoms.

**Homeopathic**: such as nux vomica, ipecacuanna, cocculus, petroleum and sepia (6-12c potency) are of benefit.

**Acupuncture point** called *Neiguan*; other points commonly used include: St 36; St 40; P 6; Ren 12; Ren 13; and Kidney 21.

### Other tips:
Try to eat dry plain crackers, biscuits or dry toast on first rising in the morning. A little serving of honey and yogurt may also help soothe the stomach. Sucking on lollipops can help with low blood glucose.

If the blood sugars are low, try to eat small meals regularly throughout the day. Snacks such as nuts may be worth considering. You may require extra chromium nutrients in your diet.

The production of hydrochloric acid in the stomach may be low; you may need to support this deficiency with a digestive enzyme supplement.

Slippery elm powder before meals can help to soothe mucous membranes.

Consuming liquid drinks such as banana smoothies may be recommended if it is difficult to keep solid food down.  Sip on barley water or baking soda (bicarbonate soda) drinks.  If you can't face solid foods, try soups and energy / nutrient dense veggie juices.

Take your time getting out of bed, don't sit up to quickly. You may feel better if you raise the bed sloping downwards slightly.

Some ladies may feel better after smelling freshly ground coffee beans.

Drink herbal teas throughout the day such as: ginger; peach leaf; fennel; chamomile; spearmint; and raspberry leaf. Stewed grated apple with a pinch of cinnamon may also help.  If appetite is poor you could try: Swedish bitters, and herbs like: calamus (sweet flag), gentian, ginseng and papaya leaves.

Avoid greasy, fatty foods.

*Medical treatments* for morning sickness may include anti-emetic medications such as: Metoclopramide, Maxalon, Phenergan and Zocor. A carbohydrate solution called Emetrol can also be considered to reduce nausea; also anti-histamine medications such as Promethazine have also been used.

*Heartburn* – some women experience heartburn during pregnancy. This occurs due to the increased levels of hormones, particularly progesterone, which reduces the effectiveness of the sphincter between the stomach and the oesophagus. To reduce getting heartburn: eat small regular meals, avoid very spicy and fatty foods, and don't lie down immediately after eating. When sleeping try slightly elevating the top end of the bed.

If heartburn occurs try taking some slippery elm powder after the meals. Sipping on herbal teas such as: anise seed; chamomile; fennel; meadowsweet; parsley and peppermint before or between meals may also help.

## Muscle cramps

Leg cramps are more likely to become problematic after the first trimester and often occur at night. Doing gentle stretching exercises, rotating the feet and ankles help to move the circulation; pregnancy massage can benefit the removal of waste products out of the muscles and improve circulation. Muscle cramps can be an indication of nutrient deficiencies such as: magnesium; calcium; sodium; potassium; and vitamin E. Dehydration is another potential cause factor. Be sure to remember to drink plenty of fluid; by the time you feel thirsty you may already be dehydrated. Back ache is also very common to have during pregnancy. Acupuncture point UB 32 (inserted under the skin, parallel to the sacrum and taped into place) may help to alleviate back aches.

## Gestational Diabetes

This is a form of diabetes that occurs during pregnancy. This condition may be caused by the hormones that are produced by the placenta affecting the activity of insulin that is produced by the pancreas gland.

This condition occurs in approximately 3 to 8 percent of pregnancies. There are a number of factors that increase the risk of developing this condition. These include being over 30 years of age, a family history of diabetes type 2 and being overweight prior to conceiving.

The blood sugar levels may rise to high, and this may contribute to an increase in the baby's birth weight. The baby may be born with low blood sugars that can potential cause problems during the delivery.

If the baby's birth weight is over 9 pound 14 ounces this is called *Macrosomia*. During the pregnancy the woman's blood levels are monitored. If the initial results appear suspect then a full glucose tolerance test (GTT) may be recommended to gain a more accurate reading. This involves drinking a sugar solution and having a blood test approximately one hour after, to yield the result.

Symptoms may include: Excessive thirst, frequent urination, dizziness and increased fatigue.

***Natural treatments to support gestational diabetes may include:***
Eat small meats often throughout the day; avoid high sugar, and simple carbohydrate foods.
***Nutrients*** such as: chromium; biotin; co enzyme q 10; manganese; lipoic acid; B-complex vitamins (esp. B1, B3, and B6); magnesium; Vitamin C; taurine; potassium; vanadium; and zinc.

***Phytonutrients***: Spirulina, an alternative to simple sugar sweeteners is the extract stevia (approximately 100 times sweeter than normal table sugar). Avoid aspartame (artificial sweetener) products.

***Herbs*** such as: bitter melon (momordica charantia); cinnamon; codonopsis; panax ginseng; gymnemia (gymnema sylvestre); goat's rue; fenugreek; jambul (syzygium jambolanum); morinda officinalis; and bilberry (vaccinium myrtillus) may benefit.

# Stretch marks

Stretch marks (also known to be referred to as 'stretches', 'life marks' or 'badges of honour') are wavy-like stripes that may appear on the abdomen, buttocks, breasts, and thighs. Usually the stretch marks start out reddish in colour and may gradually fade to a white colouration.

These marks occur because of rapid weight gain, which is typical during pregnancy. Deep layer tears to fibres in the skin develop due its over-stretching. Normally when stretch marks appear they may become permanent though tend to become much less noticeable over time.

Here are a few preventative measures that may be considered to minimise them from happening: Apply topical creams/moisturisers such as: Aloe vera; apricot; almond; grape seed; cocoa butter; Vitamin E; zinc cream; collagen-elastinhysates; gota cola (centella asiatica); wheat germ; sorbolene; glycerine; and virgin olive oils into the relevant areas on daily bases, particularly the abdomen, buttocks, breasts and thighs.

**Essential oil anti-stretch mark formula**

Blend together six (6) tbsp of almond oil; two (2) tbsp wheat germ oil; two (2) tbsp olive oil; forty (40) drops mandarin oil; twenty (20) drops chamomile oil; twenty (20) drops lavender oil.

Mix together in a bottle and leave blended oils for four (4) days to settle. Apply the massage oil to the thighs, abdomen, and breasts once to twice daily from the fifth (5th) month of pregnancy.

**Supplement with nutrients** such as: Vitamin A (mild dosages); Vitamin E; essential fatty acids; mucopolysaccharides; proline; lysine; copper; niacin; calcium fluoride (tissue salt); and zinc.

**Homeopathic remedies**: Calcarea flourica 6x, and silica 6x.

# Chloasma (Melasma)

This is a pigment condition of the skin that occurs in most pregnant women, and more commonly in those with a darker complexion. The pigment changes usually occur on the cheeks, forehead, nipples, nose, and upper lip areas. Some women taking hormone therapy or on the contraceptive pill can also develop Chloasma. Treatment for this pigment change is largely unsatisfactory; fading of the colouration usually occurs over time. In extreme cases, bleaching agents have been used with moderate success.

# Varicose veins / Haemorrhoids

Varicose veins and haemorrhoids occur because of increased pressure put on the circulation (chronic venous insufficiency) by the growing uterus and increased weight. You can help to avoid them by not putting on excessive weight whilst pregnant and by avoiding constipation. When sitting avoid crossing your legs or ankles, elevate your feet and legs but avoid sharp edges pressing into the ankles or calves because this will impede circulation. You are more likely to have these conditions if they occur in other family members. If you have varicose veins, wearing support stockings and exercise (contraction of leg muscles pushes pooled blood back into the circulation) may be recommended. Severe varicose veins can cause leg ulcers to form that are often difficult to resolve.

*Acupuncture points* used to help varicose veins may include: Lver 3; Liver 8; and Sp 10.

*Foods* such as blueberries may be beneficial and Vitamin C with bioflavonoids can strengthen the blood vessel walls. Make sure that you are eating plenty of fibre containing foods.

**Herbal remedies** to treat varicose veins and haemorrhoids may include: gota kola (centella asiatica); horse chestnut (aesculus hippocastanum); butcher's broom (ruscus aculeatus); bilberry (vaccinium myrtillus); and buckwheat (fagopyrum esculentum). Topical application of witch hazel cream can also be beneficial. Other nutrients such as: Vitamin A; Vitamin B complex; Vitamin E; bromelain; proanthocyanidin; and zinc may also be considered.

# Foods to Avoid During Pregnancy

*Listeriosis* – is caused by the bacterium Listeria monocytogenes. It can grow and multiply at the temperature of a typical fridge i.e. around 4-5 degrees C. Listeriosis infection can cause miscarriage, premature labour, stillbirth or the baby may develop the symptoms of listeriosis soon after birth, which can be serious. Symptoms are usually very mild, like a mild flu, with slightly raised temperature and general aching. Listeria infection usually results from eating contaminated foods which include: raw milk; soft ripened cheeses; ice cream; raw meat; chicken; fish; smoked fish; seafood; and precooked meat and pates. Raw vegetables can also be contaminated so make sure you wash or peel them before eating. Foods in the refrigerator should be stored sealed and away from other foods such as salad vegetables; when handling foods and utensils be stringent at washing your hands.

*Toxoplasmosis* – is caused by the parasite Toxoplasma gondii. If contracted in the first trimester of pregnancy it can cause birth defects. Toxoplasmosis contamination can occur in many of the same foods as listeria. Cat faeces is also a major source of contamination. Wear rubber gloves when handling a cat litter tray and wash your hands immediately afterwards. Other animals and birds can carry toxoplasma. Soil can be contaminated also, so if coming in contact with soil such as gardening, wash it off to remove all traces.

*Salmonellosis* – is caused by Salmonella bacterium of which there are over 200 varieties. Eggs often contain salmonella so you should avoid raw eggs or foods containing raw eggs. Be sure to read food labels. You can eat eggs as long as they are well cooked. Salmonella contamination can also occur with uncooked meats, chicken, fish, and deli meats. During pregnancy, contracting salmonella rarely has a detrimental effect on the baby directly. However, the symptoms experienced by the mother such as high fever, vomiting, diarrhoea, and dehydration can cause preterm labour or miscarriage.

# Labour

***'The moment of truth has arrived – no guts – no glory'***
The first stage of labour starts with onset of regular contractions and ends with full dilation of the cervix. The second stage is the actual delivery of the baby. In normal labour, the first stage lasts around 14-23 hours on average for first time mums and 5-13 hours for mothers who have delivered children previously. The second stage, on average, lasts 40 minutes for the new first time rookies (primigravidae) and 20 minutes for the more experienced mothers that have seen it all before (multigravidae). While excessively rapid labour can be uncomfortable for the mother and cause distress to the baby, delayed labour is the bigger problem as the baby is at risk of hypoxia (lack of oxygen) if the placenta separates before delivery or if there is compression of the umbilical cord in the birth canal.

*Acupuncture points* used close to term – to support cervical effacement and perineal elasticity: from 38 weeks of pregnancy – UB 32 to move lower abdomen QI and other Sacral points; Liver 3 and Ren 4 to target the Cervix; and UB 35 for the perineum.

Acupuncture points to help promote contractions – LI 4; Sp 6: to help ease contractions – GB 34. To reduce threatened Miscarriage – Du 20; Kidney 3; Kidney 9; Yin Tang; Ht 7; Ht 9; and P 6. For a delay of more than 20 minutes in delivering the placenta (where the option of synthetic oxytocin has not been exercised) points may include: LI 4; Sp 6; GB 21; UB 60 and UB 67 are effective in expelling the placenta and breastfeeding the newborn can stimulate natural oxytocin and hasten delivery of the placenta or a twin.

*TCM formula* used to prevent miscarriage, to correct malpresentation and to help ensure a smooth labour is – Bao Chan Wu You Tang.


## After the Birth

Prolonged or retained lochia is the discharge of remaining uterine products; blood, necrotic tissue, and mucus following childbirth, mainly from the placental site. This is a cleaning process. Normal lochia is deep red for 4-5 days (Lochia rubra), fading to clear pink for 6-10 days (Lochia serosa), then to a light straw colour (Lochia alba) for 1 week or so. The discharge is initially sterile before being colonised by bacteria. Lochia should not persist beyond about 3 weeks but can continue to discharge for as long as 2 months or, conversely, not flow, indicating that the retained products are not being cleared from the uterus, which can lead to infection.

Postpartum haemorrhage (bleeding) after childbirth is a potentially very dangerous situation which can occur if the uterus is exhausted from a long and difficult labour and is unable to contract adequately to compress the blood vessels and prevent loss of blood. Blood loss in excess of 500ml is defined as postpartum bleeding. Another cause of postpartum bleeding can be due to some portion of the placenta not expelling resulting in continued blood loss. Severe blood loss can result in collapse as the brain is denied sufficient blood flow and oxygen. If loss of blood is very severe necrosis of the pituitary gland can occur causing a causing known as Sheehan's syndrome.

There are a number of conditions that lead to excess bleeding, the main ones include: uterine atony; inertia due to prolonged labour; over-distension; fibrotic uterine muscle; placenta praevia; abruptio placentae; or general anaesthesia. Medically, ultrasound may be required if any placental tissue is retained, if so, curettage may need to be carried out. Anti-haemorrhagic medication may be needed to settle the blood loss. In TCM, Chinese formulations such as: Jiao Ai Tang is used to nourish blood and stop uterine bleeding and Du Shen Tang is used to augment to Qi and stabilise collapse, reduce dizziness, and syncope following heavy blood loss.

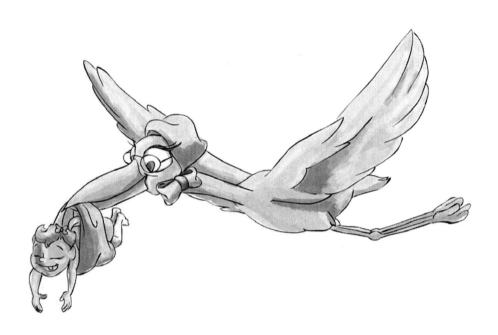

# Chapter 16

# *Surgical procedures to preserve fertility*

## For Women

### Embryo Cryopreservation – *'Where have all the children gone'?*

If a woman has a partner or is willing to accept donor sperm, she can have mature or immature eggs removed from her ovaries, fertilised via standard IVF and frozen for later implantation in her uterus. Embryo freezing has a relatively good success rate. The negative aspect, though, is that it can take 4 to 5 weeks to finish the necessary round of ovary-stimulating hormones and harvest eggs. If you are needing to undergo chemotherapy due to a diagnosed cancer, you may not have the luxury of a lot of time as chemo can cause damage to the reproductive system.

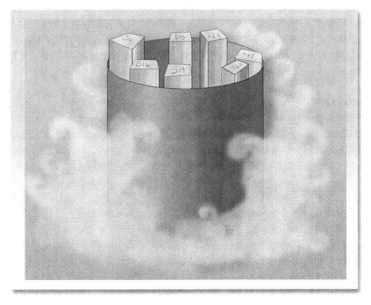

**Cryopreservation**

### Oocyte (unfertilised egg) cryopreservation

If you don't have a partner at present and don't wish to opt for donor sperm, you can freeze your unfertilised eggs to be used at a later time. When you have decided it's time to try to have a baby, the eggs are then thawed, fertilised and implanted in your uterus. However, this procedure is still relatively new and eggs are less likely to survive freezing than embryos. Those that go through with this procedure are said to have about a 3 to 6 per cent chance of a successful fertilisation into embryos that result in full-term pregnancy, though advancements in this procedure are improving.

### *Ovarian tissue cryopreservation*

This procedure is also still in its experimental stages, though the idea behind it is to preserve ovarian tissue and the thousands of immature eggs it contains. In this way, you have many eggs to attempt conception with when you are ready for pregnancy.

There are several ways to do this procedure. The easiest is to remove one ovary, cut it into strips and freeze them. The strips are later transplanted back into the pelvic or arm regions, and the woman is given ovary-stimulating hormones to produce eggs, which are then fertilised and implanted in the uterus. Another method is to freeze the entire ovary, then transplant it back in place later for egg harvesting. The down-side to this method is that it is still difficult to store whole organs because of ice crystal damage during the cooling process.

### *Oophoropexy*

This involves temporarily tying the ovaries out of the way (often behind the uterus). This surgical procedure may be called for during times when radiation therapy is required to treat a cancer near the site of the ovaries. Radiation can cause detrimental effects on fertility. This surgery does not work with chemotherapy.

### *Radical Trachelectomy*

This surgery may be used to replace having a hysterectomy performed, which would be goodbye to naturally bearing children. This procedure may be offered to a women who is in the very early stages of cervical cancer and can opt to only have the malignant area removed from part of the cervix, leaving the uterus intact.

### *Gonadotropin-releasing hormone analogues (GnRH)*

Girls who haven't yet reached puberty tend to have higher fertility rates after undergoing cancer treatments with chemotherapy than women whose reproductive organs are already matured. GnRH analogues are hormone-blocking and may be given in conjunction with the chemo to temporarily suspend the reproductive system into a state of pre-pubescence or temporary menopause to hopefully maintain fertility once treatment with chemo has finished. Mixed results to date have been observed with the use of these drugs, though, it may be an option if time is limited or if eggs retrieval is not as viable giving the time restraints. More information on GnRH is discussed in previous chapters.


## For Men

### *Sperm banking*
A male can have his sperm frozen for safekeeping until he's also ready to start a family. The sperm is later thawed and can be placed in his partner's uterus for fertilisation to occur. The success of this procedure depends largely upon the quality of the sperm.

### *Testicular tissue preservation*
The procedure can be used for men who produce sperm but the sperm quality may not be that great. Testicular tissue preservation is still in relatively early stages of development, though it may provide some hope by surgically removing testicular tissue, which contains immature sperm, freezing it, and then injecting fledgling sperm back into the testes when pregnancy is desired.


## The Future of Assisted Reproductive Medicine

### *Science fiction or science fact*

#### *'To boldly go where no man or woman has gone before'!*

No, I don't want to discuss *Star Trek* right now, but rather what may lie ahead in the not so distant future for the science of 'baby-making' medicine. The information that is discovered in relation to knowledge of science and medicine doubles every year. This is fuelled by innovative and imaginative thinking to continually stretch the boundaries and understanding of human awareness and endeavour. The constant pioneering research into finding new and better ways of improving reproductive medicine is an ever-evolving process. Life in general seems to be moving at such a rapid pace nowadays, that any revolutionary breakthrough in thought and technology is quickly replaced with the next latest and greatest step in the evolutionary chain. Though, being new does not necessarily always equate to being better! Just because we can do something, doesn't mean it has to be done!

The next leap forward into the unknown in regards to treating infertility problems in the future involves several areas that are heading into the minefield of numerous ethical and moral issues. Is science and technology now dabbling in the realm of 'Frankenstein Medicine'? Or is the necessary and logical response to forge forward, conquer new frontiers, and enlighten the world to a different way of thinking to maintain the future survival of the human race? Only the future will tell!

There are several notable areas that are looming on the horizon of this new era that we are now entering:

- *Embryo egg harvesting*
- *Embryonic stem cell research*
- *Human cloning technology, and*
- *Artificial sperm and egg production from marrow stem cells*

- *In vitro maturation (IVM)*: the era of 'drug-free' IVF is coming. This technique involves extracting immature eggs and maturing them without the use of over-stimulating drugs. At present it is estimated that 6 per cent of IVF drug users develop serious side effects. This new procedure will hopefully increase pregnancy success rates and help to improve healthier embryos. Older women appear to be the ones that would greatly benefit from IVM.

- *Somatic cell nuclear transfer (SCNT):* cloned human embryos generated from skin cells. Nuclei are removed from mature egg cells of healthy young women, DNA called fibroblasts are retrieved from the male using skin biopsy and inserted into the egg to create human blastocysts.

- *Rho GTPase proteins:* scientists have identifies two important proteins called Rac 1 and RhoA that are necessary for the embryo's ability to implant into the mothers womb lining. The first protein stimulates cells in the womb lining to move and allow the embryo to invade and implant properly while the second inhibits this. The controlled balance of these two proteins is critical for successful implantation of the embryo. Now there is new understanding of how this process works, future drug development is in the pipe line to help keep these Rho GTPases molecules to balance; this will offer greater hope at increasing the success of embryo implantation rates.

- *Synchotron:* scientists at the Monash University in Melbourne (Australia) have discovered a ground-breaking way of determining the maturity of a women's eggs. By utilizing a giant microscope to look at molecular structures using a high-powered infrared beam, we can now show why immature eggs differ from mature eggs due to indentifing varying fats and protein compositions. With future refinement of this fingerprinting 'maping' technology, classifying the stage of an eggs maturaty will considerably improve egg screening for their viability prior to undergoing fertilization in IVF procedures.

These are just some of the areas that will be explored in the future. But we will have to wait until the next edition of the book to discuss these topics!

## What if fertility treatments don't work?

Where do you draw the line and say enough is enough when undergoing fertility treatments and things are not working out? This is a very difficult question to give a cut-and-dried answer to as every individual's circumstances are very different from another's. Saying when to give up on conception is like saying how long is a piece of string.

Many factors need to be weighed up to consider how far you are willing to go in order to become a parent. For some the line may be drawn at 2 years of trying, for others it may be 20. The age of the woman is particularly of importance when considering what options remain open that you can pursue.

Moving forward with your life when pregnancy occurs is usually a smooth transition in most people's lives. But how does one move forward and let go when you are stuck in limbo with no child of your own to love and cherish, to complete the gap in your life?

Like all major events and crossroads throughout your life, we find a way to adapt and carry on. At the time it might seem impossible to imagine how you will survive, as the hurt and heartache is so deep, but you do. Life finds a way to move on.

There are many different types of families that we can be a part of. If the traditional biological family unit doesn't come to fruition, there are many other roads you can travel to have children. Do not close your mind off to seeking third party assistance such as utilising:

* ***donor eggs or sperm*** – donated from a third party source

* ***gestational carriers*** – using your biological embryo but having another woman carry the pregnancy on your behalf to term

* ***surrogates*** – when another woman is both the egg donor and pregnancy carrier

* ***embryo adoption***

* ***child adoption*** (local and overseas)

* ***fostering***

Every country and state has differing laws, legislation and red tape that need to be investigated before you decide to pursue these routes to parenting. In the back section of this book I have provided some contact associations, organisations and websites that you can utilise to gain more information about these particular areas.

# Chapter 17

## *Success Stories*

These are a few examples of letters that I have received from couples who wished to share their baby-making experiences. The following stories were written to show other couples who may be going through similar circumstances, that there can be a pot of gold at the end of their rainbow. These reality stories are only a few of the many different journeys that couples have gone through, the common link being that all have had unquenchable desire to be parents. Each story may have a particular relevance to what you may be personally going through. There are two things to remember in this battle against infertility and that is *you are not alone* and *miracles do happen!*

### *'Two's Company, Three is Perfection'*

We started our baby-making quest a little over four and a half years ago. When we made up our minds to start a family I was 39 years old and my husband Anthony was 41. We realised that we were both late starters in the game, but nevertheless we didn't expect that it was going to be such a big problem to have a baby. We initially tried to conceive the old-fashioned way for nearly 2 years and during this time nothing ended up happening. We thought that there must be something seriously wrong why I wasn't falling pregnant.

As we were both not getting any younger we decided to seek advice from my gynaecologist to see if he could shed some light on our dilemma. After having a number of tests done, from blood, sperm samples, ultrasounds and ovulation monitoring, it was concluded that both myself and my hubby had some problems that had showed up that could be the cause why we were childless.

Firstly, my husband's sperm analysis came back indicating that the count and motility were both quite poor. I was diagnosed as having a condition known as Polycystic Ovarian Syndrome, which was affecting my menstrual cycle and ovulation. Given both our medical findings, my gyno's opinion was that we would probably have about as much chance of winning the national lottery as we would conceiving naturally with our current problems (he said this in a very nice tactful way but the reality of it all was still deflating!). His recommendation was to consider trying a medically assisted procedure called ICSI to improve our chances of having a baby.

As it has been over two thousand years since I have last heard of an 'Immaculate Conception' occurring I didn't think that I had the time to sit and wait to see if I was to be the lucky one to be next. Well, we discussed our options and proceeded with the treatments. I was loaded with Clomid to stimulate the ovaries in hope that I still had some viable eggs that could be fertilised. I realised at my age that the eggs would be getting a bit furry around the edges anyway, but we had to try before my ovaries turned to fossils!

In total we attempted 5 cycles of this procedure, but for some reason or another none of them took. The ICSI procedures were spaced out over 10 months. As you could imagine we were both feeling very frustrated by this stage and our relationship and love life was to say the least beginning to suffer.

The whole process of having to rearrange work schedules and lining up in the specialist's office with a room full of other women in the same situation was stressful. Waiting for my number to be called began to feel a lot like a cattle call, blindly being led here and there, having to take this drug and that drug, have this test and that test done. I couldn't understand why we weren't having any luck. It was really starting to get disheartening and I was running out of faith. Emotionally we were both only hanging on by a very fine thread.

One day I was having lunch with a close friend of mine and as ladies do we were chatting about many things. The topic got on to health and she mentioned that she went to see a naturopath who helped her immensely with her problems and was said to have great results treating reproductive conditions. The following week I ran into a couple of other friends and lo and behold it turned out that they were also visiting this same naturopath. The way they spoke of this man sounded like he was the 'second coming'. I thought to myself, someone or something must be trying to send me a sign, this is too coincidental.

I told my husband about my conversations with my friends and we both agreed we didn't have anything to lose, so decided to go and talk to this guy. Our first consultation with Jason was in September 2002. We took along our medical tests and wondered if he may have answers for us. By the end of our first visit I felt so enlightened and comfortable with this person that I somehow knew in myself that this must be destiny and he could be the one to help us. I also tuned in to listen to Jason give health advice on talk-back radio.

We started our treatment with a course of natural medicines that included a nutritional supplement, a herbal tonic (I call my *magic potion*) Jason made specifically for me, and some homeopathic drops. About two and half months later my husband went back to have a sperm test done and I had a blood test done to check my hormones to see if they were behaving. Anthony's sperm results showed an amazing improvement: the count had almost quadrupled compared to previous tests and the motility was much better also. My hormone test also looked really good compared to previous ones and the menstrual cycle was the best one I can recall having in years, that's if you consider having menstrual periods as a good thing!

We both felt that our general health had also improved, we had more energy and I have to say our libidos had also lifted another notch, not a bad side-effect to have! The following month we timed our intercourse on particular days Jason had advised, now that I had a more accurate ovulation date to work around. At the end of that month I noticed that I felt a bit different than usual and timidly did a pregnancy test to confirm my suspicions. A tiny blue line appeared on the urine stick that morning and I nearly fell over in disbelief. Could this really be happening?

Nine months later I gave birth to our beautiful baby boy, Zack. The pregnancy and delivery all were textbook.

The words 'thank you' don't come close to the remarkable thing that I believe Jason Jackson has done for us. My husband was the last of his family's line of descendants; having a child now allowed his family's lineage to continue.

Not only have our lives changed forever, the rippling effects that have come from having our miracle baby have continued to other family members.

Jason, you have given us a priceless gift that can never be repaid, all the gold in China doesn't come close to what we owe you.

Jason Jackson has helped give us the world and filled our empty arms. If there is a fertility god then for us Jason is it.
***Cecily and Anthony***


### *'And Baby Makes Glee'!*
Our little boy came into the world on 26 July 2002. We both agree that this was the most joyous experience.

We were late starters, not marrying until 34, and then enjoying a year together before trying for a baby. We had a couple of reasons why a pregnancy may not come easy for us but our attitude at the time was ... 'Oh well, if we don't fall pregnant, it is not meant to be ... we will just have to accept it'. This comment seemed quite reasonable before we had difficulty conceiving. Once things weren't going to plan there was no way we were going to 'accept it' until we had tried every option. Apart from our age, there was also Caroline's misfortune of undergoing cancer treatment (radiation and chemotherapy) in her youth, which meant that a pregnancy may not be possible.

After going through the usual process of elimination with medical and fertility checks we ended up in the fertile, however, 'unexplained' category. We then followed the usual medical path finally trying IVF. It was September 2001 when my friend told me about Jason Jackson's fertility successes so we had our first consultation with Jason on Caroline's birthday, 2 October. Two months later Caroline was pregnant. It seemed incredible that the answer to our problems was so simple. We were supposed to be having another IVF procedure in January so we were all too pleased to cancel it.

The pregnancy went smoothly and we now have a beautiful boy. We recommended Jason to two other women who were having fertility troubles and they too have fallen pregnant.

We consider ourselves very fortunate to have found Jason. There are some people in this world that you just cannot repay for what they have done for you and we thank Jason from the bottom of our hearts.
**Caroline and Shayne**


### 'Inconceivable'

My name is Leona and I am now 33 years old. My husband and I decided to start a family. We were successful just before Christmas 2000. The excitement we both felt was the best Christmas surprise. Then I started bleeding at six weeks five days and had to go to hospital on New Year's Eve. After many blood tests and an ultrasound, we were told how common miscarriages were. So we tried again and fell pregnant. An ultrasound and blood test confirmed all was OK.

Regular blood tests were taken checking my HCG levels and progesterone levels. We got to eleven weeks and one day I again started light bleeding. The ultrasound finding was no heartbeat and I was admitted for a curette on the 23rd April 2001. The results from the test showed an abnormal chromosome. So both Dom and I had full chromosome tests, all of which came back normal.

It is hard to write down what is going through your mind, your feelings. When can you get excited about being pregnant? We waited a few months before trying again and on the 17th September 2001 it was confirmed through a blood test that we were pregnant again. Third time lucky!

We are a healthy couple. I have never been a smoker and I do not drink alcohol, tea, coffee or Coke. I drink plenty of water, eat healthy food and used to walk regularly. I was told to take it easy as the pounding while walking may not be good for me. I worked five days a week in a Child Care Centre. My obstetrician kept a close eye on me and I had regular blood tests and scans. We got to eight weeks and the ultrasound again showed no heartbeat – back to hospital again for another curette. This is not the way it was supposed to be for us.

A scan was taken whilst not being pregnant to exclude any abnormalities in my uterus, ovaries and kidneys. No abnormalities were found, all being within normal limits. Then more tests were taken checking for every possible aspect; all came back within normal ranges. I was found to have Gilbert's disease, which I have been told is not an actual disease. It relates to your liver and it has no effects on pregnancy. My obstetrician asked Monash IVF if there were any recommendations to be had from them, although apparently there was no real problem to fix.

Possibly something was happening to my blood when I became pregnant so I was told to take one Cartia (low-strength aspirin) tablet a day. I am not a fan of taking anything and it is very rare for me to even take a Panadol tablet, but if it might help you will try anything.

Friends say things happen for a reason but that is no comfort when it keeps happening to you and there is no problem to fix. Life goes on and you stay positive, knowing there are people less fortunate than yourself. I have my health and I am very much loved. We tried again with blood tests confirming we were pregnant on the 3rd June 2002. This time I took progesterone pessaries. After many blood tests and scans we made it to thirteen weeks and all seemed to be going well. We had passed the twelve-week mark.

You'd think we could get excited and share this news as our dream was finally coming true. But at the thirteen week scan all was not well as no heartbeat could be detected. Back to hospital! I didn't think there was much more they could test me for but they did. Trying to get blood from me is not any quick or easy thing, as my veins tend to shut down. Again all the tests came back within the normal range. We had now reached the point where so-called conventional methods were not working.

Doctors were being sympathetic but were still not able to shed any light on why the miscarriages were happening. At this point we just wanted to know why. My obstetrician recommended Naturopath Jason Jackson; he had not mentioned this before, as we did not have a problem falling pregnant. My husband and I went and spoke with Jason and he looked at our health, background and lifestyle. Jason worked in with the recommendations of my obstetrician with me taking the Cartia tablet daily. I was then placed on a tonic, multi-vitamin, Omega oils and Vitamin C. Jason also recommended two different tablets for my husband. We fell pregnant that month, which took us by surprise. I still see Jason regularly when I am running low on my vitamins. I still have to take one Cartia tablet daily and I took progesterone pessaries till 13 weeks.

I see my obstetrician regularly and my scans to date have all been positive, as have been my blood tests. Everyone to date is pleasantly surprised to see how well we are going with this pregnancy and ask what we have done differently. The answer to this is we have seen a Naturopath. I am presently 24 weeks pregnant and I could not be better. I have been well and it is nice to feel bub kick and to have that reassurance from inside. I take each day as it comes and I am well aware that there are no guarantees about tomorrow.

I have been told that my case is unusual and although miscarriages are common, four in a row with no diagnosed medical problem is not. So we are staying positive that it will be fifth time lucky. This is one very much wanted new life and will be loved more than you could possibly imagine.

I sincerely thank everyone involved to get us to this stage, as we are well aware that pregnancy does not come easily to everyone. Life is a precious gift. Never give up on something that is important to you. Sometimes it takes trying something new to get to where you want to go.

P.S. Hi. It is now 12th February 2007. I find myself writing again, updating my little story. I am happy to say my pregnancy went full term. I was amazed to sail through such an easy pregnancy without one sick day. I am now 37 years old and have two healthy, active boys. Mitch was born in June, weighing 9lb 4oz. Mitchell was perfect in every way. We could not have been happier. We had been blessed with a precious little boy. Our life with Mitch was just a wonderful dream. I did go back to Jason when were thinking of having another baby. Could we do it again? I never stopped taking my vitamins but I wanted to go back on the tonic. We did not want to change what seemed to work for us.

We did fall pregnant again. Although I did find it hard to tell anyone or get my hopes up that we could possibly breeze through another perfect pregnancy. Having Mitch certainly helped my way of thinking. However, I do know all too well what can happen. There are no guarantees of what tomorrow will hold. We were blessed for a second time. Evan was born when Mitch was 18 months old. Evan has an amazing personality and a very unique character. We have truly been so blessed. The boys are now three and a half and two. Life is busy and wonderful. We are grateful and thankful. There was a time when we thought, could we actually have a child? The past is in the past for me. I am not a person who dwells on or talks about the unlucky start we had in having a family.

My husband and I are more than aware of the challenges facing many couples out there. We have a happy ending to our life story. I will say, going to Jason helped us and we could not be happier. Maybe through reading this story it can give a little hope to another couple wanting to fall pregnant. As I have said before sometimes it takes trying something new to get you where you want to go. We are currently working on number three.
*Leona*


### 'Getting that baby'

A couple of years ago, I came across an article in my local paper, about Jason Jackson and his success in helping couples to conceive. At the time I had been trying for several months to fall pregnant, without success, so I decided to see Jason. It was only a matter of weeks before I too, was pregnant. It was actually during my pregnancy that I most valued my visits with Jason. He took

the time to talk to me about the different stages of pregnancy and with his help I had the most wonderful pregnancy. In May 2002, I gave birth to my beautiful and healthy 4.18kg son. I can't thank Jason enough for helping my husband and me to have our family.
*Helen*


### *'Getting back on the horse'*

After three years of trying for a family, going through the heartache and expense of IVF and all the early morning 3-hour trips to Brisbane, we were finally on the way, but we had double the excitement with twins. Everything was going well until 23 weeks when I went into premature labour. I was flown down to the Mater Mothers' Private Hospital where I stayed in labour for 7 days; what an experience that was, one I will definitely not go through again.

The staff at the Mater hospital where absolutely fabulous, but unfortunately my babies would not hold out and I had to deliver; they were both too young to pull through. Everyone told us that the best cure for when you suffer the loss of a child is to have another straight away, but when you have trouble conceiving this adds to the heartache.

I then received my monthly Queensland Fertility Group Newsletter, where I read an inspiring story about a couple who had been on a real rollercoaster, through years of IVF and miscarriages and then their family asked if they would go and see a Naturopath. They decided they would try anything although they had no faith in natural therapies. After visiting Jason Jackson and taking the prescribed tonics and tablets they were blessed 2 months later with the news they were to become parents at last.

I quickly phoned Jason Jackson myself and we got down there for a consultation the next week. Before I knew it I was taking horse-sized tablets and trying to stomach the worst-tasting tonics out. It actually took us nine months to be successful in falling pregnant. Our excitement was then dulled by the fear of going into premature labour again, and sure enough at 20 weeks and after having fortnightly checkups with my local doctor, my cervix was beginning to open once again.

Jason sent me some tablets to try and strengthen things up and I was then sent for bed rest at 26 weeks until 37. This was successful and I managed to deliver a healthy 8-pound baby girl after being induced one day after my due date. I am now 12 weeks into my third clinical pregnancy and couldn't be happier, although the nerves are yet to start all over again. So for anyone who is ready to give up on having a child due to being too emotionally and physically drained from other treatments, do your body a favour and go and see Jason; you may or may not be successful but at least while you are going through the whole process of trying to get pregnant the natural treatments are making you overall healthier and Jason's wealth of knowledge and empathy for

couples enduring this baby-making marathon made all the difference in our success of having a baby.
*Tracey*


### *'Empty cradle'*
My husband and I live in Sydney and were married for 20 months before we decided to start a family. We had heard so many stories from friends and colleagues about problems they had experienced falling pregnant, but we thought we are young, healthy and have a good family history of child bearing so we would be ok. Naturally we felt confident and ready to start the ball rolling!

To our delight, we fell pregnant during the first month of trying. We thought it was easy and now we could plan for our child and the changes we would need to make before the big day!

During my 7th week of pregnancy, I woke with flu-like symptoms and felt dreadful. Unfortunately this continued for a couple of days and as my flu worsened my pregnancy feelings seemed to have faded a little. By the third day, I rushed to my GP and ask to have an ultrasound to make sure the baby was ok. This was organised for the following day and to our amazement we saw that we had a twin pregnancy! As the ultrasound continued, the nurse discovered that one sac was empty and the second sac had a baby but no heartbeat could be detected. We knew from this time, that the pregnancy was non viable and that I was to be scheduled for a D and C.

Nothing can prepare you for these emotions and no answers could be given as to why it happens. We didn't want to be scheduled for further tests that were offered and we just decided that we would try again, as this wasn't meant to be our time. Again, we fell pregnant in the first month. This time everything seemed different and I really felt that this was it; we were going to have a healthy pregnancy.

All was going well until the 8th week when one morning I started to see some physical signs that the pregnancy could be threatened. Before I could get to my obstetrician in the afternoon, I was experiencing a full miscarriage and was admitted again for another D and C.

By this time we were starting to lose hope of ever having a baby and couldn't even bring ourselves to discuss trying again. At the same time as I was recovering from the second miscarriage I had heard of a friend who had been experiencing similar problems with pregnancies and was recommended to Jason Jackson. I decided to wait and see what their outcome was and as soon as I heard the good news and that they were past three months at least, I thought this could really be the answer for me too.

So off I went to visit Jason. The appointment went really well and I felt many of my questions and concerns were answered. I left his clinic, feeling renewed hope and excited about trying to conceive again. Not to mention, I was stocked up with plenty of vitamins and a tonic to ensure this pregnancy would work!

Following Jason's instructions, we fell pregnant again in the second month. I called Jason to tell him, and from then on I knew I had someone by my side monitoring my progress and confident that we would succeed.

Even though I lived in Sydney and only physically visited Jason's clinic a couple of times during the pregnancy, it was successful and we now have a beautiful baby girl born last year.

For anyone considering starting a family, I recommend they visit Jason for a check up and a chat. If I was aware of his success rate earlier on, I may have avoided the disappointments and heartaches experienced for so long.

Well done Jason and we look forward to next time!!
*Catherine and Brendon*

*P.S. And there was a next time – after trying for number two together Catherine and Brendon returned for some advice and now have a very handsome baby boy also!*


### 'Stolen joy'
We decided to start a family and I was very lucky to conceive the first month of trying. Unfortunately this ended in tragedy as our son died at 33 weeks gestation due to placenta abruption. (This is when part or the whole of the placenta tears away from the abdomen wall.) After a little while we decided to try again and with how easy it was the first time we did not think we would have any trouble.

How wrong we were! To cut a long story short, after six years of everything from medications such as Clomid etc. and numerous IVF attempts including ISCI (which is where they insert the semen into the eggs), we had no success.

I had heard very good things about Jason Jackson through my mother who had met a friend of Jason's whilst playing golf. I was reluctant to see Jason as I had already spent a year with another herbalist with no luck.

Anyway, out of sheer desperation we went and saw Jason. I and my husband answered a series of questions and then Jason gave us some tablets to take and he also made up a mixture for me to drink. I will not tell you any lies when I say that the mixture was terrible to drink but to our surprise the very first month after taking the tablets and mixture we found out we were expecting our son (Connor) who turned 4 on 30th November 2003.

I have never used contraception since 1992 and the very month I started taking the tablets and mixture Jason had given us we conceived. We decided to try for number two and without much success on our own we again turned to Jason for help. He again made us up a mixture and a course of tablets and yes, again within a month I was pregnant again. Unfortunately we lost this baby at 14 weeks due to other complications which we did not know about at the time.

I have recommended Jason to a number of people I have met through the IVF circles and all of them have had success after seeing Jason. I would have no hesitation in recommending Jason as we will always be indebted to him as he has helped us achieve a dream we started believing might not ever happen.

*Julie*

## 'Maybe baby'

I was introduced to Jason 4 years ago after suffering severe endometriosis for 10 years and unfortunately having 3 miscarriages. In the 10 years of pain and sadness with the miscarriages, I had seen several specialists and had also been seeing another naturopath for 3 years. By the time I had met Jason I guess I was a bit sceptical about naturopathic medicine but was desperate for help.

Jason was a ball of life and made me feel like there was still hope. After spending a good hour and a half talking with Jason, I walked out of the clinic with a bag of goodies and hearing Jason saying, 'that on average with other patients it may take 3 months or so before you could expect to be pregnant'.

Two and a half months later our son Bailey was conceived, and at 35 years of age, I have never felt so healthy. Bailey was born on 24th April. Three and a half years later after trying by ourselves with no success and suffering another miscarriage, we went back to Jason and asked him for his help. Four months later I called Jason with the good news: our second baby is due in May 2004.

Thank you, Jason, for making our dreams come true.

*Wendy, Dane and Bailey*

## 'Helping the Stork'

My husband and I have been trying to conceive a child for many years; I have been on the merry-go-round of drugs and IVF treatments with sadly no success. I felt that I was rapidly running out of time and options. Visiting Jason Jackson has opened up a whole new world of alternative possibilities and renewed hope.

I am ecstatically happy to say that we now have a beautiful healthy child with the assistance of Jason's treatment program. He truly changed not only our lives but countless others, and I'm sure he can also help to change yours. THANK YOU, THANK YOU, THANK YOU.

*Sarah Jane*

## 'Expecting miracles'

I heard of Jason Jackson through a girlfriend of mine who successfully maintained two pregnancies and now has two beautiful girls after being on Jason's fertility program, previously having had several miscarriages.

My story: I first sought Jason's advice in December 2002 after trying to fall pregnant for eight years. The only thing I ever wanted in my life was to be a wife and mother; for whatever reason I had everything but motherhood. I was a flight attendant for 15 years and of course found anything I could to blame for my inability to fall pregnant. I decided to then start studying Naturopathy part time in 1991, graduating in 1998. Throughout this whole time and for some time thereafter I sought anyone and everyone to help me help myself to fall pregnant.

Both my husband and I had many investigations and it was found that I had one blocked fallopian tube and an inter-uterine fibroid which was causing the shape of my uterus to be somewhat distorted. My husband and I then went through 3 stimulated cycles of IVF and then 2 frozen embryo cycles, all of which were unfortunately unsuccessful. We and my wonderful doctor then decided that we would have the fibroid removed. My doctor performed such a wonderful job and apart from a little scarring in my uterus all looked well. We then decided to give IVF a break and investigated overseas adoption which we are still very committed to.

As mentioned previously I sought Jason's advice in December 2002 only putting a small amount of pressure on him stating, 'I just know you are going to be my miracle worker'. I was on Jason's herbs for three months. I am now almost 18 weeks pregnant and all looks to be going well. I was also having acupuncture and spiritual healing as well and truly believe that finding Jason was what I needed to finally fulfil our dream.

I will be forever grateful to all who have helped us. To Jason I will say, 'thank you for being my miracle worker'. I have referred many couples to see Jason over the past few years who found Jason's treatment program to be very successful.

**Fiona Newcome-Wright (Naturopath)**

*P.S. Fiona and her husband are now the proud parents of a healthy baby boy. Fiona came back for help trying for bubby number 2, and I'm proud to say she got her wish come true, again!*


## 'I Dream of Baby'

My name is David and my wife Michelle and I started to try for a family seven years ago when we were both aged 35. We initially tried to conceive a baby for just over a year with no result. We live in a remote part of the country in central Australia and have very little medical amenities near us. Occasionally I need to venture into the big smoke for work and as it had been some time since my wife and I had been trying for a baby we thought it best that we seek out some medical assistance to investigate why things were not happening.

The doctor went through our medical histories and advised that some diagnostic tests would be warranted. I have worked on the land most of my life as a farmer and labourer, so the doctor suspected that my sperm may have been affected by my work environment as I have been exposed to pesticide chemicals and machinery fumes.

When I was younger I recall having an accident when a horse gave me a fair kick in the private parts, which I thought may have caused some long-term damage that may have been a reason behind the problem. The doctor also performed a physical exam on me and found that I had a varicose (varicose vein) in the testes that may also be a potential cause.

The first sperm test I had done showed that I only produced a sperm count of 1.8 million sperm, the motility was very average, and the abnormalities were at 87 per cent. This result was not good and the chances of conception would be 'buckley's and none', the normal way with these types of readings.

My wife Michelle also had many investigations done and all her results came back as being OK. The doctor recommended that the best chances for us to have a baby would be to try a procedure called ICSI, as having poor sperm quality was less important to have success than with other procedures.

Well, due to our remote living arrangements, getting to an IVF clinic was a very difficult task for us as the closest one was still several hundred miles away. But because the desire to have a family was so important to us we endured the long trips in hope of a result. To cut a long story short, in total we had one IVF and five ICSI procedures performed, but none of them took.

During this time the sperm counts never improved over 8 million. Some of the tests showed some improvements in motility, but the abnormality amount remained always over the 80 per cent mark. Our dreams of having a baby were not looking like it would become a reality.

To be honest we were both getting very disappointed with these constant failed attempts. I was really starting to feel a bit neurotic and inadequate as a male not being able to father a child to my wife, and Michelle was developing severe anxiety attacks from the ongoing dramas of trying to make a baby. Our lives at this point resembled a badly scripted soap opera saga. If there is a place called Purgatory (hell's waiting room) then I think we had found it.

Many of our friends were all having children during the same time we were also trying. We were becoming quite envious that others could have something that we didn't. The green-eyed monster showed its ugly head more than a few times. The grass looked much greener on the other side of the fence! I think that we would have sold our souls to the devil to have a baby to get us out of this living nightmare.

When Michelle and I both turned 41 we really thought that was it, and tried to be philosophical about things that for some reason or another kids just weren't meant to be for us. But it was still a bitterly hard pill to swallow regardless! A relative of ours had been to Brisbane and said they went to see a Naturopath for a health problem they were having and was very happy with the result. I was very ignorant about what a Naturopath was, living out in the sticks. I had great visions of a voodoo witch doctor mixing up some wicked brew in a cauldron.

We eventually decided after much procrastination that we needed to change tack to have one last chance at this. We went to Brisbane to see this Naturopath who was Jason Jackson and there were no witch's cauldrons to be found!

Jason was absolutely wonderful; he went through our histories, did some additional investigations and explained to us what he thought the problems were and what his plan was to hopefully correct them. He prescribed some natural medicines for us and I was to get a sperm test done in three months to check on the progress of the treatment, in the event that Michelle hadn't fallen pregnant during this time.

We religiously did what Jason advised and three months later I had my sperm test done. The doctor read out my result and I thought that there must have been some mix-up with the specimens. The sperm count increased to 220 million, the motility was over 70 per cent, and the abnormalities were down to 50 per cent. This result was more than 20 times better than any other result I have had done; it blew me away!

This good news really motivated us again to think we may have a chance at this. That following month my wife was quite late with her periods, which are usually very regular. We had stocked up on pregnancy test kits in the hope we may actually get to use them. On 26th March 2004, the pregnancy test confirmed a positive result, a sight I didn't think we would get to see. My wife and I looked at each other like stunned mullets in disbelief. I got on the phone to Jason to tell him the great news, still in a daze from the magnitude of the result.

Jason got us sorted out with some changes in supplements to help with the pregnancy and sent everything we needed to us. The pregnancy went extremely well and our baby boy Michael was born 15th November 2004. They say 'It ain't over until the fat lady sings'; in our case she was definitely starting to clear her throat, so we consider ourselves very lucky. Reflecting back on our journey now Michelle and I took more beatings than Sylvester Stallone did in his *Rocky* movies; like Rocky we felt down and out, absorbing hit after hit, back against the rope but saving just enough will to hang in there and ultimately win the epic fight in the final round by knock-out!

I recall a particular conversation that we had when seeing Jason. I personally found the way in which he simplified the complexities of infertility very refreshing and I wished that other people that we had sought advice from before could have explained things to us in a similar way that Jason has. Jason also does a lot of work with professional athletes, getting them in peak condition for major sporting events. He told us that the preparation process we were also doing was comparable to how an athlete fine-tunes their preparation before they compete. The training regime and nutrition requirements are tailored toward achieving a certain goal. We also are tailoring our preparation to achieve a certain goal. The better the preparation the best chances we will have when we also 'take our crack at winning the title'. Being a sports nut to me this made logical commonsense!

Help comes in many forms and to us Jason Jackson is a saint. He helped us achieve something in 4 months that through more than 5 years of other avenues did not. Before we saw Jason we were given little to no hope at all of having a family of our own; he has changed all that for us. He is a true champion of the people, thank you from the bottom of our hearts.
***David and Michelle***


### 'Failure to launch'
I am a 32-year-old female with two boys, 3 years 2 months, and 22 months. We conceived very easily with the boys; however, whilst trying for our third child, my husband and I encountered difficulties. After trying to conceive naturally for a few months I felt a sharp pain on my left side down in the pelvic region. This came out of the blue one day about 24 hours after we had tried to conceive. I saw my GP and I was referred to an obstetrician. Following that I had a laparoscopy and hysteroscopy, but both found no evidence of any abnormalities or cause of the pain. We kept trying for a series of months, some with and some without the pain occurring.

Eventually after 11 months of trying to conceive, my obstetrician prescribed Clomid to be taken as one tablet from day 2-6 of my cycle. I felt awful on this, mood swings, very angry, highs and lows and I didn't ovulate after the first month of taking this drug. Combined with the pain on my left side, my obstetrician found that I was only having random ovulation. I would get the tests done on day 21 of my cycle and I'd see the doctor on day 9 to check for dominant follicles. For the majority of months, from March to October there were no dominant follicles. We were described as 'unexplained infertility'.

I took myself off Clomid after 2 months as I didn't agree with what it was doing to my system and moods. I did actually ovulate in the second month of taking this drug. We were considering IVF at this stage when a friend told me about

Jason Jackson. I was a little sceptical as I had never tried natural medicine before. But I thought at this stage, what have I to lose? Within 5 weeks I found out that I was pregnant, much to our utter amazement and utter disbelief after having tried unsuccessfully for 14 months using traditional medicine.

Coincidentally, I am not the first person my friend has recommended to Jason. Apparently she has spoken to 3 other friends and we are all now happily pregnant or have delivered healthy babies after seeking Jason's advice. I'm sure that without Jason's assistance and sympathetic ear we may not have been so fortunate. You are a marvel!
*Name withheld*


### *'Houston...we have a problem'!*
Our first child was conceived on our first wedding anniversary and came as a huge surprise. I had just gone off the Pill and we had begun to discuss starting a family. I remember feeling so incredibly blessed. When our son turned two we decided it was time to welcome another child into our lives. Six months later we were once again celebrating our good fortune, calculating due dates and sharing our joy with family and friends. At eight weeks we had our first miscarriage, a blighted ovum the doctor told us. One month later I was rushed into surgery to remove an ectopic pregnancy that had been missed. The doctor told me it was very rare for this to happen and that I was lucky to be alive, as I could have bled to death. I didn't feel lucky; I had lost my right fallopian tube and another precious child.

Somewhere inside me I lost some of the confidence I had been feeling about my marriage, my life and myself. I had some very lonely, empty feelings at this time.

It was hard to accept the way things were going for us. After a while we got back up, counted our blessings for the child we already had and continued on.

The following year for Mother's Day I got a wonderful gift, confirmation that at last another baby was on the way.

I breathed a huge sigh of relief and began to feel hope that our plan for a family would be realised. Three days later my confidence drained away as I began to bleed. After this it seemed we just weren't able to conceive at all. The next couple of years became a pretty much a blur of doctors, fertility drugs, timed intercourse, temperature charts and month after month of disappointment and tears. The treatments made me feel constantly moody; I was having erratic cycles, abnormal bleeding and PMT three weeks out of every month. A horrible feeling developed deep inside along with unbelievable tension within our marriage. I just started to shut down from the pain.

We eventually turned away from traditional medicine and found a naturopath who specialised in fertility. I pinned my hopes on constant reassurances and a foul-tasting tonic for two years with no improvement until I finally got to the point where I was a complete wreck emotionally and physically. I just couldn't understand why we couldn't achieve something that was meant to be so natural. No one could tell us what was wrong or how to get out of this nightmare. Then we found Jason.

I remember walking into his office with my husband and thinking 'We've tried everything, you might have helped other people but you can't possibly help us.' I actually really liked Jason from the start in spite of my hopeless mood. He was just so, well … likeable. He joked with us and put us both at ease but he also gave us his complete attention, understanding and real empathy. I liked that he treated both of us, even when I told him that the doctors had told us that I was the problem.

He made us feel like we were in this together. I walked out of his office already feeling healthier than when I came in. I had more tonics to take as well as various vitamins and nutritional supplements.

Six months later we agreed we were certainly doing better emotionally and feeling a lot healthier. Then two months later, success. There were two little blue lines on the pregnancy test. I couldn't speak, I just cried. After my husband, the second person I told was Jason. He sounded genuinely pleased but not at all surprised. I got the feeling that he got this kind of phone call all the time.

More tonic, supplements, care and support to get us through those first few months. I glowed through the whole nine months, had a fantastic labour and we now have a second beautiful son who sleeps, eats, laughs and fills our hearts with absolute joy.

Recently my husband jokingly requested that I stop telling people who ask how our little miracle happened, about Jason. 'I had something to do with it too you know,' he reminds me. 'I know, honey,' I tell him. But we both really know that when love and a really wanted child just weren't enough there was somebody there who really knew how to help.
***Name withheld***


***Email –'The pursuit of happiness'***
Hi Jason,

Yes, I believe I am another success story of yours. My beautiful baby boy is in this world I believe because I came to your clinic for help.

I first visited you in April last year to get help with my PCOS and get my hormones into a regular pattern … partly because I was getting married this past February and wanted to feel good and have my cycle under control so my day could be planned for everything!

When I first came to see you and we went through my symptoms and talked, you told me that if I wasn't pregnant within three months then we would need to look further and possibly look at more than PCOS. Well, I went away from the visit with tablets and tonic in hand and after the first shot of the tonic the next morning was about to give it all up! But I persisted and the taste got better … about 6 weeks later (due to another irregular cycle) I was back for another visit … more tonic and tablets in hand as I left …

I was due to come back mid to late July but with my engagement party raging I lost track of the days and all of a sudden it was the first week of August and I hadn't been to visit you for the third time as my period hadn't come … when the engagement party was over, I had an urge of sickness the next Monday and thought I was suffering from a release of anxiety and stress that had been building up … it was the next day I found out I was 6 weeks pregnant!!!! My wedding in February consequently was all postponed for another day …

Our baby – Jake – was born on 3rd April this year and he is absolutely gorgeous! Any doctor who saw me for the first time during my pregnancy was amazed that with PCOS I had fallen pregnant so quickly … I told them all that it was my naturopath's fault!!!

I am forever grateful for your wonderful help and am proud to be a success story of yours – I will be coming back to your clinic as soon as we are ready to have our next baby as you are my best chance for me extending my family.
*Kristy*


### *'From Tragedy to Triumph'*
My husband Greg and I were thrilled when we discovered that I was pregnant after a couple of years of trying. We were very good and waited till I was 14 weeks to let everyone know. Everyone was just as thrilled as we were. Little did we know we would be calling everyone back only one week later to tell them I had been diagnosed with breast cancer! That was the 23rd April 2004 – I was 15 weeks.

In the week that followed I had surgery to remove the lump and 23 lymph nodes. The surgery was a success and my doctor was happy with the outcome but the cancer had shown up 6 lymph nodes, which meant chemotherapy. At first my doctor wanted me to wait till my baby was 30 weeks, then deliver early before starting further treatment, but the night before I got out of hospital, my Oncologist came to visit me and said that if I waited I would only have a 20 per cent chance of survival. I had a 60 per cent chance of survival if I started chemo straight away – this is based on all cancer survivors over a 5-year period. Because I was 16 weeks I could not terminate, I had to let nature take its course. My doctor, as well as the nurses in my ward told me that my baby would more than likely die. So, after spending one of the worst nights of my life, lying in my hospital bed listening to my heart pound in my chest worrying about what might happen, I decided to get on with it and see what would happen.

At 19 weeks I had my first chemo treatment. My Obstetrician, who was fantastic, was with me that first night monitoring Tegan (my little girl). She had a fine strong heartbeat. I cannot begin to describe what it felt like to have that poison pumped into my arm and had no idea what it was going to do to me or my baby. It wasn't a pleasant feeling, I can tell you that. Felt like ice was speeding up through my veins and I could taste it. It tasted like I was sucking on coins. The next day I was very tired, a little sick, but mostly worried because Tegan didn't move. Finally 3 days later I felt her shift and knew she was ok. Shortly after my first treatment, I went to visit Jason Jackson my naturopath. I had meant to see him about my pregnancy the day I was diagnosed, but somehow didn't get round to it. Jason prescribed a course of tablets that would not only help me feel better but would give my baby a fighting chance.

I would get very sick after each chemo treatment; I was barely able to move and was very tired. My mother, who would move in for a week every 3 weeks, would force me to eat good food and make me drink the required 3-4 litres of water a day. I would sleep a lot because I tired very easily, for example, if I did a load of washing I would have to lie down for a while.

The treatments were every three weeks and I would always pick up a little in the last week just in time for the next lot of chemo. But I seemed to do very well, compared to other people I would speak to who were going through the same treatment. I had regular scans to check on Tegan and there were never any problems, always the correct weight and length. My doctors were always impressed at how well she was doing at every visit, and while none of them believed in naturopathic supplements I was taking, they didn't stop me. (I would have liked to see them try!). I truly believe that my baby wouldn't have been born healthy (and beautiful) if I hadn't had Jason's help.

Originally Tegan was to be born at 30 weeks, but because she did so well, she was born by caesarean on the 10th September 2004 at 34 weeks. She weighed 1879 grams (4 pounds 3oz), a very good size for a premmie baby.

From day one she surprised everyone by how strong she was. She stayed in the oxygen crib for only one night then moved to the section in the nursery they call the 'fat farm' soon after. She pulled her feeding tube out twice by herself so eventually the nurses gave up and fed her by bottle only. She stayed in the hospital for only 2 weeks and came home on my 30th birthday.

I had 6 treatments while I was pregnant and 4 treatments after Tegan was born, finally finishing on 24th November. It had been a very long pregnancy. Three weeks after my last treatment my hair started to grow back, (much quicker than it normally does), and I started my radiotherapy treatments. This was very different to chemo. Firstly it didn't make me sick but it did make me very tired. Secondly, I would travel to the hospital daily except weekends and public holidays. I had 30 treatments all up so they stretched over Christmas and finished on 2nd February. Mum moved in again and stayed with me for a couple of weeks after I finished because I was just too tired to get up to Tegan through the night and Greg had to get up for work every day. The skin in the treated area had burnt quite badly; this would take a few months to settle. By the end everyone was exhausted and very glad it was all over, especially me.

Since February Tegan has continued to grow and prosper, gaining weight and meeting every milestone head on. I have continued to get stronger and stay positive every day. I have also continued to see Jason and he has prescribed different mixtures and supplements to help me through every stage of recovery, and is helping me to stay healthy and hopefully this will never happen to me again. Recently, I had my first lot of tests to check if everything is ok, and of course it is!

Many thanks to all my doctors, Jason Jackson, my friends, my family, my husband and of course my beautiful baby girl – who probably saved my life.
*June*


### 'Great expectations'
Finding good advice these days is difficult. As my fiancé and I met later in life we were both 41 when we decided to try to have a family. Everybody was telling us something different and we were torn between the medical and herbal fields. When we met Jason Jackson he made us feel completely at ease and immediately we felt confident enough to be guided by his expertise.

Jason has an extensive knowledge of both medical and naturopathic fields and tailored an easy plan for us as individuals, taking into consideration our lifestyle and general health. After 3 months we were blessed with a pregnancy and the entire journey has been a 'dream run'. I could not have asked for better health during the 9 months or a better result in the end product – a perfectly healthy little boy.

Thank you, Jason, for your compassion, guidance and expertise – we are forever grateful.
*Jen, Ron and baby Mathew*


### 'When your cheese slips off your cracker'!
My name is Andrew and I have been compelled to share some of my life history with you in the hope that my experience can help others that are pursuing parenthood.

After finishing high school I went to work for my father's large construction company as a builder's apprentice. At the same time I also started at university doing a Business degree as my father was keen for me to take over the family business when he was ready to retire. During my final year of uni I met my now wife Sharon at one of the many parties that I frequented during that time. In hindsight I think I did a little too much partying and not enough studying, but I did get to meet the love of my life. I finally graduated with my Business degree (luckily!) and Sharon and I got married three years later. During my school and uni years I also participated in a number of sports in particular rugby and cycling were I competed at a national representative level.

My father has since retired and I have taken over the reins managing his construction company going from a blue-collar worker to a white-collar worker responsible for hundreds of contractors and work sites.

At the age of 35 Sharon and I thought it was time to start our own family and keep the family legacy going. After about a year of trying we had no success. My younger brother Brad had just told us the news that his wife Jenny was expecting and I remember he had the biggest grin on his face when he announced he was going to be a dad. Thinking to myself at the time, if Brad could father a child and there weren't any other relatives that had fertility problems in our family that I knew about, then it was just a matter of time until we too could spill the same news.

Another six months went by, the workload was getting more and more, I was putting in ridiculously long hours at work, and the intimacy between Sharon and I was becoming less and less. Finally, it was decided that we go see a gyno specialist to see if there was really a problem or not. Sharon had blood tests and a laparoscopy done to rule out any internal issues. Her results come back perfect. The gyno then focused his attention on me. He said that it would be best if I provided a sperm sample for analysis … not my finest hour by the way.

I felt sick to the stomach to think that the problem all along was me. We had to know, so I provided the sperm sample, took it into the clinic and went back to work, all the time praying it would be all right. Two days later we got a call from the fertility clinic asking to schedule an appointment to discuss the results. Straightaway we knew there must be something wrong … if the results were good then they would have told us on the phone then and there.

We made an appointment as soon as possible. That night I could not sleep, I tossed and turned thinking how could there be a problem. Was it from playing too much sport, some kind of chemical exposure from the work sites, overstressed from work, partying to hard? … My mind was racing; the list of possibilities was endless.

We fronted up at the gyno's office; the result we dreaded to hear was bad, really bad, no traces of any sperm at all were found in the sample. The first thought I had was, the result must be completely wrong, it can't be true. The doctor asked me to get a blood test to see if that could enlighten us more to what may be going on. I had the blood test done and the results showed that my testosterone levels were lowish, but a hormone called FSH was a bit on the high side, which was explained to me as meaning that the sperm weren't being nourished enough to grow properly. It's amazing what new terminology I was learning by now. The doctor explained as a matter of deduction the results pointed to several possible leading causes.

Testicular failure (similar to female menopause) (that sounded horrifying!), drug use (to be truthful was a possibility), extreme stress response (also a big possibility), a severe infection like the mumps (I didn't know) or an endocrine gland dysfunction particularly of the testes, adrenals, hypothalamus and/or pituitary glands (I know about the testes, for the other ones I had no idea what they were!).

The doctor explained that there were several options that could be tried to hopefully get some sperm forming. One option was to firstly do another sperm test to confirm the original test, number two option was hormone therapy, which was said to have mixed results, or number three a testicular biopsy to remove some deeper testicular tissue to see if any sperm was forming at all. If all other options proved futile then option four was to consider possible donor sperm to be used with Sharon's eggs in an ICSI-IVF procedure. Options two, three and four didn't sound like ideal choices to me, so I took the chicken option number one to confirm the original sperm test. The result came back the same!

I was young, healthy, an accomplished athlete, ran a successful company, and had a beautiful wife; I was in the prime of my life, I thought I was bullet proof. But this situation dropped me to my knees – life had thrown a curve ball I wasn't expecting, I felt mentally exhausted and emotionally started to shut down. Weeks went by and I was getting more and more depressed, not a good thing when you have a big company to run. I was busier than a one-legged Irish River Dancer; I had no time for this crap!

The doctor referred us to have couples counselling (code for 'shrink') to discuss my emotions. I stubbornly and flatly refused. I wanted to feel pissed off because I thought that I may be permanently sterile. The doctors wanted to chop up my 'family jewels' (testes) in a remote attempt to scrounge for some remnants of sperm, and now they wanted to label me as a 'nut case' as well; life at that moment was just 'peachy'. Reflecting back on things now my reactions were so immature and self-absorbed, counselling may have been an option that could have helped me cope better but I couldn't see past my own self-pity.

Several months later, Sharon came to me and said she was speaking to a work colleague about natural medicines being used to help with fertility. The notion sounded a bit airy-fairy to me but I had to try and be open minded for Sharon's sake. We booked an appointment with Naturopath Jason Jackson who was recommended to us. I started to do some reading and looked up every website on the internet to research as much information I could to better prepare; it was doing my head in.

We went for our meeting. I have to admit Jason really knows his stuff; I threw at him some very tough questions, and for every question I asked he gave an honest and intelligent answer. Truthfully, I walked into that first meeting thinking that this was going to be a waste of our time. By the end, I felt like the weight of the world was being lifted off my shoulders. Jason recommended it was worth giving some natural remedies a try; if worse came to worse the other medical treatments were still options if it had to come to that. I needed to be on the treatment for several months as it can take at least 72 days to start producing new sperm. This option sounded much less invasive than the other alternatives I was faced with, so I gave it a try.

Three months later I had more blood tests and another sperm analysis done. The results came back very promising; the testosterone levels were much better, the FSH had dropped down, and the big news was that they found some sperm in the sample. The sperm numbers were still not very good and the motility was also ordinary, but the result was encouraging and going in the right direction. Jason was thrilled to see this improvement.

Two and a half months later Sharon's period was late. I tore down to the chemist to get a pregnancy test kit and my heart was pounding. Sharon did the test and after a breath-holding wait those magic positive little lines showed up. What a feeling! Who could imagine looking at a tiny piece of plastic that had just been peed on could fill your heart with such joy. We rang Jason straight away to give him the good news. He was really happy for us. Sharon's pregnancy was excellent and on the 13th September 2006 our precious baby girl Amy was born. We have not experienced happiness like this. We are so fortunate to have found Jason, not to say that if we pursued the medical options that we wouldn't have become parents in the end. But Jason's approach is something special; he has certainly made a believer out of us and to top it all off I got to save some potentially very unpleasant trauma to my balls. We will see Jason again soon when we try for number two.
*Andrew and Sharon*


### 'The road less travelled – how far are you willing to go'
Over the years I have personally seen thousands of couples that have come to me for a variety of health and reproductive problems. There is one particular couple that will leave a lasting impression with me until the day I die.

I first saw this particular couple several years ago now, but their life story has me in tears every time I think of them. As we were going through our initial consultation, the couple explained to me what had been going on prior to seeing me. Collectively the lady has had no less than 34 medically assisted reproductive procedures performed on her over a period of 12 years, in their attempts to have a baby. They had tried everything from multiple IVF interventions, ICSI, SUZI, GIFT, and Artificial Insemination (AI) using her partners and donor sperm, and so on. My mind boggled how anyone could go through all that anguish!

The couple were both 48 years of age (so there weren't too many more shopping days til Christmas)! They were both surprisingly in exceptionally good health particularly considering what they had been through. Through all the medical investigative work-ups prior to this, no identifiable cause was to be found, though the male's sperm analysis showed slightly low levels in sperm count and motility, though it was not low enough to explain why they shouldn't be able to conceive naturally.

Throughout all these procedures to try to have a child, only 3 out of the 34 attempts carried beyond the first trimester and only one made it to 24 weeks.

Before I had seen this couple they had virtually travelled to the four corners of the globe in their frantic search to have a child of their own to love and nurture.

They continued to explain their tragic story. After all the unsuccessful medical outcomes the couple decided to pursue a different path and applied to adopt a child overseas. To avoid the rigmarole of bureaucratic red tape they packed their bags and moved to Mexico for 6 months in an attempt to speed up proceedings. In the final weeks before the legal matters were to be settled their whole world fell apart once again as the supposed agency they were dealing with shot through with some $100,000 dollars (Australian) of their money, leaving no trace.

As you would imagine, both of them had been to hell and back; not only had they collectively spent and lost a king's fortune, their hearts would have felt like they were torn from their chests after enduring such an emotional marathon just to end up back at the very beginning. No more attempts were made for several years because the despair and wretchedness of it all had almost been the end of them both.

One day a friend of theirs came to see me also for fertility-related issues and she subsequently fell pregnant. She begged her friends to also try again. Nearly a full year later the couple found a splinter of lingering hope and courage and possibly out of curiosity they came in to talk with me. After hearing their astonishing history and plea for help I wondered what the hell I could do for these people that they hadn't already gone through before. Rather than become overwhelmed with the complex nature of the situation I thought we should get back to basics and try simply to build a strong foundation plan of improving both their pre-conceptual health.

The one irony in all this was that approximately 3 months after the time I first saw the couple I received a phone call from the woman's partner to inform me that they had performed a pregnancy test and came up with a positive result. The lady could not speak on the phone, as she had not stopped crying all day, due to a mixture of pent-up emotional strain and happiness. We quickly proceeded to take some active measures to support her body in the hope of not miscarrying. I am proud to say that they had a beautiful, healthy child as a result of their love and affection for each other.

Their testimonial shows how an optimistic attitude and persistent determination can sometimes get you what you want, particularly when you are fighting against the odds. This couple did get their fairytale ending and are now living happily ever after, as are many other couples who I have been humbled and privileged to help over the years and witness their dreams come true. Hopefully there will be many more to come in the future.

# A Final Word

# *'You Never Know What Can Happen'*

There are four foundation principles that I strictly adhere to when assisting couples in the preparative stage of trying to conceive and making babies.

1) Protect the genetic load of both the egg and sperm where possible;
2) Stabilise the immune systems – to avoid incompatibility problems;
3) Improve the lymph and circulation flow to the reproductive organs; and
4) Bring balance and harmonise the various hormone systems of the body.

I have found that when all these areas are synergistically functioning correctly the major battle of achieving successful conception has already been won.

A female's reproductive system sadly does have a limited shelf-life, even with all this current knowledge and technology at our disposal. Even Moses himself couldn't hold back the parted sea forever. What goes on outside of the body may not necessarily reflect what may be going on inside. Your biological age and physiological age are not the same. For example, a woman in her thirties may have irregular menstrual cycles and reduced ovarian reserves and go through premature menopause, therefore having a physiological reproductive age of a woman much more her senior. Whereas another woman may still be regularly menstruating and still have relatively good ovarian reserves well into her fifties, thus having the reproductive physiological age in comparision to other women more her junior. Both genetics and environment will play major dictating roles in where you may fit into this equation.

Statistically speaking, **'the longer the duration of the infertility has been, the lower the chances each month of getting pregnant will be – no matter what the tests show'.** The closer women get to the menopausal years, generally the higher the FSH levels become, therefore more follicles are lost resulting in a smaller amount of viable eggs available for fertilisation.

**'When it comes to fertility <u>TIME</u> may be your greatest nemesis!'**

If I can leave you with one last piece of advice, *'please don't let the clock beat you'.* There are many wonderful fertility-boosting therapies available that may hold the key that ultimately solves your problem to help you to conceive; don't delay in giving them a try. I have witnessed some amazing things happen over the years. Just at my clinic alone I have had at least sixty forty-eight year olds and more than a few fifty-year-old women who have given birth for the first time from natural conception after being given little to no chance. By adopting a pre-conception and pregnancy natural fertility program you can greatly stack the odds of success more in your favour and widen that window of opportunity.

Personally, I place little faith in by-the-book statistics. Even though I have quoted some throughout the book for illustration purposes, they should be viewed as a general guide rather than solid indisputable facts that are etched in stone; statistics can change, don't become a lost statistic. Just through my experiences dealing with health and reproductive issues, I love to see it when people defy the laws of statistics and make the improbable possible – it happens every day; it's never over until it's over, and even then there are other possible avenues to parenthood.

***Remember the 3 'P' golden rules:***

1) **Preparation**
2) **Persistence**
3) **Perseverance**

***'Even in your darkest hour the light of hope can still break through.'***

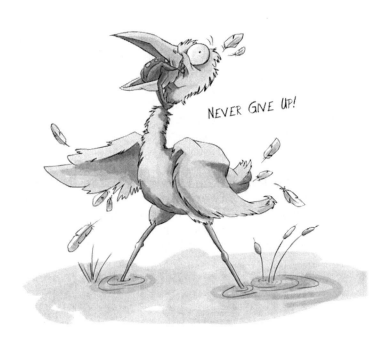

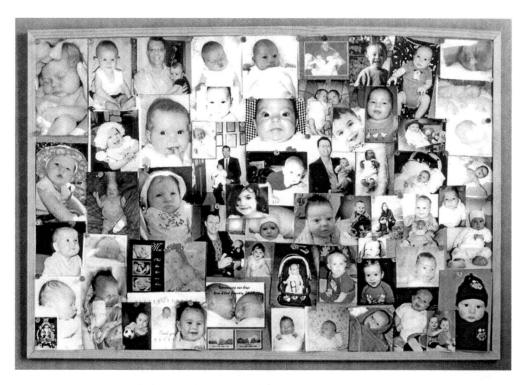

A photo collage of just some of the babies that Jason Jackson's natural fertility program has helped bring into the world.

# Twelve things to do to help improve fertility

1) Go off any contraceptive pills or devices 3 to 6 months prior attempting conception

2) Limit or discontinue all unnecessary drugs/medications (under doctor's advice).

3) Males should avoid over heating on the testicles, consider wearing loose-fitting clothes and boxer undershorts.

4) Consider adopting a pre-conception health program for both sexes 3 to 6 months prior to trying to fall pregnant.

5) Eat a good well-balanced diet, substitute with live organic wholesome foods where possible. A high quality multivitamin/mineral supplement designed for reproduction health may be recommended.

6) Nutrients of particular importance for male reproductive health may include: zinc; Vitamin B12; Vitamin C; Vitamin E; selenium; L-carnitine; L-arginine; taurine; folic acid; and Co Q 10.

7) Herbs of particular importance for male reproductive health may include: tribulus; panax and Siberian ginseng; damiana; withania; saw palmetto; horny goat weed; maca root; morinda officinalis; oats; muira puama; rhodiola; shativari; and schisandra.

8) Nutrients of particular importance for female reproductive health may include: folic acid; zinc; Vitamin E; Vitamin C; essential fatty acids; Vitamin B complex (especially B6 and B12); Vitamin A (low dose); selenium (low dose); magnesium; and iron (if required).

9) Herbs of particular importance for female reproductive health may include: false unicorn root; true unicorn root; vitex; paeonia; shativari; tribulus; dong quai; liquorice; black cohosh; cramp bark; raspberry leaf; and wild yam.

10) If natural conception has not occurred after a full year of timed, unprotected intercourse, consider seeking further advice from your gynaecologist and/or natural therapist regarding tests and treatment options.

11) Avoid excessive exposure to STRESS, heavy metals, electro-magnetic fields, chemicals and other pollutants.

12) Further investigations such as: sperm analysis; blood work of hormone function; ultrasounds; and physical examinations may need to be considered to rule out any underlying medical condition that may be affective fertility.

# Support Groups and Other Contacts

**The Australian and New Zealand Infertility Counsellors Association**.
Website:  www.swin.edu.au/hosting/anzical/ANZIChome.htm

**Access – Australia's National Infertility Network.**
PO Box 959
Parramatta NSW 2124
Tel: (02) 9670 2380
Fax: (02) 96702638
Email: info@access.org.au
Website: www.access.org.au

**Oasis Infertility Support Inc.**
GPO Box 2420
Adelaide SA 5001
Tel: (08) 8223 7434
Email: oassissupport@chariot.net.au
Website: www.users.chariot.net.au/~oassisup-port

**Genesis Infertility Support Group**
Box 1574
Booragoon WA 6154
Tel: (08) 9375 7572
Website: www.users.bigpond.com/genisiup-port

**Friends of Queensland Fertility Group**
GPO Box 1271
Brisbane QLD 4001
Email friendssqfg@rocketmail.com
Website: www.geocities.com/hotsprings/2952

**Donor Conception Support Group of Australia**
Po Box 53
Georges Hall NSW 2198
Email: dcsg@optushome.com.au/dcsg

**Australian Multiple Association**
Po Box 105
Coogee NSW 2034
Email: amba_national@yahoo.com.au
Website: www.amba.org.au


**Endometriosis Association**

28 Warrandyte Rd.
Victoria 3134
Tel: (03) 9879 2199
Fax: (03) 9879 6519
Email: info@endometriosis.org.au
Website; www.endometriosis.org.au

**Polycystic Ovarian Syndrome Association of Australia**
PO Box 689
Kingswood NSW 2747
Tel: (02) 8250 0222
Email: info@posaa.asn.au

**Quit – The National Tobacco Campaign**
Tel: (02) 6289 1555
Email: quitnow@health.gov.au
Website: www.quit.info.au

**Saliva Testing**
ARL Laboratories 119-123 York St
Sydney NSW 2000
Tel: (02) 9267 7889
Fax: (02) 9264 1653

**Foresight Association**
Foresight, The UK Association for the Promotion of Preconception Care
Contact: Foresight
16/133 Rowntree St Birchgrove NSW 2041
Tel:/Fax: (61-2) 9818 3734
Website: www.wellnesscentre.com.au

**The American Infertility Association (New York)**
666 Fifth Avenue, Suite 278
New York, NY 10103
(212) 764-0802
www.americaninfertility.org

www.fertilinet.com

**Fertilitext**
www.Fertilitext.org

**American Society for Reproductive Medicine**
1209 Montgomery Highway
Birmingham, AL 35216-2809
(205) 978-5000
www.asrm.org
**Complementary Medicine**

**Australian College of Nutritional & Environmental Medicine**
13 Hilton St
Beaumaris VIC 3193
Australia
Tel: 03 9589 6088
www.acnem.org

**Australian Integrative Medicine Association**
Locked Bag 29
Clayton VIC 3168
Australia
Tel: 03 9594 7561
www.aima.net.au

**British Holistic Medical Association**
59 Lansdown Place
Hove
East Sussex BN3 1FL
United Kingdom
Tel: 01273 725951
www.bhma.org.uk

**The American Association of Naturopathic Physicians**
www.naturopathic.org

**British Society for Allergy, Environmental and Nutritional Medicine**
PO Box 7
Knighton
Powys LD7 1WF
United Kingdom
Tel; 01547 550378
www.bsaenm.free-online.co.uk

**Greenslopes Naturopathic Clinic**
Jason Jackson N.D.
615A Logan Road
Greenslopes Brisbane QLD 4120
Australia
Tel: 07 339 77 882
jason@jacksonhealth.com
www.naturopathic.net.au
www.jacksonhealth.com.au
www.brisbanebabymaker.com.au


**Infertility Support and Preconception Care**

**Access: Australia's National Infertility Network**
PO Box 959
Parramatta NSW 2124
Australia
Tel: 02 9670 2380
www.access.org.au

**British Infertility Counselling Association**
69 Division St.
Sheffield S1 4GE
United Kingdom
Tel: 0114 263 1448
www.bica.net

**Fertility UK – The National fertility Awareness & Natural family planning service**
www.FertilityUK.org

**RESOLVE: The National Infertility Association**
www.resolve.org

**CHILD: The National Infertility Support Network**
Charter House
43 Leonard's Road
Bexhill-on-Sea
East Sussex TN40 1JA
United Kingdom
Tel: 01424 732361
www.child.org.uk

**Fertility NZ**
Po Box 34151
Birkenhead
Auckland
New Zealand
Tel: 0800 333 306
www.fertilitynz.org.nz

**Fertility Society of Australia**
Waldron Smith Management
61 Danks St.
Port Melbourne VIC 3207
Tel: 03 9645 6359
www.fsa.au.com


**Foresight**
28 The Paddock

Godalming
Surrey GU7 1XD
United Kingdom
Tel: 01483 427839
www.foresight-preconception.org.uk

**Issue: The National Fertility Association**
114 Lichfield St.
Walsall WS1 1SZ
United Kingdom
Tel: 01922 722888
www.issue.co.uk

**New Zealand Infertility Society**
PO Box 34
151 Birkenhead
Auckland
New Zealand
Tel: 04 795 952
www.nzinfertility.org.nz

**Andrology Australia – male factor information**
www.andrologyaustralia.org

**Fertility Society of Australia**
www.fsa.au.com

**The International Council on Infertility
Information Dissemination, Inc
Inciid**
(General information source on infertility)
www.inciid.org

**Infertility Treatment authority**
www.ita.org.au

**Australian Polycystic Ovarian Syndrome Association**
www.posaa.asn.au
www.pcosupport.org


**Miscarriage support**

**Miscarriage support and information**
www.sands.org.au

**Fertility Plus Miscarriage Support &
Information Resources**

www.fertilityplus.org/faq/miscarriage/resourses.html
**Pregnancyloss.info**
www.pregnancyloss.info/

**Women's Health Organisation Queensland**
www.womhealth.org.au

**The National Infertility Network (US)**
www.resolve.org

**Environmental Causes of Infertility**
www.chem-tox.com/infertility/

**Canadian Infertility Network**
www.infertilitynetwork.org

**EIN: electronic infertility news**
www.ein.org/brnews.htm

**IVF Australia**
www.ivf.com.au

**IVF support list**
www.group.yahoo.com/groups/IVF/

www.ivfconnections

**Friends of Queensland Fertility Group Inc**
www.friendsqfg.org.au

**SELNAS-USA (Gender Selection Calendar)**
www.SELNASUSA.com

**Software that can help track your fertility cycles**
WWW.tcoyf.com and WWW.cyclewatch.com

**Adoption**

**Gladney**
www.adoptionsbygladney.com

**Spence-Chapin**
www.spence-chapin.org

**The national adoption information clearing house (NAIC)**
www.calib.com/naic

www.adoption.com

**Overseas adoption**
www.holtintl.org

**Donor eggs**
www.eggdonor.com
www.awomansgift.com
**www.sherinstitute.com**

**Sperm Bank – shopping for sperm**
www.xytex.com

Two internet sites that have information on sperm tests are:
WWW.babyhopes.com and WWW.completefertility.com

**General information and chat room site**
www.essentialbaby.com.au
www.nextgenfertility.com
**www.haveababy.com**

**Erectile Dysfunction**
www.TheWeekend.com.au

**Ovulation & Pregnancy Test Kits**
www.lullabyconception.com.au

# References and Recommended Reading

Airola, P. Every Woman's Book. Health Plus Publishers. Arizona, USA, 1991

Atkins, Robert C. Dr. Atkins' Vita-nutrient Solutions (Nature's answer to drugs). A Fireside Book, Simon and Schuster. NY, 1999

Barbieri, Robert L., Domar Alice D. & Loughlin Kevin. Six Steps to Increase Fertility: an Integrated Medical and Mind/Body Approach to Promote Conception. Simon and Schuster, New York, 2000.

Billings, E. & Westmore, A. The Billings Method. Anne O'Donovan, Melbourne, 1980

Balch, Phyllis A. & James F. Prescription for Nutritional Healing. (Third edition). Avery, Penguin, Putnam Inc, NY. 2000

Bensky, D. & Gamble, A. Chinese Herbal Medicine Materia Medica. Eastland Press, Seattle, 1986

Berman, Annarosa. Sex at 6pm, a personal journey through IVF. New Holland Publishers, Australia, 2006

Bisset N G. ed. Herbal Drugs and Phyto Pharmaceuticals. Medpharm Scientific Publishers, Stuttgart, 1994.

Blumenthal M. et al, eds. The Complete German Commission E Monographs: Therapeutic Guide to Herbal Medicines. American Botanical Council, Austin, 1998.

Boericke's Materia Medica with Repertory. Jain Publishers Pty Ltd. New Delhi (India) 1991.

Bone, Kerry. A Clinical Guide to Blending Liquid Herbs (Herbal Formulations for the Individual Patient). Churchill Livingston (UK), Elsevier (USA) 2003.

Bone, Kerry. Clinical Applications of Ayurvedic and Chinese Herbs. Monographs for the Western Herbal Practitioner. Phytotherapy Press. Warwick, Qld. 1996.

Bone, Kerry & Mills, Simon. Principles and Practice of Phytotherapy. Modern Herbal Medicine. Churchill Livingston, Harcourt Publishing Ltd, 2000.

Bradford, Nikki. Natural Fertility. (How to maximise your chances of conception). Hamlyn (Great Britain) London, 2002.

British Herbal Medicine Association's Scientific Committee: British Herbal Pharmacopoeia. Bournemouth, 1983 BHMA.

Cabot, S. Women's Health. Pan Books, Sydney. 1087.

Caton, Helen. The Fertility Plan. (A Holistic Program for Conceiving a Healthy Baby). A Fireside Book. Simon and Schuster. 2000.

Chan, Catherine. Fertility Seminar and Workshop Booklet. Ourimbah, NSW, 2002

Chopra, Deepak & Simon, David. The Chopra Centre Herbal Handbook. Natural Prescriptions for Perfect Health. Rider, Ebury Press, Random House, Inc, USA. 2000.

Chevallier, Andrew. Encyclopaedia of Medical Plants. (revised edition). Dorling Kindersley Pty. Ltd. London. NSW 2001.

Cronin, Kim. Woman to Woman. Managing Your Hormones Safely and Naturally. Interactive Presentations Pty. Ltd. Brisbane. 2002.

Davies, S & Stewart, A. Nutritional Medicine, Pan Books. London. 1987

Drake, K and J. Natural Fertility Control, Thornsons, UK, 1984

Domar AD et al. Impact of group psychological interventions on pregnancy rates in infertile women. Fertil Steril 2000; 73:805-11

Fisher, Leslie. The Clinical Science of Mineral Therapy. The Maurice Blackmore Research Foundation, NSW. 1993

Flynn, A.M. & Brooks, M. Natural Family Planning, Unwin, London.1984

Furse, Anna. Your Essential Infertility Companion. Thorsons, Harper Collins Publishers, London, updated edition 2001.

Grieve, M. A Modern Herbal. Penguin, UK, 1977.

Haas, Elson. M. Staying Healthy with Nutrition. (The Complete Guide to Diet and Nutritional Medicine). Celestial Art Publishing, California 1992.

Hannerley, Milton and Kimball, Cheryl. What to do when the Doctor says it's PCOS (Polycystic Ovarian Syndrome). Fair Winds Press, USA. 2003.

Hollingsworth, Elaine. Take Control of Your Health and Escape the Sickness Industry. 9th edition, Hippocrates Health Centre of Australia, Empowerment Press International, Mudgeeraba, Qld, Aust, 2006.

Indichova, Julia. Inconceivable: A Woman's Triumph over Despair and Statistics. Broadway Books, New York. 2001.

Jansen, R.P.S. Ovulation and the Polycystic Ovary Syndrome, Australian and New Zealand Journal of Obstetrics and Gynaecology, 34: 277-85 (1994).

Sex, Reproduction and Impregnation: By 2099 We Won't Confuse Them, Medical Journal of Australia; 171: 666-7 (1999)

Jansen, Robert. Getting Pregnant. 2nd edition (A Compassionate Resource to Overcoming Infertility and Avoiding Miscarriage), Allen and Unwin, NSW. 2003.

Kittel, Mary & Dr. Metzger, Deborah. Stay Fertile Longer - Planning Now for Pregnancy When You're Ready- in Your 20s 30s and 40s or Today. Published by Rodale Ltd UK 2003 Pan McMillan Ltd.

Kovacs, Gabor and Smith, Jane. A Patient's Guide to the Polycystic Ovary. Its effects on Health and Fertility. Hill of Content, Melbourne 2001.

Lauersen, Neils H, M.D.,PhD., & Bouchez, Colette. Getting Pregnant. What you need to know right now. Fireside of Simon & Schuster Inc, New York, USA, 2000.

Leridon, H. Human Fertility: The Basic Components. University of Chicago Press, Chicago, USA. 1977.

Lewis, Randine PhD. The Infertility Cure. Little, Brown & Company. 2004.

LLewyn-Jones, D. Getting Pregnant, Ashwood House Medical, Melbourne. 1990

Luminare-Rosen, Carista. Parenting Begins Before Conception: A Guide to Preparing Body, Mind and Spirit for you and your Future Child. Rochester: Healing Arts Press, 2000.

McLean, Sandra. Late Babies. Having a Baby after 35. Bantam (Division of Random House), Brisbane, Australia, 2004

Meletis, D. Chris, Better Sex Naturally. Harper Collins, NY. USA. 2000

Medi Media Australia, Pty. Ltd. The Australian Edition (MIMS) Twenty-seventh edition, St. Leonards. NSW. 2003.

Meletis, Chris N.D., & Brown, Liz. Enhancing Fertility. Overcoming obstacles to conception through healthy diet and natural medicine. Basic health publications, Inc, North Bergen, NJ. 2004

Meyers-Thompson, J. & Perkins, S. Fertility for Dummies. Wiley Publishing Inc. New York. 2003

Mills, S. Dictionary of Modern Herbalism , Thornsons, UK. 1985.

The Essential Book of Herbal Medicine, Arkana, UK. 1991

Mosby's Handbook of Herbal Supplements and their Therapeutic Uses. Mosby, Elsevier Science, St. Louis, Missouri. 2003.

Murray, M.T. Healing Power of Herbs. 2nd edition. CA: Prima Publishing 1995.

Murray, M.T. & J. Pizzaro. Encyclopaedia of Natural Medicine Revised 2nd edition, CA: Prima Publishing 2002.

Naish, F. The Lunar Cycle, Nature and Health Books, Australia and New Zealand.

Natural Fertility, Sally Miller Publishing, Sydney, 1991

Naish, F. and Roberts, J. The Natural Way to Better Babies, (Preconception Health Care for Prospective Parents). Random House Australia 1996.

Neuberg, Roger. Infertility. Tests, Treatments and Options. Thorsons Harper Collins Publishers, London 1991.

Osiecki, Henry. The Physician's Handbook of Clinical Nutrition. (6th edition). Bio Concept Publishing. Eagle Farm, Qld. 2001.

The Nutrient Bible (5th edition) Bio Concept Publishing , 2002.

Payne, Niravi B. & Lane Richardson, Brenda. The Fertility Solution: A Revolutionary Mind-Body Programme to Help you Conceive. London: Thorsons, 2002

Priest, Judy & Atwell, Kathy. Drugs in Conception, Pregnancy and Childbirth. (Updated and fully revised). Thornson. Harper Collins. London. 1996

Price, Cathine & Robinson, Sandra. Birth – Conceiving, Nurturing and Giving Birth to your baby. Macmillan, Sydney 2004.

Reiss, Fern. The Infertility Diet: Get Pregnant and Prevent Miscarriage. Newton, MA: Peanut Butter and Jelly Press, 1999.

Rand, Victoria M.D., Ohlson, Melissa, M.S.,RD, & Shaffer Bev. Healing Gourmet Eat to Boost Fertility. McGraw-Hill. New York. 2006.

Sharkey, Ruth. Fertile Fathers, Published by Ruth Sharkey, Nerang Qld. 2003.

Sharkey, Ruth. Mother Nature's Help for Infertile Couples 2nd edition. Published by Ruth Sharkey, Aust. Castleview Pty. Ltd. 2001.

Sharkey, Ruth. Ruth Sharkey's Guide to Natural Conception. Castleview Pty Ltd, Tasmania, Aust 2004.

Shealy, C. Norman M.D., Ph.D. Alternative Healing Therapies. (The Complete Illustrated Encyclopedia of). Element Books Ltd, Penguin Australia, 1998.

Shettles L.B. & Rorvik, David. How to Choose the Sex of your Baby. (A complete update on the method best supported by scientific evidence). Harper Collins Publishing 1999. Original, Doubleday Inc. 1984 (USA) First published.

Siber, S. J. Why are Humans So Infertile? How to get Pregnant with the New Technology: New York: Warner Books 1990.

What Forms of Male Fertility Are There Left to Cure? Human Reproduction 10: 503-4. 1995.

Spencer, John. W. & Jacobs, Joseph. J. Complementary and Alternative Medicine. An Evidence Based Approach. Mosby Inc. 2003.

Stone, L. The Family, Sex and Marriage in England 1500-1800. London: Weidenfeld and Nicholson , 1997.

Stoppard, Mirianm Dr. Conception, Pregnancy and Birth. (The childbirth bible for today's Australian parents), Dorling Kindersley Camberwell, VIC, Aust, 1993 & 2000.

Thorn, Gill. Not Too Late, Having a Baby after 35. Practical Parenting, Bantam Books Great Britain 1998.

Tomlins, Jacqueline. The Infertility Handbook: A Guide to Making Babies. Allen and Unwin. NSW 2003.

Trattler, Ross and Jones Adrian. Better Health through Natural Healing. (How to get Well without Drugs or Surgery), 2nd edition. McGraw-Hill, Hinkler Books Pty. Ltd. Vitoria 2001.

Trickey, Ruth. Women, Hormones & the Menstrual Cycle: Herbal and medical solutions from adolescence to menopause. Allen & Unwin, NSW. Fully revised and updated edition 2003.

Watanabe, H. Shibuya T. eds.: Pharmacologic Research on Traditional Herbal Medicine, Amsterdam, 1999, Harwood Academic Publishers.

Weiss, R. F. Herbal Medicine. Stuttgart, Germany: Hippocrates Verlog, 1985.

Werbach, M.R. & Murray, M.T. Botanical Influences on Illness. 2nd edition: CA; Third Line Press 1994.

Werbach, M.R. Nutritional Influences on Illness. 2nd edition: CA: Third Line Press 1996

Weschler, Toni. Taking Charge of your Fertility: The Definitive Guide to Natural Birth Control, Pregnancy Achievement and Reproductive Health. London Vermillion, 2003

West, Zita. Fertility & conception. The complete guide to getting pregnant. Dorling Kindersley (a Penguin company), London, 2003

Winston, Robert. Infertility. (A sympathetic approach to understanding the causes and options for treatments). Vermilion. Random House. London. 1996.

Winston, R. Getting Pregnant. 2nd edition, I ANAYA publishers, London,1989

White, Ian. Australian Bush Flower Essence. Bantam Books NSW. 1999

# Glossary

**Abortifacient**: a substance which can cause abortion.

**ACE inhibitor**: a class of drug used in the treatment of high blood pressure.

**Acidophilism**: a type of bacteria present in yoghurt. Used to re-establish normal bowel flora.

**Adrenals**: glands situated above the kidneys, which are involved in stress response.

**Adhesions**: scar tissue, usually from earlier surgery or infection that can obstruct the movement of egg or sperm.

**Agglutination**: when sperm clump together, rather than moving freely.

**Agonist**: a synthetic hormone that briefly stimulates the pituitary gland to release follicle stimulating hormone (FHS) and luteinising hormone (LH), but then suppresses their production.

**Aldosterone**: a hormone secreted by the adrenals, responsible for the maintaining of electrolyte balance in the body.

**Amenorrhea**: where a woman has no menstrual periods.

**Amnionitis:** inflammation of the amniotic membrane.

**Anaerobes:** organisms that survive in the absence of oxygen.

**Androgens**: male sex hormones-testosterone is the main androgen in men and androgens are also present in small amounts in women.

**Andrologist**: a specialist in male reproductive health.

**Aneuploidy**: an incorrect number of chromosomes that results in abnormalities.

**Anovulation**: where a woman does not ovulate.

**Antagonist**: a synthetic hormone that immediately stops the pituitary gland releasing (FHS) and (LH).

**Antibodies:** substances formed by the body in response to the presence of antigen/allergen.

**Antihypertensive**: a substance used to reduce high blood pressure.

**Antiphospholipid**: antibodies that may be associated with tiny blood clots forming in the blood vessels of the placenta, and which may be associated with miscarriage.

**Anti-sperm antibodies**: antibodies that can attach to the head or tail of the sperm and in sufficient numbers make it difficult for the sperm to fertilise the egg.

**Artificial insemination (AI);** when sperm is inserted into the vagina or uterus, normally with a syringe or catheter; AI may be artificial insemination by husband (AIH) or artificial insemination by donor (AID) also known as donor insemination (DI).

**Artificial thaw cycle**: a treatment protocol using thawed embryos and some low level drug treatment to prepare the uterus to accept a pregnancy.

**Asherman's syndrome**: a condition where the sides of the uterus start to grow together, usually as a result of scarring from previous infection or surgery, and cause damage to the endometrium.

**Aspermia**: where a man has no semen.

**Assisted hatching**: a process of artificially puncturing the outer shell of an embryo to help it hatch.

**Asthenozoospermia**: where the sperm is weak and has poor motility.

**Azoospermia**: where a man has no sperm.

**Basal body temperature**: the temperature of the body which can be tracked to assist in identifying whether ovulation has occurred.

**Benzodiazepine:** a class of tranquilliser (eg. Serapax, Valium).

**Beta-blocker**: a drug used to treat high blood pressure.

**Bicornuate uterus**: a congenital condition in which both the inside and outside of the uterus are divided.

**Bifidus**: a type of bacteria present in yoghurt, used to re-establish normal bowel flora.

**Biochemical pregnancy**: where a blood test shows evidence of raised human chorionic gonadotropin (HCG) levels, but there is no ongoing clinical pregnancy.

**Blastocyst:** the stage of the embryo, about five days after it has fertilised, when it usually implants into the lining of the uterus.

**Blighted ovum**: where there is a gestational sac, but no evidence of a foetus.

**Calcium channel blocker**: a drug used to treat high blood pressure.

**Carcinogen**: a substance that can cause cancer.

**Cardiovascular**: of the heart and blood vessels.

**Catheter**: A fine plastic tube used for transferring embryos and for other procedures.

**Cerebral palsy**: spastic paralysis

**Cervical mucus**: mucus secreted by the cervix around the time of ovulation to help the movement of sperm.

**Cervicitis**: inflammation of the cervix.

**Cervix**: the neck of the uterus.

**Cetrotide**: a brand name of a gonadotropin-releasing hormone-antagonist.

**Chlamydia**: a micro-organism that can be sexually transmitted and may cause infection and adhesions in the pelvis.

**Chromosomes**: thread-like structures that appear in pairs in human cells and carry genetic material.

**Cilia**: fine hair-like structures in the fallopian tube that help move the egg.

**Cleavage**: the process by which a fertilised egg divides.

**Clomid**: Brand name of the drug Clomiphene.

**Clomiphene**: a drug that increases the natural production of follicle stimulating hormone (FSH).

**Clomiphene cycle**: a treatment protocol involving low level follicle stimulation using the drug Clomiphene.

**Coeliac condition:** sensitivity to gluten, leading to malabsorption of fats.

**Colitis**: inflammation of the colon (lower bowel).

**Comparative genome hybridisation (CGH)**: a new technique for assessing the embryos before they are transferred, a form of pre-implantation genetic diagnosis.

**Complete abortion**: where all the products of conception have passed out of the body naturally after a miscarriage.

**Congenital defect**: a defect present from birth.

**Corpus luteum**: the structure that remains after the egg has left the follicle, which is responsible for producing progesterone to support a pregnancy in its early stages.

**Corticosteroid**: a hormone formed by the adrenals, or a similar synthetic derivative.

**Crohn's disease**: inflammation of the intestines.

**Cryptorchidism**: a condition where the testes do not descend into the scrotum:

**Curette**: a procedure to remove tissue from the uterus usually referred to with 'dilation' – a 'D and C'.

**Cyst**: a sac or structure containing fluid or other matter.

**Cystic fibrosis**: a serious genetic disorder that affects the development of the lungs.

**Cytomegalovirus (CMV)**: a virus that can be transmitted via semen.

**Cytoplasm**: the part of an egg that surrounds the nucleus into which the sperm is injected in the process of intracytoplasmic sperm injection.

**Depo provera**: a long acting injectible contraceptive.

**Dilation**: an 'opening', usually referring to the opening of the cervix in order to perform a curette – a 'D and C'.

**Dioxin;** a toxic product released during the manufacture of organochlorines.

**Diuretic**: a drug used to promote the flow of urine.

**Diverticulitis**: inflammation of small pockets in the large intestine.

**Down regulated protocol**: a treatment protocol involving the gradual suppression of natural hormones with a Gn RH-agonist and the stimulation of follicles with a follicle stimulating hormone (FHS).

**Down's syndrome**: a genetic disease caused by an extra chromosome 21, also known as Trisomy 21.

**Dysmenorrhea**: a condition in which a woman has painful periods.

**Ectopic pregnancy**: where a pregnancy forms outside the uterus, normally in the fallopian tube.

**Egg pick-up**: the commonly used term for ovum pick-up.

**Ejaculate**: the seminal fluid that is expelled from the penis during ejaculation.

**Ejaculatory duct**: part of the male reproductive system attached to the seminal vesicle.

**Embryo**: a fertilised egg.

**Embryo transfer (ET)**: the process of transferring an embryo that has been created 'in vitro' in the uterus.

**Endocrine gland**: a ductless gland which releases a hormone directly to the bloodstream.

**Endocrinology**: the study of hormones.

**Endometriosis**: a condition in which endometrial tissue grows in places other than the uterus.

**Endometritis**: a condition in which the endometrium becomes inflamed.

**Endometrium:** the lining of the uterus which sheds as menstruation (period).

**Endorphins**: the body's natural pain killers, appetite suppressants, mood enhancers.

**Epididymis**: a part of the male reproductive system in which sperm are sorted and nourished.

**Epididymitis**: a condition where the epididymis becomes inflamed.

**Episiotomy**: a surgical cut made in the perineum to enlarge the birth outlet.

**Erythrocytes**: red blood cells.

**Fallopian tube**: part of the female reproductive system, connecting the ovaries to the uterus.

**Fibroid**: a non-cancerous tumour that can form in the uterus.

**Fimbria:** tiny finger-like structures at the open end of the fallopian tube that 'pick-up' the egg once it has been released from the ovary.

**Flare protocol**: a treatment protocol that involves less suppression of natural hormones and takes advantage of the body's flare of (FHS) and (LH) caused by the agonist before it becomes suppressive.

**Foetus:** an unborn infant after the embryonic stage (i.e. after approximately two months).

**Foetal alcohol syndrome**: a condition that newborn babies are born with as a result of excessive alcohol intake by the mother during pregnancy.

**Follicle**: a sac in the ovary that contains an egg.

**Follicle stimulating hormone (FSH)**: a hormone produced by the pituitary gland – in women it stimulates follicles on the ovaries to grow and in men it stimulates the production of sperm in the testes.

**Follicular phase**: the first part of the menstrual cycle, before ovulation.

**Fragile X syndrome**: a syndrome of impaired functioning in males, which often causes retardation.

**Fundus**: the main part of the uterus, particularly the top area away from the cervix.

**Fungicide**: a fungus-destroying substance.

**Gamete**: sperm or egg.

**Gamete intrafallopian transfer (GIFT)**: a procedure where eggs are retrieved mixed with sperm and then inserted into the fallopian tube.

**Genetic engineering**: the manipulation of genetic material in an attempt to produce superior offspring.

**Germ cells**: sexual reproduction cells in males and females – sperm, ova.

**Gestation**: the period between conception and birth.

**Gonadotropin releasing hormone (GnRH)**: a hormone produced by the hypothalamus that regulates the production of (FSH) and (LH).

**Gonadotropin releasing hormone-agonist**: see agonist.

**Gonadotropin releasing hormone-antagonist**: see antagonist.

**Gonal F**: a brand name of synthetic follicle stimulating hormone.

**Gonorrhoea**: a bacterial infection that can be sexually transmitted.

**Haemoglobin:** the red pigment of blood, which carries oxygen from the lungs to the rest of the body.

**Haemophilia**: a sex-linked genetic disease of the blood.

**Hepatitis B and C**: infectious diseases that cause inflammation of the liver.

**Herbicide**: a substance used to kill plants (notably weeds).

**Herpes**: a sexually transmitted viral disease.

**Hirsutism**: an excessive growth of hair.

**Homeostasis**: the process of maintaining constant conditions within the body.

**Hormone**: a natural chemical substance passed into the blood that stimulates organs to action.

**Huntington's disease**: a genetic disorder that is associated with deterioration in functioning, often in one's 30s and 40s.

**Human chorionic gonadotropin (HCG)**: a hormone secreted by the placenta during pregnancy, the presence of which shows up on a pregnancy test; also sometimes given as luteal support under the brand name Pregnyl or Profasi.

**Human immune-deficiency virus (HIV)**: a sexually transmitted virus that causes acquired immune deficiency syndrome.

**Hydrocephalus**: the enlargement of an infant's head by the accumulation of cerebrospinal fluid.

**Hydrosalpinx**: when fluid develops on the fallopian tubes because of a blockage.

**Hyperemesis**: severe vomiting in pregnancy.

**Hyperprolactinemia**: where too much prolactin is produced by the pituitary gland.

**Hypoglycaemia:** low sugar levels in the blood.

**Hypothalamic anovulation**: where there is no ovulation because the hypothalamus doesn't produce sufficient gonadotropin releasing hormone (GnRH) or the pituitary doesn't respond to stimulation with GnRH.

**Hypothalamus**: a part of the brain that controls the pituitary gland, and which is responsible for producing (GnRH).

**Hysterosalpingogram (HSG)**: an x-ray procedure for examining the endometrial cavity and internal outline of the fallopian tubes.

**Hysteroscopy**: an exploratory procedure for examining the uterine cavity using a fine telescope-like instrument similar to that used for a laparoscopy.

**Idiopathic infertility**: where the cause of infertility is unknown.

**Immunobead test**: a test carried out on sperm to check for the presence of anti-sperm antibodies.

**Immunosuppressive:** a substance that adversely affects the function of the immune system.

**Implantation**: where an embryo embeds itself into the lining of the uterus.

**Impotence**: where a man is unable to maintain an erection.

**Incomplete abortion:** where the products of conception do not pass out of the body naturally after miscarriage.

**Intracytoplasmic** sperm injection (ICSI): a technique for injecting a single sperm into an egg.

**Intramural fibroid**: a fibroid that grows within the uterus wall.

**Intrauterine contraceptive device (IUD)**: a device inserted into the uterus as a method of contraception.

**In vitro**: in a test tube.

**In vitro fertilisation**: the process of fertilising an egg in a laboratory.

**In vivo**: in the living body.

**Isthmus:** the part of the fallopian tube closest to the uterus.

**Karyotype**: a systemised diagram of chromosomes.

**Klinefelters syndrome**: a genetic condition in which a man has an extra X chromosome.

**Kremer test**: a test that examines the interaction between sperm and cervical mucus.

**Laparoscopy**: a surgical operation on the abdomen.

**Leucocyte**: a type of white blood cell.

**Leuprolide**: the brand name of a GnRH agonist.

**LH surge**: the increase in luteinising hormone that occurs in women just before ovulation.

**Listeria**: a bacteria found in some foods that is very occasionally associated with pregnancy.

**Long protocol**: another name for a 'down regulated' protocol.

**Lucrin (leuprolide)**: a brand name of GnRH agonist.

**Luteal phase**: the second half of the menstrual cycle, after ovulation.

**Luteal support**: drugs given to help maintain the endometrium after an embryo transfer.

**Luteinising hormone (LH)**: a hormone secreted by the pituitary gland – responsible in women for ovulation of the mature follicle from the ovary.

**Lymphocyte**: a type of white blood cell.

**Mastitis**: fever and flu-like symptoms sometimes experienced during breastfeeding – not necessarily due to infection

**Menstrual cycle**: a woman's reproductive cycle that involves the growth of follicles, release of eggs from the ovary, and the preparation of the lining of the uterus (the endometrium) to receive the eggs, normally about 26-34 days in length.

**Microgynon:** the brand name of an oral contraceptive pill usually prescribed at he beginning of a stimulated treatment cycle to assist programming.

**Microsurgical epididymal sperm aspiration**: a microsurgical procedure for retrieving sperm.

**Mid-luteal serum progesterone**: a blood test performed around day 21 of a woman's menstrual cycle to assess levels of progesterone.

**Miscarriage**: when the foetus is lost before it is viable.

**Missed abortion**: when there is a gestational sac and evidence of the foetus, but no heartbeat.

**Monosomy**: where there is only one chromosome.

**Motility**: the ability of sperm to move.

**Mullerian duct disorders**: congenital defects of the female internal reproductive ducts which can result in abnormalities to the uterus and vagina.

**Myoma**: a benign (non-cancerous) tumour of the muscle wall of the uterus, the same as a fibroid.

**Myomectomy**: a surgical procedure performed to remove a fibroid/myoma.

**Myometrium**: the muscle wall of the uterus.

**Natural thaw cycle**: a treatment protocol that involves tracking natural ovulation and transferring a thawed embryo.

**Neonatal**: of newborn babies (first four weeks of life).

**Neurological**: of the nervous system.

**Nucleic acid**: DNA/RNA – the stuff of genetic material.

**Oestradiol**: the main naturally produced oestrogen.

**Oestrogen**: female sex hormone responsible for stimulating growth.

**Offal/organ meats**: products including kidney, heart, tongue, liver etc.

**Organochlorines**: insecticides which break down slowly are stored in fatty tissues in living creatures and persist in the environment.

**Organophosphates**: insecticides which break down more quickly than organochlorines.

**Oligomenorrhea**: where a woman has menstrual cycles longer than 35 days.

**Oligoovulation**: where a woman has infrequent ovulation.

**Oligozoospermia (oligospermia)**: where there is a reduced number of sperm in the ejaculate, 'a low sperm count'.

**Oocyte**: an egg.

**Orchitis**: an inflammation of the testes.

**Orgalutran**: a brand name of a GnRH-antagonist.

**Ovarian cysts**: a sac filled with fluid found in the ovary.

**Ovarian hyper stimulation syndrome**: a condition where the ovaries become enlarged and fluid is released into the abdominal cavity.

**Ovary**: female reproductive organ responsible for producing eggs.

**Ovulation**: the release of eggs from the ovaries.

**Ovulation induction**: where drugs are used to induce ovulation.

**Ovum (ova)**: an egg (eggs).

**Ovum pick-up**: where eggs are surgically retrieved form the ovaries, usually by transvaginal follicle aspiration.

**Pancreatitis:** inflammation of the pancreas.

**Pap smear:** a test done to determine the presence of cancer cells or other abnormal cells in the cervix.

**Pelvic inflammatory disease (PID)**: an infection of the reproductive organs in a woman

**Perinatal**: the period shortly before, during, and after the birth.

**Perineum**: muscle and tissue bridge between genital organs and anus.

**Pessaries:** a small tablet of a drug, in this case progesterone that is inserted into the vagina.

**Pituitary gland**: a gland controlled by the hypothalamus which is responsible for the production of (FSH) and (LH) and other hormones.

**Placenta**: the organ by which an unborn infant receives nourishment from its mother.

**Polycystic ovarian syndrome (PCOS)**: a condition in women where there is a higher than normal production of the male hormone androgen, causing a range of symptoms that may affect fertility and often causes ovulatory difficulties.

**Polycystic ovaries (PCO)**: where a number of small cysts form on the ovaries, which may or may not affect fertility.

**Polyp**: a benign (non-cancerous) growth of tissue.

**Post-coital test (PCT):** a test used to determine sperm-mucus problems, increasingly replaced by the Kremer test.

**Postnatal/postpartum**: after birth (as in postnatal depression).

**Pre-implantation genetic diagnosis (PGD)**: a technique for identifying genetic abnormalities in embryos before they are transferred into the uterus.

**Pregnyl**: a brand name of a synthetic human chorionic gonadotropin (HCG).

**Premature ovarian failure (POF):** where a woman stops ovulating before the age of 40, also known as a premature menopause.

**Primolut**: a brand name of a progestogen.

**Products of conception**: the gestational sac and foetal tissue remaining after a miscarriage.

**Profasi:** a brand name of a synthetic (HCG).

**Progestagen:** a progesterone-like substance sometimes used to regulate menstrual bleeding.

**Progesterone:** a key female hormone secreted by the corpus luteum and responsible for supporting a pregnancy in its early stages.

**Prognyova:** a brand name of oestrogen.

**Prolactin:** a hormone that stimulates the production of milk, disturbances of which can impair ovulation.

**Proliferative** phase: the first half of the menstrual cycle before ovulation.

**Proluton:** a brand name for a progesterone injection.

**Pronuclei**: the cells that form after a fertilised egg has divided.

**Prostatitis**: infection of the prostate gland.

**Protocol:** the combination of drugs and procedures for an IVF treatment cycle.

**Prothrombin**: one of several blood clotting factors.

**Puregon**: a brand name of a synthetic follicle stimulating hormone.

**RDA**: recommended daily allowance, the dose required to prevent a frank deficiency state.

**Recurrent miscarriage**: generally defined as three or more miscarriages in a row with no successful pregnancy in between.

**Retrograde ejaculation**: where part of the ejaculate moves backwards into the bladder.

**Rubella (German measles)**: a disease which can cause developmental abnormalities in an unborn baby if contracted by the mother during pregnancy.

**Salpingitis**: inflammation of the fallopian tubes.

**Salpingogram**: an x-ray procedure used to examine the fallopian tubes.

**Scrotum**: pouches of skin containing the testicles.

**Secretory phase**: the second phase of the menstrual cycle, after ovulation.

**Secondary fertility**: when a woman cannot conceive after having already having had a pregnancy.

**Semen**: the fluid produced at ejaculation.

**Seminal vesicles**: male sex organs that contribute to the development of semen.

**Septate uterus**: where a barrier (a septum) divides the uterus into two.

**Short protocol**: another name for a flare protocol.

**Sickle cell anaemia**: a genetic disease of the blood.

**Sonohysterogram:** an ultrasound procedure for examining the endometrial cavity and internal outline of the fallopian tubes.

**Speculum**: an instrument inserted into the vagina, used for pap smears, embryo transfers and inseminations.

**Sperm (spermatozoa)**: the male reproductive cell.

**Spermatogenesis:** the formation of sperm.

**Spermicide**: a chemical used with a condom or diaphragm as a contraceptive.

**Sperm-mucus penetration test**: a technique for examining the interaction between sperm and cervical mucus (also known as the Kremer test).

**Subcutaneous**: under the skin.

**Submucous fibroid**: a fibroid that grows inwards in the uterine cavity.

**Subserous fibroid**: a fibroid that grows on the outside of the uterus.

**Surrogacy:** when a woman carries a baby for someone else.

**Synarel**: a brand name of a GnRH-agonist.

**Syphilis**: bacteria that can be sexually transmitted.

**Tay Sachs disease**: a serious genetic disorder affecting the brain.

**Testes (testicles)**: the two male sex glands.

**Testicular biopsy:** a surgical procedure where a small amount of tissue is removed from the testes to diagnose a fertility problem or to retrieve sperm.

**Testosterone:** the main sex hormone secreted in the testes and necessary for the development of sperm, also found in women in smaller quantities.

**Tetraozoospermia:** where sperm are malformed or misshapen.

**Thalassemia:** a genetic condition that affects the blood.

**Thrombosis**: clotting of blood in an artery or vein.

**Thyroid stimulating hormone**: a hormone produced by the pituitary gland that activates the thyroid gland.

**Translocation:** where part of a chromosome is knocked off and attaches to another chromosome.

**Transvaginal follicle aspiration**: a technique for retrieving eggs during an IVF treatment cycle.

**Transvaginal ultrasound scan:** a technique for examining a woman's internal reproductive organs often used to monitor the development of follicles and the endometrium.

**'Trigger' injections:** an injection of human chorionic gonadotropin (HCG) that activates ovulation.

**Trimester:** pregnancy is divided into three trimesters – first, second and third – each is of three months duration.

**Trisomy**: where there is an extra chromosome.

**Tubal patency**: the extent to which the fallopian tubes are open.

**Ultrasound follicle aspiration:** the medical term for ovum (egg) pick-up.

**Urethra**: a tube which transports urine out of the body and in men is part of the sperm transport system.

**Uterus**: the womb, where a pregnancy develops.

**Uterus didelphus**: where there are two separate cavities in the uterus.

**Vagina**: the passage from the uterus to the vulva.

**Vaginismus**: a condition where the muscles in the vagina spasm and make intercourse painful or difficult.

**Varicocele**: small varicose veins that develop on the testes.

**Vas deferens:** part of the male reproductive system that connects the epididymis with the seminal vesicles.

**Vasectomy**: a male sterilisation procedure.

**Vasography:** an x-ray procedure performed to examine the penis and testes.

**Vasovasostomy (vasoepididymostomy)**: the reversal of a vasectomy.

**ZIFT**: assisted conception procedure – Zygote Intra Fallopian Transfer.

**Zona pellucida**: the outer shell of an egg.

**Zygote**: a fertilised egg before it divides for the first time.

# Figures – Illustrations

458

# About the Author

*Jason Jackson N.D. is one of Australia's leading naturopath experts in reproductive health and infertility. He is recognised as an authority in the fields of nutrition and herbal medicine.*

*Mr Jackson is a graduate of the Australian College of Natural Medicine with further studies at the Queensland Institute of Natural Sciences. He holds Diplomas of Applied Sciences in Naturopathy, Homeopathy, and Herbal Medicine. Jason is a fully accredited and registered member of multiple professional organisations.*

*For over 16 years Mr Jackson has studied and practised Naturopathic Medicine and worked in research and development of natural medicine manufacturing. He has lectured extensively on numerous health topics in Australia and overseas and is a very popular talkback radio host. Jason also appears regularly in the media and contributes articles to respected health and wellbeing magazines and journal publications.*

*With a broad foundation of clinical experience, Mr Jackson offers a wealth of up-to-date, informative knowledge in all aspects of natural health care, with particular specialisation in fertility and reproductive disorders.*

*Jason Jackson is the Director and chief Naturopath of the Greenslopes Naturopathic Clinic with his team of dedicated Alternative health care professionals. Mr Jackson's background also involves being in the nursing, sporting and fitness industries.*

*Consultations – if you would like to have a consultation (either in person or by telephone), then please feel free to phone or e-mail the clinic for appointment reservation; fertility-enhancing natural supplements are also available to order.*

*For more information please contact:*

*Greenslopes Naturopathic Clinic*
*615A Logan Road, Greenslopes, Queensland, Australia, 4120.*
*Tel: 61+ (07) 3397 7882 / Fax: (07)3324 0516*
*Email: jjackson.gnc@bigpond.com*
*    jason@jacksonhealth.com*
*Website: www.naturopathic.net.au*
*    www.jacksonhealth.com.au*

# 'The Must-Have Book for anyone who is considering Treatment options for Reproductive Problems'

*Making Babies* is a thorough and comprehensive compilation of up-to-date scientific research, blended with a wealth of informative, practical knowledge, and is packed full of relevant self-help information that has something to suit everyone.

This book has been combined to offer you a 'warts and all' overview of both the medical approach to reproductive dysfunctions and the effective benefits that holistic, natural medicines and conventional, orthodox medicine can have on influencing your reproductive health, general wellbeing and gender selection.

*Making Babies* is an easy-to-read guide that covers in-depth descriptions of all the major medical and complementary therapies from acupuncture, diet, clinical nutrition, herbal medicine, homeopathy, medically assisted technology, surgical procedures, IVF, prescription medications and much more.

This book is essential reading that will assist in preparing and educating you on the various causal factors, medical conditions and all the very latest in treatment protocols. Some of the topics covered include: endometriosis; miscarriage prevention; PCOS; PMS; fibroids; menstrual dysfunction; hormone imbalances; male reproductive disorders; pregnancy support; and fertility boosting techniques.

Learn of new and traditional methods that are available today that can improve both you and your partner's pre- and post-conception health care and optimise fertility success.

*Making Babies* is an invaluable guide that can assist you to resolve your reproductive problems and help you to manage your way through the complexities of the infertility maze.

*Jason Jackson runs a successful Natural Medicine practice from Brisbane, Australia.*

*He has lectured and consulted extensively on numerous health topics throughout Australia and overseas. Mr Jackson specialises in reproductive health and infertility and is recognised as one of Australia's leading Naturopaths in this area and is an authority in the field of Clinical Nutrition and Herbal Medicine.*
*Jason has appeared widely in the media and his encyclopaedic knowledge of Alternative and Complementary Medicines has been greatly sought after.*

*The phenomenal success of Jason Jackson's Natural Fertility Programmes has not only helped thousands of couples all over Australia but has reached clients from around the world.*

LaVergne, TN USA
20 December 2009

167657LV00003BA/38/P

9 781921 406683